Management of Facial Asymmetry

Pushkar Mehra • Larry M. Wolford
Editors

Management of Facial Asymmetry

Current Principles and Practice

Springer

Editors
Pushkar Mehra
Oral and Maxillofacial Surgery
Boston University Medical Center
Boston, MA, USA

Larry M. Wolford
Oral and Maxillofacial Surgery
Texas A&M University College of Dentistry
Baylor University Medical Center
Dallas, TX, USA

ISBN 978-3-030-44970-4 ISBN 978-3-030-44971-1 (eBook)
https://doi.org/10.1007/978-3-030-44971-1

This Springer imprint is published by the registered company Springer Nature Switzerland AG
The registered company address is: Gewerbestrasse 11, 6330 Cham, Switzerland

Acknowledgments

Acknowledgment by Pushkar Mehra
This book would not have been possible without guidance from my friend and mentor, Larry Wolford. The time spent with him during my fellowship was the most positive experience in my evolution as a surgeon.

I dedicate this book to: my parents, Drs. Mahendra and Sheila Mehra for being there unconditionally at every stage of my life and for working very hard to make sure that their children got every opportunity; my younger brother Gautam, for unselfishly supporting and putting up with me; all my students and residents, for inspiring me; my department faculties, who make me look better than I actually am; my friends, for being there during all good and bad times; my daughter, Zaara, who is the sunshine of my life—you make me so proud; and, my wife, Deepika—I would not be where I am if you had not come into my life. You have made me a better person, and your sacrifices have allowed me to be successful professionally. Thank you so much for teaching me the importance of being a good father and husband.

Acknowledgment by Larry M. Wolford
It was an honor to be asked to produce this book with my very good friend, Pushkar Mehra. The year he spent with me in fellowship was one of the most productive (and fun) years of my entire career in Oral and Maxillofacial Surgery. He is an exceptionally gifted leader in our specialty.

This book is dedicated to my parents, Dr. Donald and Wilma Wolford. They taught me hard work, kindness, and respect for others. Also, my older brother Gary, whom I followed through school and residency; my younger sister Jean, who lost her life to breast cancer; my wonderful children, Dax, Dallas, Demi, Dylan, and Dash; and most of all, I dedicate this book to my wife, Denise, who guided our children, managed our practice, made many personal sacrifices, and provided love and support so that I could be successful today. I thank all of you in this journey.

Contents

Contributors

Eduardo Arias Division of Plastic, Reconstructive and Cosmetic Surgery, The University of Illinois at Chicago, The Craniofacial Center, Chicago, IL, USA

Marianela Gonzalez Carranza Department of Oral and Maxillofacial Surgery, Texas A&M, Dallas, TX, USA

Kristopher R. Cooper Department of Oral and Maxillofacial Surgery, University of Pittsburgh, Pittsburgh, PA, USA

Bernard J. Costello Department of Oral and Maxillofacial Surgery, University of Pittsburgh, Pittsburgh, PA, USA

Myles Davidson Private Practice, Mid-Kansas Oral & Maxillofacial Surgery, Wichita, KS, USA

Brian B. Farrell Private Practice and Director of Fellowship Program, Carolinas Center for Oral and Facial Surgery, Charlotte, NC, USA

Department of Oral and Maxillofacial Surgery, Louisiana State University Health Sciences Center, New Orleans, LA, USA

G. E. Ghali Louisiana State University Health Sciences Center-Shreveport, Shreveport, LA, USA

Willis Knighton Health System, Shreveport, LA, USA

Daljit S. Gill Great Ormond Street Hospital NHS Foundation Trust and UCLH Eastman Dental Hospital, London, UK

Cesar A. Guerrero Private Practice in Houston, TX, USA

David C. Hatcher School of Dentistry, Department of Orthodontics, University of Pacific, San Francisco, CA, USA

Orofacial Sciences, School of Dentistry, University of Pacific, San Francisco, CA, USA

School of Dentistry, University of California, Los Angeles, CA, USA

Dept. of Surgical & Radiological Sciences, School of Veterinary Medicine, University of California, Davis, Los Angeles, CA, USA

Samuel Liu Department of Oral and Maxillofacial Surgery, University of Pittsburgh, Pittsburgh, PA, USA

Portland, ME, USA

Caitlin B. L. McGraw Portland, OR, USA

Elena V. Mujica Sta Rosa Maxillofacial Surgery Center, Caracas, Santa Rosa, CA, USA

Farhad B. Naini Kingston Hospital NHS Foundation Trust and Queen Mary's Hospital Sidcup, King's College Hospital NHS Foundation Trust, London, UK

Pravin K. Patel Division of Plastic, Reconstructive and Cosmetic Surgery, The University of Illinois at Chicago, The Craniofacial Center, Chicago, IL, USA

Daniel E. Perez Oral and Maxillofacial Surgery, UT Health San Antonio, San Antonio, TX, USA

Shikha Rathi Department of Orthodontics, University of Pacific, San Francisco, CA, USA

David Szalay Oral and Maxillofacial Surgery, UT Health San Antonio, San Antonio, TX, USA

Paul S. Tiwana Department of Oral and Maxillofacial Surgery, The University of Oklahoma, Oklahoma City, OK, USA

Timothy A. Turvey Department of Craniofacial and Surgical Services, University of North Carolina at Chapel Hill, Chapel Hill, NC, USA

Jennifer E. Woerner, DMD, MD, FACS Shriners Hospital for Children, Shreveport, LA, USA

Larry M. Wolford Departments of Oral and Maxillofacial Surgery and Orthodontics, Texas A&M, University College of Dentistry, Baylor University Medical Center, Dallas, TX, USA

Diagnosis and Patient Evaluation

Paul S. Tiwana and Myles Davidson

Abstract

Facial features are more symmetric in certain people compared with others, yet facial asymmetry of different degrees is present in every individual. While one person's asymmetry may be noticeable only to their eye, others have asymmetry which greatly affects their daily lives. Regardless of the perceived severity of one's asymmetry, each person will form their own opinion about the relevance of their unique facial features. Functional, psychological, and social barriers are just a few of the ramifications that can result from an individual's perception of their facial symmetry, or lack thereof. In addition to history and physical with thorough history of the present illness, facial asymmetry workup requires a detailed clinical assessment of the patient. This assessment should include extraoral and intraoral examination, with particular attention being given to the orbits, chin, skull base, position of the glenoid fossae, and ramus condyle unit. Adjunctive craniofacial imaging, dental study models, and computer-aided surgical simulation (CASS) may be used to aid in diagnosis and treatment planning. Facial asymmetry may be absolute in nature or involve a number of known sources of pseudo-asymmetry. Furthermore, age considerations related to growth and development of craniofacial structures should play a role in evaluation of any pediatric patient.

Keywords

Facial asymmetry · Pseudo-asymmetry · Ramus condyle unit · Condylar hyperplasia · Condylar resorption · Cleft lip and palate · Growth assessment

P. S. Tiwana (✉)
Department of Oral and Maxillofacial Surgery, The University of Oklahoma, Oklahoma City, OK, USA
e-mail: Paul-tiwana@ouhsc.edu

M. Davidson
Private Practice, Mid-Kansas Oral & Maxillofacial Surgery, Wichita, KS, USA

P. Mehra, L. M. Wolford (eds.), *Management of Facial Asymmetry*,
https://doi.org/10.1007/978-3-030-44971-1_1

Introduction

One should resist any temptation to evaluate symmetry as simply right versus left, as facial asymmetry can occur in all planes of three-dimensional (3D) space. The combination of vertical, transverse, and anteroposterior (AP) positional changes can make it difficult to pinpoint the extent of an asymmetry. Furthermore, asymmetry may be isolated to one anatomic area of the face or involve multiple tissues and regions. Bones such as the mandible, maxilla, nasal bones, zygomas, orbits, and cranial bones may all be involved. Soft tissue structures affected may include the skin, vascular and lymphatics systems, nasal and auricular tissues, salivary glands, muscles, and nerves. While easy to overlook on an extraoral exam, alveolar bone and abnormalities in the dentition may contribute to, or even be the cause of, a noticeable asymmetry. Finally, the mandibular ramus condyle unit and temporomandibular joints (TMJs) are a unique combination of both soft and hard tissues which commonly contribute to facial asymmetry. Abnormal development or function of the tissues in the ramus condyle unit frequently leads to asymmetry in the surrounding bony, soft tissue, and dentoalveolar structures.

When a patient presents for treatment of facial asymmetry, proper diagnosis and treatment, if indicated, are paramount to obtaining an optimal outcome. The most crucial step in this process is often the surgeon's thorough evaluation of a patient's chief complaint. Without correct diagnosis of the etiology of facial asymmetry, appropriate treatment will be difficult to render. Initial workup for any facial asymmetry should consider medical history, historical timeline and progression of the condition, facial and oral evaluation, imaging, laboratory studies, and any indicated study casts or virtually generated computer models.

Beyond diagnosis, however, there are multiple factors that will influence the final result. A surgeon's experience and technique may render even correctly diagnosed etiologies challenging to treat. Regardless of a provider's experience and skill, some sources of asymmetry are simply more difficult to manage than others. Greater levels of difficulty will always make management of an asymmetry more challenging. While treatment plan execution can parallel the ability of the surgeon, many factors unique to the patient will also influence outcomes. Because facial growth abnormalities often present in developing children, remaining growth potential should be factored into every child who is evaluated. Opinions about management of the growing facial skeleton vary among practitioners, but failure to incorporate future growth into a treatment plan will negatively affect long-term surgical outcomes. Additional factors unique to each patient, such as their expectations and medical comorbidities, can alter even the most skillfully performed surgical procedures. These factors should be carefully considered and managed on a case-by-case basis.

Etiologies of facial asymmetry may be genetic, developmental or growth related, neuromuscular, iatrogenic, or acquired secondary to trauma, pathology, and infection [1]. The mandibular ramus condyle unit, in particular, is a region of the craniofacial skeleton that can be associated with most of these causes and frequently plays a role in many common facial asymmetries. Etiologies of facial asymmetry also include a large number of both congenital and developmental conditions. Several of these conditions such as craniosynostosis, hemifacial microsomia, and abnormalities of the TMJ will be reviewed in greater detail in later chapters. The focus of this chapter will be on initial diagnosis and patient evaluation in commonly encountered sources of facial asymmetry.

Clinical Assessment

Facial Assessment

Facial asymmetry can be evaluated using a combination of clinical examination, facial photographs, and craniofacial imaging. Oftentimes, clinical assessment is utilized as the first method of diagnosis. Photography and craniofacial imaging, however, serve as important ways to verify clinical assessments and document baseline records for progression over time and postoperative comparisons. Clinical assessments should be performed in the frontal, sagittal, and axial planes. Importantly, evaluation in these planes relies on relatively symmetric cranial base anatomy. Conditions such as craniosynostosis, hemifacial microsomia, and pathology or trauma affecting the orbital and midface regions will distort landmarks used in establishing baseline asymmetry [2–4]. Furthermore, head positioning should always be one of the first considerations when evaluating symmetry. Patients will oftentimes compensate for asymmetry with posturing of the head to mask cosmetic and functional sequelae of abnormal anatomy. Both the Frankfort (a line connecting the tragus of the ear with the bony infraorbital rim) and interpupillary planes should be kept parallel with the floor to ensure accurate facial analysis.

Frontal Evaluation

The frontal view allows analysis of facial symmetry in both vertical and transverse dimensions. Analysis is facilitated with horizontal lines drawn through the pupils and inferior portion of the earlobes. Generally, these lines are combined with a vertical line in between the medial palpebral fissures, approximating nasion, which is extended inferiorly through the mandibular border [5]. This established vertical reference allows comparison of transverse deviations in structures including the nose, mandible and chin, maxilla, and dental midlines. As previously highlighted, cranial base asymmetries causing vertical dystopia in the orbital or auricular regions will influence these reference planes and should be considered as part of each workup. A slightly different method of evaluating transverse relationships utilizes the rule of fifths. The transverse width of the face is divided into five zones based on vertical lines drawn through the outer helix of each ear and the medial and lateral ocular canthi. Each of the five zones created should be approximately equal to the width of an eye [6].

Most commonly associated with upper facial asymmetry is craniosynostosis, whether isolated or syndromic. Unilateral coronal synostosis and unilateral lambdoid synostosis can cause deflections of the skull base by more than 14 degrees resulting in significant orbital and mastoid asymmetry and may even result in lower

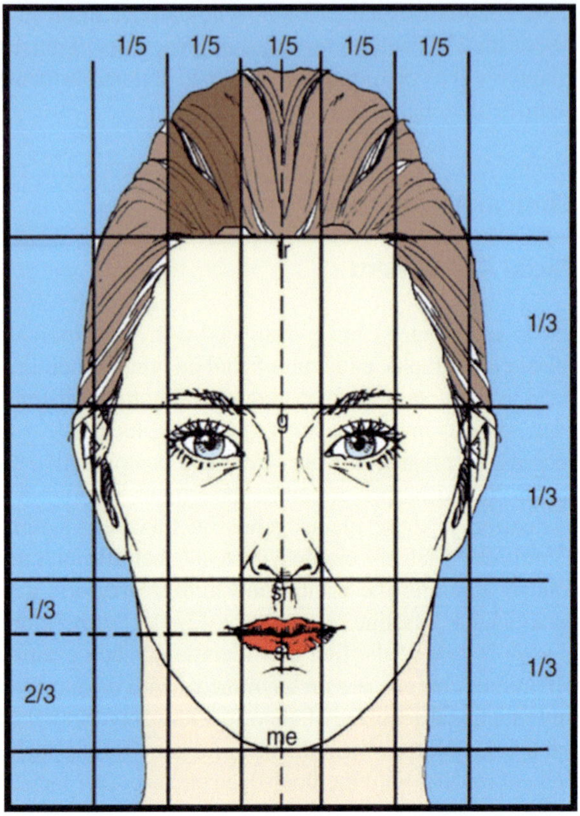

Fig. 1 Division of the vertical face between trichion (Tr) and soft tissue mention (Me). Facial "thirds" are produced with horizontal lines transecting soft tissue glabella (g) and subnasale (Sn). Evaluation of horizontal facial symmetry also depicted through the "rule of fifths"

facial asymmetry as childhood growth continues [7]. The syndromic forms of craniosynostosis such as Apert's syndrome may cause bilateral upper and lower facial deformity secondary to cranial base synostosis and synchondrosis. Symmetric deformity of the middle third of the face is also characterized by other genetic conditions such as mandibulofacial dysostosis which may result in variable orbitozygomatic hypoplasia and soft tissue deficiencies. Various pathological conditions such as fibrous dysplasia or tumors may also significantly contribute to facial asymmetry.

Vertical dimensions of the face are contained within the total facial height as measured from trichion (Tr) to soft tissue menton (Me). As depicted in Fig. 1, horizontal lines through soft tissue glabella (G) and subnasale (Sn) further divide this region into convenient upper, middle, and lower facial "thirds." The relative proportion of the upper, middle, and lower thirds is approximately 30%, 35%, and 35%, respectively [8]. Variability in these facial thirds will be noticed as facial morphologic change from mesocephalic to more asymmetric brachycephalic and dolichocephalic facial types [9]. Additional vertical comparisons can be made with measurements inferiorly from an interpupillary reference line, provided no orbital dystopia is present. Relationships of structures including the malar prominences, mandibular angles and inferior borders, chin, alar bases, oral commissures, and dentoalveolar canting as related to the maxillary canines can all be studied. Holding a tongue blade flat against the maxillary canines for comparison to the interpupillary plane is an alternate method to quickly assess dentoalveolar canting.

Profile Evaluation

Studying the contours of the face from a profile view will allow comparison of the angles and projections between the right and left facial halves. Positioning the head as shown in Fig. 2, specifically keeping Frankfort horizontal parallel to the floor, will ensure accurate assessment of relevant anatomy. The profile evaluation is generally most helpful for determining the relative anteroposterior (AP) positioning of the maxilla and mandible. Nonetheless, unique aspects of someone's profile can include landmarks from the bone and soft tissue overlying the frontal bone down

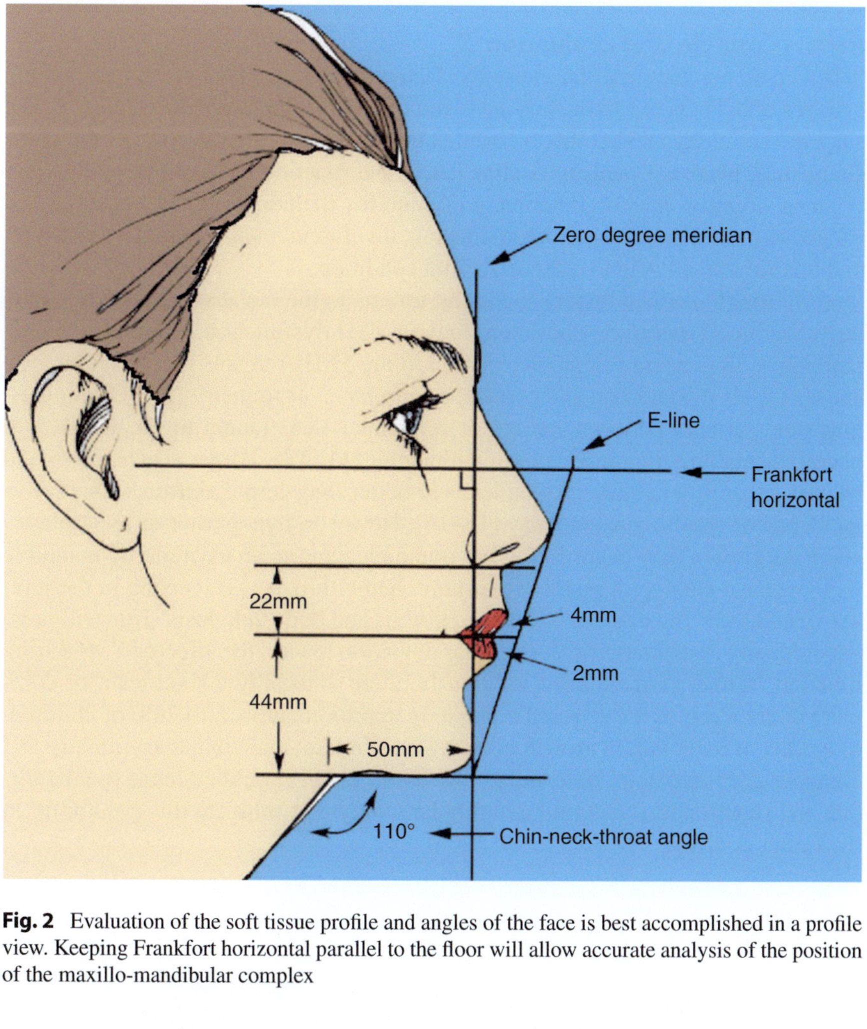

Fig. 2 Evaluation of the soft tissue profile and angles of the face is best accomplished in a profile view. Keeping Frankfort horizontal parallel to the floor will allow accurate analysis of the position of the maxillo-mandibular complex

through the soft tissue overlying the anterior neck. The nasolabial, labiomental, and chin-neck angles, for example, often correlate with skeletal abnormalities associated with class II and class III patients. Projection of the malar eminence and superior orbital rims can indicate underlying bony asymmetries which often differ between individuals and occasionally may be asymmetric in the same individual due to developmental, pathologic, or traumatic history.

Axial Evaluation

Asymmetry of prominent facial structures including the chin, mandibular condyles and body, nasal bones and cartilage, malar regions, and bony orbits can be visualized with relative ease in the axial plane. Clinically, this can be performed by standing behind the patient and looking down, or by standing in front and viewing the patient's projection with the head tilted back. The specific origin of any asymmetry can then be determined through adjunctive clinical history and radiographic exams.

Ramus Condyle Unit Evaluation

Whether or not they are the causative factor or simply affected by surrounding changes, the TMJs are frequently involved in facial asymmetry. Regardless of the suspected etiology of TMJ involvement, a thorough clinical evaluation of the joints should take place to establish baseline health and function. Assessment of clicking/popping, crepitus, pain on function, joint mobility including maximal opening and excursive movements, deviation on opening, myofascial pain, headaches, earaches, and tinnitus can all help to categorize joint condition.

A thorough medical history including trauma to the facial skeleton may be the most beneficial tool to diagnosis etiology of TMJ dysfunction. While many TMJ pathophysiologies are idiopathic, trauma to the TMJs remains the most common cause of their dysfunction and contribution to facial asymmetry [10]. Oftentimes, however, patients may not realize or remember that trauma to the joints ever occurred, making diagnosis more challenging [11, 12]. Larger regenerative and healing capacity in children often leads to better long-term function with a lower incidence of resulting asymmetry [13–16]. However, hypoplastic or hyperplastic condylar growth may occur following trauma leading to an asymmetric mandible with occlusal canting at rest. Furthermore, hemarthrosis and scarring in the joint may lead to varying degrees of reactive fibrous and bony ankylosis. This will present clinically as asymmetric mandibular deviation toward the affected TMJ during function. While, as mentioned previously, there is usually a significant or complete remodeling of the affected condyle in approximately 15 to 20% of children, a significant reduction in growth occurs with resultant mandibular asymmetry and compensatory maxillary deformity [17]. Every effort should be made to rehabilitate and function the fractured mandibular condyle to mitigate this possibility to the extent possible.

Conditions resulting in condylar resorption, whether unilateral or bilateral, will present with multiple abnormalities on clinical assessment. Juvenile idiopathic arthritis (JIA) and degenerative disease can create notable pain and dysfunction in the TMJs. While JIA will often be diagnosed from existing systemic involvement, TMJ involvement has been reported to range from 11% to as high as 87% [18–20]. When involved, many of these patients go on to develop degeneration and internal derangements. Clinically, dysfunction can range from mild stiffness to a retrognathic presentation with decreased opening and partial ankylosis [21].

Idiopathic condylar resorption is another condition resulting in progressive resorption of condylar mass. By definition, it cannot be attributed to rheumatoid or osteoarthritis and is most commonly seen in 15- to 30-year-old females [22–24]. Although etiologies for the condition have included increased trauma/loading, avascular necrosis, and estrogen hormonal influences, the cause of this resorption remains largely unknown [24–27]. Because this condition nearly always occurs bilaterally, it does not result in extensive asymmetry between the right and left mandibular condyles. Patients will, however, have extensive changes noted to their occlusion and profile evaluation. Progressive anterior open bite, increasing overjet, and class 2 occlusion with a retruded chin will all be observed. Regardless of the etiology of condylar resorption, appropriate imaging should play a role in diagnosis and treatment planning. Magnetic resonance imaging (MRI) remains a valuable adjunct to the TMJ clinical exam. MRI of the TMJ is valuable for its ability to detect synovitis, joint effusion, marrow edema, and bony morphology [28, 29]. Skeletal scintigraphy and serial plain film studies can also be helpful to ensure that premature treatment is not rendered during an active resorption process [30, 31].

In contrast to resorptive processes, condylar hyperplasia (CH) is an accelerated and progressive overgrowth of one or both of the mandibular condyles. Many different etiologies have been suggested including trauma, infection, condylar loading, hormones, heredity factors, and alterations in growth factors [32]. Classification systems and treatment algorithms for CH have helped to organize its treatment with predictable outcomes [33–36]. Figures 3, 4, and 5 illustrate the clinical presentation of this condition and the asymmetry it can produce. Depending on the number of TMJs involved, clinical assessment will yield either a unilateral or bilateral progressive class 3 relationship with possible dental crossbite and mandibular midline shift [37].

The classic congenital abnormality of the ramus condyle unit remains craniofacial/hemifacial microsomia. While controversy exists as to its causality, one generally accepted explanation put forth by Poswillo is thought to be related to in utero infarction of the stapedial artery [38]. Similar abnormalities can be seen in the genetically based Goldenhar syndrome or oculo-auriculo-vertebral syndrome which

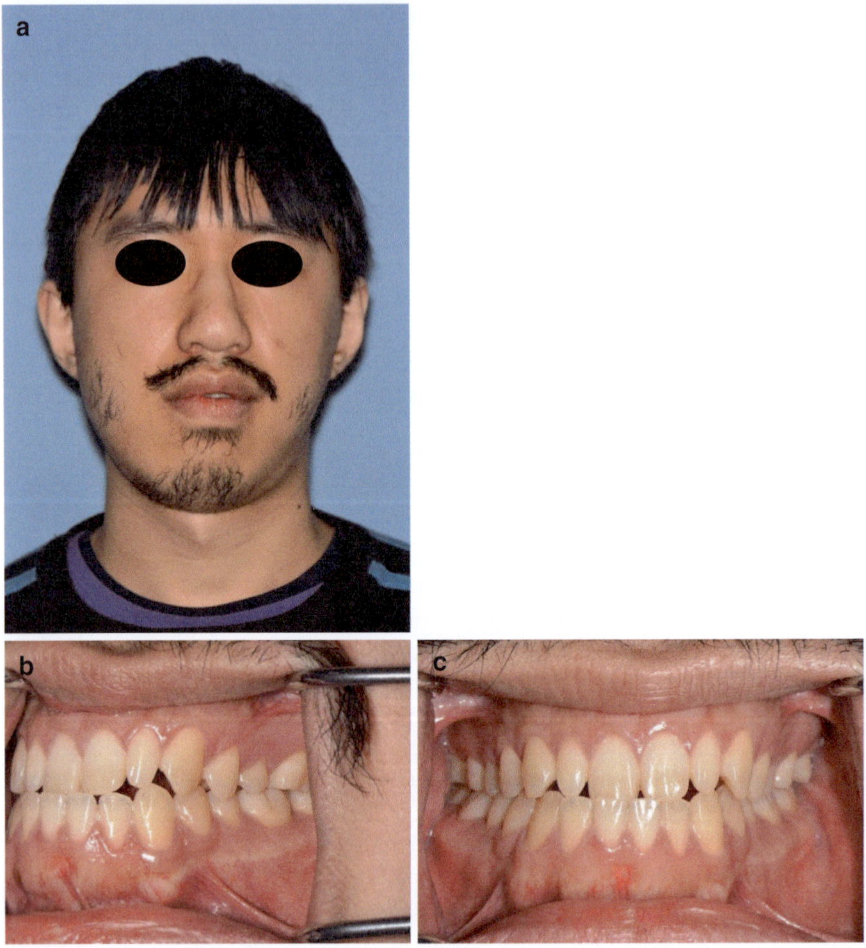

Fig. 3 (**a**) A 26-year-old patient with unilateral left condylar hyperplasia. (**b**, **c**) A characteristic ipsilateral class 3 malocclusion with a mandibular midline shift away from the affected condyle is seen on preoperative intraoral evaluation

causes anomalous development of units in the first and second branchial arch. Regardless of the etiology, numerous classification schemes have been developed to describe the aberrant anatomy of the ramus condyle unit. Clinically useful classifications as described by Kaban usually describe the degree of hypoplasia of the affected mandibular ramus and condyle as well as the position/degree of hypoplasia of the glenoid fossa [39]. While a unilateral deformity as shown in Fig. 6 is more common, it can also present bilaterally.

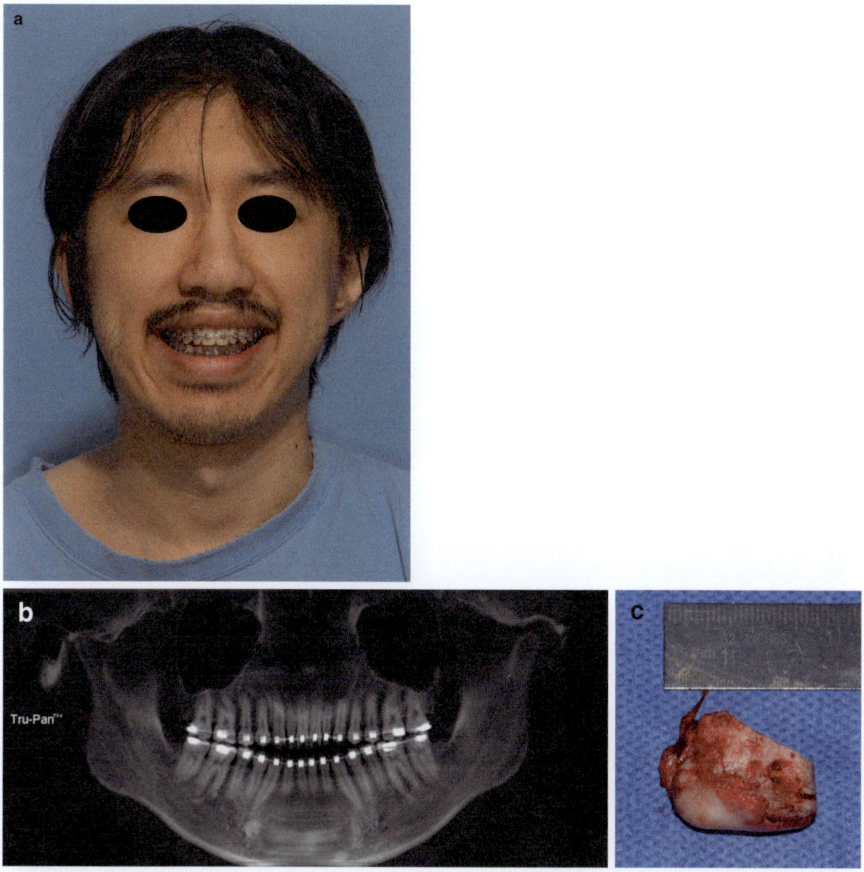

Fig. 4 (**a**, **b**) The same 26-year-old patient following a left high condylectomy and initiation of orthodontic therapy. (**c**) The left condyle specimen obtained during the high condylectomy procedure

Timeline of Symmetry Changes

During evaluation of facial asymmetries, it is important to consider the speed at which progression of an abnormality has developed. The high prevalence of TMJ etiology or involvement in asymmetrical changes has previously been highlighted. Generally, asymmetry of TMJ origin will develop over a period of weeks to multiple months. Idiopathic condylar resorption, condylar hyperplasia, osteochondroma, and other TMJ pathology are just several examples of conditions which lead to asymmetries in this manner. Alternatively, rapid changes in symmetry of the face or mandible should be worked up for recent trauma, infection, or neuromuscular etiologies.

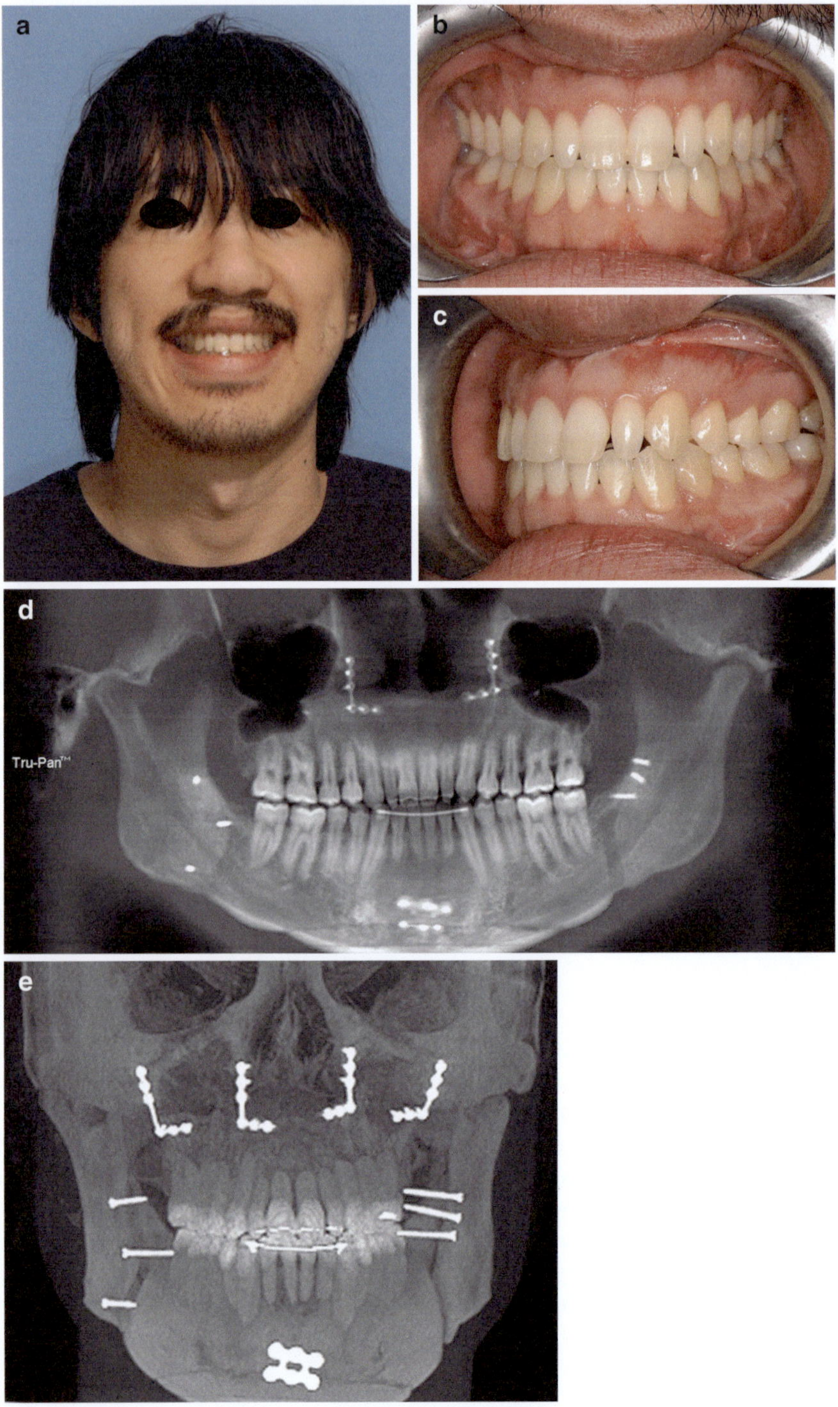

Fig. 5 The same 26-year-old patient following orthognathic surgery. (**a**) Restoration of facial symmetry was achieved following surgery. (**b**, **c**) Intraoral exam illustrating correction of the previous class 3 malocclusion and midline discrepancy. (**d**, **e**) Postoperative imaging confirms establishment of symmetric dimensions to the condylar-ramus subunits

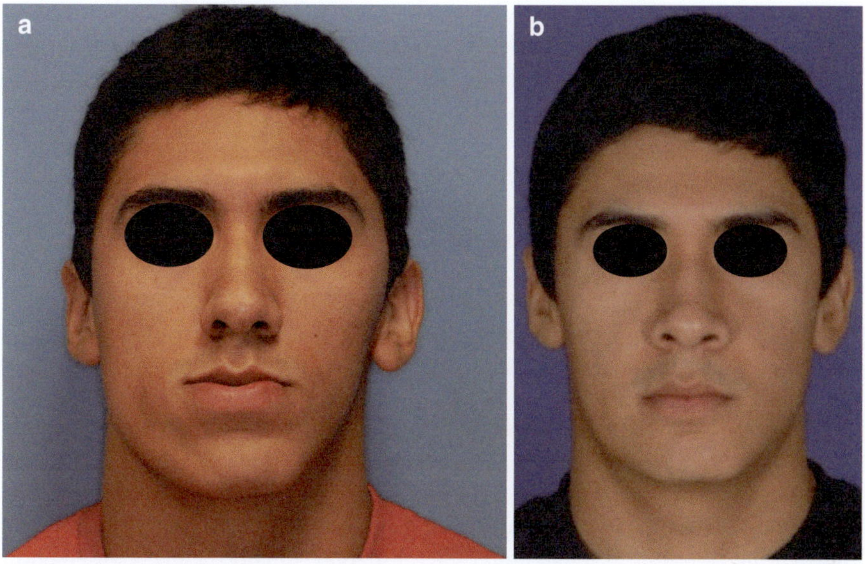

Fig. 6 (**a**) Unilateral facial asymmetry in a patient with left hemifacial macrosomia. Marked asymmetry of the left mandibular body and ramus is evident. The patient underwent a right mandibular sagittal osteotomy, left vertical ramus osteotomy with left angle bone graft, reversing wedge genioplasty, and three-piece Le Fort 1 with incorporated yaw to address his facial asymmetry. (**b**) Postoperative restoration of facial symmetry

Furthermore, age of onset often provides clues about particular abnormalities. While conditions such as craniofacial microsomia will be identified early in life, irregular condylar growth and resorptive processes are particularly common in the teenage years. While not all sources of facial asymmetry can be correlated with age, understanding some of these tendencies can greatly assist your efforts to determine a diagnosis and treatment plan.

Oral Assessment

Similar to extraoral evaluation of asymmetry, intraoral contributions to facial asymmetry can occur in the vertical, horizontal, and AP dimensions. The etiology of these dentoalveolar variations can be entirely idiopathic or related to habits, loss and disease of the dentition, discrepancies between CR and CO, congenital conditions, or pathology.

Idiopathic causes of dentoalveolar asymmetry commonly result in canting of the occlusal plane from unequal vertical growth of the alveolar complexes. This dentoalveolar canting is readily identified on extraoral exam in relation to the interpupillary plane as previously discussed. Additionally, unequal AP alveolar development can result in a shift of one or both of the dental midlines. Similar to idiopathic causes, long-standing pathology of the dentoalveolar region can also cause both occlusal canting and midline shifts.

Several congenital conditions which can cause extensive asymmetry of the craniofacial skeleton are hemifacial microsomia, craniosynostosis, and cleft lip and palate. While hemifacial microsomia and craniosynostosis will be discussed in detail in future chapters, the asymmetries created from cleft lip and palate should not be overlooked. Cleft lip and palate is the most common congenital craniofacial anomaly occurring in approximately 1 in 700 live births [11, 40]. Whether unilateral or bilateral, cleft lip and palate results in multiple dentoalveolar asymmetries in all dimensions. These develop due to decreased vertical and horizontal alveolar ridge development, hypoplastic or missing teeth, and reduced maxillary growth secondary to scarring from multiple childhood surgeries [11, 41–43].

Careful assessment of the dentition is also necessary during workup for facial asymmetry. Loss of tooth mass due to hypo-/oligodontia, peg-shaped lateral incisors, trauma, caries, impaction, or ankylosis can lead to poor alveolar ridge development, canting of the occlusal plane, and dental midline shifts away from the facial midline. An additional source of dental midline shifting, specifically seen in the mandible, is a discrepancy between CR and centric occlusion (CO). This should be suspected if a shift of the mandibular midline away from the facial midline occurs after putting the teeth into maximum intercuspation. Finally, changes observed in the dentition can be indicative of functional habits that lead to facial asymmetry. The combination of anterior dental intrusion, flared maxillary anterior teeth, and apertognathia, for example, suggests a thumb sucking habit that may manifest with collapse of the transverse palatal dimension. Similarly, apertognathia and dentoalveolar asymmetry may be the result of a tongue thrust habit originating from an enlarged or hyperactive tongue muscle.

Study Models and Computer-Aided Surgical Planning

Dental study models offer a method to confirm and quantify the asymmetries noted on a clinical exam. Planning for surgical interventions can be performed if these models are accurately mounted on an anatomic articulator. Unfortunately, the mounting of these study models is known to have some potential inaccuracies, particularly when utilizing a facebow registration. This may leave room for errors in surgical planning and future execution [44–46]. Mounting with an occlusal plane indicator is one alternative to this potential error [47, 48]. However, obtaining an accurate occlusal registration in CR and the inaccuracies associated with traditional model surgery can all introduce error into surgical plans. Current technological innovations like virtual surgical planning and computer-aided surgical simulation are adding diversity and accuracy to the way surgeons diagnose and the treatment plan for facial asymmetries [49–51].

Pseudo-asymmetry

Absolute and relative asymmetries should be carefully differentiated during diagnosis and treatment planning. Absolute asymmetry exists when the craniofacial skeleton, dentition, or overlying soft tissues have asymmetry that is not corrected with positioning of the mandible into a CR position. In comparison, pseudo-asymmetry is present when positioning of the condyles into CR eliminates the asymmetry in question. Posturing of the mandible in this way can originate from multiple sources including malocclusion, neuromuscular dysfunction, infection, myositis, and condylar dislocation.

Malocclusion

Pseudo-asymmetry caused by a malocclusion is generally the result of premature occlusal contacts. Patients with occlusal prematurity will shift between CR and CO to achieve a more comfortable occlusal position. Clinically, this will present as a mandibular midline shift which is eliminated during positioning of the mandible into CR. The side with occlusal interference will often be in a class 3 relationship with radiographic workup confirming anterior positioning of the condyle in the glenoid fossa. More often than not, the malocclusion will result from a combination of skeletal and dental asymmetry in three dimensions of space. Occlusal equilibration, orthodontics, or orthognathic surgery can be utilized to correct this type of asymmetry.

Muscular Dysfunction

While multiple muscles can be involved, the relationship of the TMJ to the lateral pterygoid muscle helps explain its frequent implication in mandibular asymmetries of neuromuscular origin. Neuromuscular disorders, myositis, guarding secondary to pain, and trauma-related contracture are just several etiologies one should consider. Clinically, this condition will present with a similar mandibular midline shift away from the affected side. Similar to a malocclusion, this will result in an ipsilateral class 3 occlusion with a possible contralateral crossbite. Unlike a malocclusion, however, a muscular etiology tends to present more abruptly as it is oftentimes related to pain stemming from trauma or infection/inflammation.

Condylar Dislocation

Condylar dislocation can be caused by a many different etiologies. Poor muscle coordination, ligament laxity, altered eminence morphology, trauma, myospasm, prolonged opening, and connective tissue disease can all be possible causes of this condition [52, 53]. Dislocation involves displacement of the mandibular condyle past the height of the articular eminence resulting in significant malocclusion and anterior ipsilateral mandibular displacement. While spontaneous reduction can occur, oftentimes, the inability to reduce this dislocation will be a source of great pain and anxiety to the patient. Categorization and treatment of the condition is based on the acute or chronic nature of the dislocation. Acute dislocations are often managed nonsurgically with bimanual intraoral reduction or stimulation of the patient's gag reflex [54–56]. Chronic dislocations may be managed with botulinum toxin, muscle relaxants, a period of intermaxillary fixation, sclerosing agents, and autologous blood injections to decrease range of motion through fibrosis [57–59]. If chronic dislocations continue, however, surgical interventions such as lateral pterygoid myotomy or eminectomy may be indicated.

Infection

Infections can present in many facial regions. Common regions include dentoalveolar structures, salivary tissue, fascial spaces, lymphatic tissue, and overlying skin. In addition to creating a notable facial asymmetry, clinical examination will often reveal pain and tenderness to palpation, erythema, warm temperature, induration, and possible purulent discharge [60]. Most infectious causes of facial asymmetry will be acute onset in nature, and an accurate clinical history will often go a long way in helping with diagnosis. Appropriate imaging should be followed by standard principles of incision and drainage, culture and sensitivity, debridement/irrigation, removing the source of infection, and antibiotic therapy [61]. One frequently associated cause of mandibular asymmetry secondary to infection is recurrent mastoiditis in early childhood. If not adequately controlled medically, this chronic inflammatory condition may result in restricted growth of the TMJ and/or ankylosis ultimately resulting in significant asymmetry.

Age Considerations

Facial asymmetry diagnosed in the child or adolescent must take into consideration the remaining growth potential of the patient. Females have generally completed facial skeletal maturation by age 15 and boys slightly later by age 17 or 18 [62–65]. It is ideal for any patient, child, or adult to limit the number of surgeries to as few as possible. Waiting until completion of a patient's growth for restoration of facial asymmetry is one way to ensure this. While prolonging asymmetry correction may be possible in certain patients, others have abnormalities that cannot be delayed [66, 67]. Some indications for surgery prior to skeletal maturation include psychological benefit, pathology, and functional/masticatory dysfunction [10, 68]. If a patient undergoes surgery prior to growth completion, educating the patient and family about the likelihood of needing additional surgery is paramount.

References

1. Srivastava D, Singh H, Mishra S, Sharma P, Kapoor P, Chandra L. Facial asymmetry revisited: part 1 diagnosis and treatment planning. J Oral Biol Cranifac Res. 2018;8:7–14. https://doi.org/10.1016/j.jobcr.2017.04.010.
2. Sandor GKB, Habil D, McGuire TP, Ylikontiola LP, Serlo WS, Pirttiniemi PM. Management of Facial Asymmetry. Oral Maxillofac Surg Clin N Am. 2007;19:395–422. https://doi.org/10.1016/j.coms.2007.05.001.

3. Thiesen G, Gribel BF, Freita MPM. Facial asymmetry: a current review. Dental Press J Orthod. 2015;20(6):110–25. https://doi.org/10.1590/2177-6709.20.6.110-125.sar.
4. Posnik JC. Treatment planning in orthognathic surgery. In: Fonseca RJ, editor. Oral and maxillofacial surgery, vol. 3. 3rd ed. St Louis: Elsevier; 2018. p. 13–30.
5. Wolford LM. Facial asymmetry: diagnosis and treatment considerations. In: Fonseca RJ, Marciani RD, Turvey TA, editors. Oral and maxillofacial surgery, vol. 3. 2nd ed. St Louis: Elsevier; 2009. p. 272–315.
6. Sarver DM. Esthetic orthodontics and orthognathic surgery. Mosby: Elsevier Science; 1998. p. 1–60.
7. Stella JP. Evaluation of the face for aesthetic surgery. Oral Maxillofac Surg Clin N Am. 1996;8(1):1–12.
8. Farkas LG, Munro IR. Anthropometric facial proportions in medicine. JAMA. 1987;258:5–16.
9. Movahed R, Mercuri LG. Management of temporomandibular joint ankylosis. Oral Maxillofac Surg Clin N Am. 2015;27:27–35. https://doi.org/10.1016/j.coms.2014.09.003.
10. Waite PD, Urban SD. Facial asymmetry. In: Miloro M, Ghali GE, Larsen PE, Waite PD, editors. Peterson's principles of Oral and maxillofacial surgery. Connecticut: People's Medical Publishing House; 2012. p. 1393–410.
11. Proffit WR, Vig KW, Turvey TA. Early fracture of the mandibular condyle: frequently an unsuspected cause of growth disturbances. Am J Orthod. 1980;78:1–24.
12. Defabianis P. TMJ fractures in children and adolescents: treatment guidelines. J Clin Pediatr Dent. 2003;27:191–9.
13. Zhang Y, He DM. Clinical investigation of early post-traumatic temporomandibular joint Ankylosis and the role of repositioning discs in treatment. Int J Oral Maxillofac Surg. 2006;35:1096–101. https://doi.org/10.1016/j.ijom.2006.09.003.
14. Chang S, Yang Y, Liu Y, Wang J, Zhang W, Ma Q. How does the remodeling capacity of children affect the morphologic changes of fractured mandibular condylar processes after conservative treatment? J Oral Maxillofac Surg. 2018;76:1279.e1–7. https://doi.org/10.1016/j.joms.2018.01.029.
15. Theologie-Lygidakis N, Chatzidimitriou K, Tzerbos F, Gouzioti A, Iatrou I. Nonsurgical Management of Condylar Fractures in children: a 15-year clinical retrospective study. J Craniomaxillofac Surg. 2016;44:85–93. https://doi.org/10.1016/j.jcms.2015.11.011.
16. Billiau AD, Hu Y, Verdonck A, Carels C, Wouters C. Temporomandibular joint arthritis in juvenile idiopathic arthritis: prevalence, clinical and radiographic signs, and relation to Dentofacial morphology. J Rheumatol. 2007;34:1925–33.
17. Frid A, Nordal E, Bovis F, Giancane G, Larheim TA, Rygg M, et al. Temporomandibular joint involvement is associated with quality of life, disability and high disease activity in juvenile idiopathic arthritis. Arthritis Care Res. 2017;69:677–86. https://doi.org/10.1002/acr.23003.
18. Mandall NA, Gray R, O'Brian KD, Baildam E, Macfarlane TV, Davidson J. Juvenile idiopathic arthritis (JIA): a screening study to measure class II skeletal pattern, TMJ PDS and use of systemic corticosteroids. J Orthod. 2010;37:6–15. https://doi.org/10.1179/14653121042831.
19. Granquist EJ. Treatment of the temporomandibular joint in a child with juvenile idiopathic arthritis. Oral Maxillofac Surg Clin N Am. 2018;30:97–107. https://doi.org/10.1016/j.coms.2017.08.002.
20. Huang YL, Pogrel MA, Kaban LB. Diagnosis and Management of Condylar Resorption. J Oral Maxillofac Surg. 1997;55(2):114–9.
21. Sansare K, Raghav M, Mallya SM, Karjodkar F. Management related outcome and radiographic findings of idiopathic condylar resorption: a systematic review. Int J Oral Maxillofac Surg. 2015;44:209–16. https://doi.org/10.1016/j.ijom.2014.09.005.
22. Papadaki ME, Tayebaty F, Kaba LB, Troulis MJ. Condylar resorption. Oral Maxillofac Surg Clin N Am. 2007;19:223–34. https://doi.org/10.1016/j.coms.2007.01.002.
23. Hwang SJ, Haers PE, Seifert B, Sailer HF. Non-surgical risk factors for condylar resorption after orthognathic surgery. J Craniomaxillofac Surg. 2004;32:103–11. https://doi.org/10.1016/S1010-5182(03)00127-6.

24. Hwang SJ, Haers PE, Zimmermann A, Oechslin C, Seifert B, Sailer HF. Surgical risk factors for condylar resorption after orthognathic surgery. Oral Surg Oral Med Oral Pathol Oral Radiol Endod. 2000;89:55452. https://doi.org/10.1067/moe.2000.105239.
25. Gunson MJ, Arnett GW, Milam SB. Pathophysiology and pharmacology control of osseous mandibular condylar resorption. J Oral Maxillofac Surg. 2012;70:1918–34. https://doi.org/10.1016/j.joms.2011.07.018.
26. Navallas M, Inarejos EJ, Iglesias E, Lee GYC, Rodriguez N, Anton J. MR imaging of the temporomandibular joint in juvenile idiopathic arthritis: technique and findings. Radiographics. 2017;37(2):595–612. https://doi.org/10.1148/rg.2017160078.
27. Vaid YN, Dunnavant FD, Royal SA, Beukelman T, Stoll ML, Cron RQ. Imaging of the temporomandibular joint in juvenile idiopathic arthritis. Arthritis Care Res. 2014;66(1):47–554. https://doi.org/10.1002/acr.22177.
28. Cisneros GJ, Kaban LB. Computerized skeletal scintigraphy for assessment of mandibular asymmetry. J Oral Maxillofac Surg. 1984;42:513–20.
29. Kaban LB, Cisneros GJ, Heyman S, Treves S. Assessment of mandibular growth by skeletal scintigraphy. J Oral Maxillofac Surg. 1982;40(1):18–22.
30. Hayward JD, Walker RV, Poulton G, et al. Asymmetric mandibular excess. In: Bell W, Proffit W, White R, editors. Surgical correction of dentofacial deformities. Philadelphia: WB Saunders; 1980. p. 947–53.
31. Wolford LM, Movahed R, Perez DE. A classification system for conditions causing condylar hyperplasia. J Oral Maxillofac Surg. 2014;72:567–95. https://doi.org/10.1016/j.joms.2013.09.002.
32. Wolford LM, Morales-Ryan CA, Garcia-Morales P, Perez D. Surgical management of mandibular condylar hyperplasia type 1. Proc (Bayl Univ Med Cent). 2009;22(4):321–9. https://doi.org/10.1080/08998280.11928546.
33. Wolford LM, Mehra P, Reiche-Fischel O, Morales-Ryan CA, Garcia-Morales P. Efficacy of high condylectomy for management of condylar hyperplasia. Am J Orthod Dentofac Orthop. 2002;121:136–51. https://doi.org/10.1067/mod.2002.118403.
34. Wolford LM. Mandibular asymmetry: temporomandibular joint degeneration. In: Bagheri SC, Bell RB, Khan HA, editors. Current therapy in oral and maxillofacial surgery. St. Louis (MO); 2012. p. 696–725. Chapter 82.
35. Rodrigues DB, Castro V. Condylar hyperplasia of the temporomandibular joint. Oral Maxillofacial Surg Clin N Am. 2015;27:155–67. https://doi.org/10.1016/j.coms.2014.09.011.
36. Tolarova MM, Cervenka J. Classification and birth prevalence of orofacial clefts. Am J Med Genet. 1998;75:126–37.
37. Bardach J. The influence of cleft repair on facial growth. Cleft Palate J. 1990;27:76–8.
38. Shaw WC, Dahl E, Asher-McDade C, Brattstrom V, Mars M, McWilliam J, et al. A six-center international study of treatment outcome in patients with clefts of the lip and palate. Part 5. General discussion and conclusions. Cleft Palate Craniofac J. 1992;29:413–8.
39. Semb B. A study of facial growth in patients with unilateral cleft lip and palate treated by Oslo CLP team. Cleft Palate Craniofac J. 1991;28:1–21.
40. O'Malley AM, Milosevic A. Comparison of three facebow/semi-adjustable articulator systems for planning orthognathic surgery. Br J Oral Maxillofac Surg. 2000;38:1855–190. https://doi.org/10.1054/bjom.1999.0182.
41. Ellis E, Tharanon W, Gambrell K. Accuracy of face-Bow transfer: effect on surgical prediction and postsurgical result. J Oral Maxillofac Surg. 1991;50:562–7.
42. Gateno J, Forrest KK, Camp B. A comparison of 3 methods of face-Bow transfer recording: implications for orthognathic surgery. J Oral Maxillofac Surg. 2001;59:635–40. https://doi.org/10.1053/joms.2001.23374.
43. Wolford LM, Galiano A. A simple and accurate method for mounting models in orthognathic surgery. J Oral Maxillofac Surg. 2007;65:1406–9. https://doi.org/10.1016/j.joms.2005.12.047.

44. Mayrink G, Sawazaki R, Asprino L, Moraes M, Moreira RWF. Comparative study between 2 methods of mounting models in Semiadjustable articulator for orthognathic surgery. J Oral Maxillofac Surg. 2011;69:2879–82. https://doi.org/10.1016/j.joms.2010.12.030.
45. Farrell BB, Franco PB, Tucker MR. Virtual surgical planning in orthognathic surgery. Oral Maxillofac Surg Clin N Am. 2014;26:459–73. https://doi.org/10.1016/j.coms.2014.08.011.
46. Gelesko S, Markiewicz MR, Weimer K, Bell RB. Computer-aided orthognathic surgery. Atlas Oral Maxillofac Surg Clin N Am. 2012;20:107–18. https://doi.org/10.1016/j.cxom.2012.01.002.
47. Yuan P, Mai H, Li J, Ho DCY, Lai Y, Liu S, et al. Design, development and clinical validation of computer-aided surgical simulation system for streamlined orthognathic surgical planning. Int J Comput Assist Radiol Surg. 2017;12(12):2129–43. https://doi.org/10.1007/s11548-017-15585-6.
48. Liddell A, Perez DE. Temporomandibular joint dislocation. Oral Maxillofac Surg Clin N Am. 2015;27:125–36. https://doi.org/10.1016/j.coms.2014.09.009.
49. Adekeye EO, Shamia RI, Cove P. Inverted L-shaped ramus osteotomy for prolonged bilateral dislocation of the Temporomandiublar joint. Oral Surg. 1976;41(5):568–77.
50. Howe AG, Kent JN, Farrell CD, Poidmore SJ. Implant of articular Eminence for recurrent dislocation of the temporomandibular joint. J Oral Surg. 1978;36(7):23–526.
51. Ardehali MM, Kouhi A, Meighani A, Rad FM, Emami H. Temporomandibular joint dislocation reduction technique: a new external method vs. the traditional. Ann Plast Surg. 2009;63:176–8. https://doi.org/10.1097/SAP.0b013e31818937aa.
52. Fordyce GL. Long standing bilateral dislocation of the jaw. Br J Oral Surg. 1960;52:222–5.
53. Machon V, Abramowicz S, Dolwick MF. Autologous blood injection for the treatment of chronic recurrent temporomandibular joint dislocation. J Oral Maxillofac Surg. 2009;67:114–9. https://doi.org/10.1016/j.joms.2008.08.044.
54. Awang MN. A new approach to the reduction of acute dislocation of the temporomandibular joint: a report of three cases. Br J Oral Maxillofac Surg. 1987;25:244–9.
55. Fu KY, Chen HM, Sun ZP, Zhang ZK, Ma XC. Long-term efficacy of Botulinim toxin type a for the treatment of habitual dislocation of the temporomandibular joint. Br J Oral Maxillofac Surg. 2010;48:281–4. https://doi.org/10.1016/j.bjoms.2009.07.014.
56. Osborn TM, Assael LA, Bell RB. Deep space neck infection: principles of surgical management. Oral Maxillofac Surg Clin N Am. 2008;20:353–65. https://doi.org/10.1016/j.coms.2008.04.002.
57. Lypka M, Hammoudeh J. Dentoalveolar infections. Oral Maxillofac Surg Clin N Am. 2011;23:415–24. https://doi.org/10.1016/j.coms.2011.04.010.
58. Björk A, Skieller V. Growth of the maxilla in three dimensions as revealed radiographically by the implant method. Br J Orthod. 1977;4:53–64.
59. Savara BS, Singh IJ. Norms of size and annual increments of seven anatomical measures of maxilla in boys from three to sixteen years of age. Angle Orthod. 1968;38:104–20.
60. Singh IJ, Savara BS. Norms of size and annual increments of seven anatomical measures of maxilla in girls from three to seventeen years of age. Angle Orthod. 1968;36:312–24.
61. O'Reilly MT. A longitudinal growth study: maxillary length at puberty in females. Angle Orthod. 1979;49:234–58.
62. Wolford LM, Karras SC, Mehra P. Considerations for orthognathic surgery during growth part 1: mandibular deformities. Am J Orthod and Dentofac Orthopedics. 2001;119:95–101. https://doi.org/10.1067/mod.2001.111401.
63. Wolford LM, Karras SC, Mehra P. Considerations for orthognathic surgery during growth part 2: maxillary deformities. Am J Orthod and Dentofac Orthopedics. 2001;119:102–5. https://doi.org/10.1067/mod.2001.111400.
64. MacGregor FC. Facial disfigurement: problems and Management of Social interaction and implications for mental health. Aesth Plast Surg. 1990;14:249–57.

65. Kiyak HA, McNeill RW, West RA. The emotional impact of orthognathic surgery and conventional orthodontics. Am J Orthod. 1985;88(3):224–34.
66. Rustemeyer J, Gregersen J. Quality of life in orthognathic surgery patients: post-surgical improvements in aesthetics and self-confidence. J Craniomaxillofac Surg. 2012;40:400–4. https://doi.org/10.1016/j.jcms.2011.07.009.
67. Resnik CM. Temporomandibular joint reconstruction in the growing child. Oral Maxillofac Surg Clin N Am. 2018;30:109–21. https://doi.org/10.1016/j.coms.2017.08.006.
68. Singh V, Verma A, Kumar I, Bhagol A. Reconstruction of ankylosed temporomandibular joint: sternoclavicular grafting as an approach to management. Int J Oral Maxillofac Surg. 2011;40:260–5. https://doi.org/10.1016/j.ijom.2010.09.023.

Imaging and Facial Asymmetry

David C. Hatcher and Shikha Rathi

Abstract

Facial asymmetry may occur due to multiple etiologies, including developmental, pathologic, and traumatic conditions or a variable combination of these. Facial asymmetry is a radiographic or clinical sign, and not a diagnosis. The diagnostic category or etiology of a facial asymmetry can be determined by integrating three-dimensional (3D) imaging with the clinical findings and the patient's history. A large field of view such as seen with computerized tomography (CT) or cone beam CT (CBCT) scans is ideal for imaging the maxillofacial skeleton to identify or rule out the presence of a skeletal asymmetry. In the case of a skeletal asymmetry, a CBCT enables an anatomic component analysis to determine which skeletal elements are demonstrating deviant form and growth. The component analysis results are used to identify the etiology and activity status of the maxillofacial asymmetry. It is well recognized that facial asymmetry due to mandibular asymmetry is frequently associated with an underlying temporomandibular joint (TMJ) anomaly. This chapter discusses the biomechanics and morphologic alterations involved in the development of an asymmetry along

D. C. Hatcher (✉)
School of Dentistry, Department of Orthodontics, University of Pacific, San Francisco, CA, USA

Orofacial Sciences, School of Dentistry, University of Pacific, San Francisco, CA, USA

School of Dentistry, University of California, Los Angeles, CA, USA

Dept. of Surgical & Radiological Sciences, School of Veterinary Medicine, University of California, Davis, Los Angeles, CA, USA
e-mail: David@ddicenters.com

S. Rathi
Department of Orthodontics, University of Pacific, San Francisco, CA, USA

P. Mehra, L. M. Wolford (eds.), *Management of Facial Asymmetry*,
https://doi.org/10.1007/978-3-030-44971-1_2

with a focus on imaging characteristics associated with TMJ-related conditions contributing to a mandibular asymmetry.

Keywords

Facial asymmetry · 3-dimensional imaging · computerized tomography · Temporomandibular Joint · TMJ anomaly

Introduction

Facial asymmetry is a clinical phenotype that must be investigated to determine the underlying cause and activity state. Facial asymmetry signifies a size and shape difference when comparing the two halves of the face. Asymmetry severity exists along a continuum extending from very minor to major asymmetry. Minor asymmetries are usually considered within the range of normal variation, while more severe asymmetries are often an external manifestation of an underlying anomaly of the skeleton or soft tissues [1]. The diagnostic category or etiology of a facial asymmetry can be determined by integrating 3D imaging with the clinical findings and patient history.

Imaging Diagnosis of Facial Asymmetry

Any of the tissue types comprising the facial soft tissue can be the source of a facial asymmetry. These include muscle, fat, blood vessels, nerves, lymphatics, salivary glands, and epithelium. Anomalies of the blood vessels, nerves, and lymphatics may have a trophic effect on the subjacent skeleton either enhancing or diminishing skeletal growth. Congenital anomalies, such as hemifacial microsomia and a first and second branchial defect, involve hard and soft tissues. It is convenient to divide skeletal asymmetries into those associated with growth and development and those resulting from an acquired anomaly derived from any of the intraosseous odontogenic and non-odontogenic components. This imaging chapter will highlight primary skeletal asymmetries of the mandible, and this class of asymmetries is mostly derived from TMJ anomalies occurring during period of growth and development. An insult or anomaly of the TMJ occurring prior to the completion of somatic growth and development induces concurrent regional growth influence on the facial skeleton and may include the mandible, maxilla, skull base, and airway [2–12]. The severity of the regional effects are inversely proportional to age of onset and directly proportional to the severity of the joint anomaly (Fig. 1). A differential diagnosis for mandibular asymmetries is organized into a decision tree (Fig. 2) and illustrated in this chapter. Analysis of the CT or CBCT scan is the preferred technology to navigate the decision points within this decision tree, which divides mandibular asymmetries into true- and pseudo-asymmetries. With a true asymmetry, one half of the

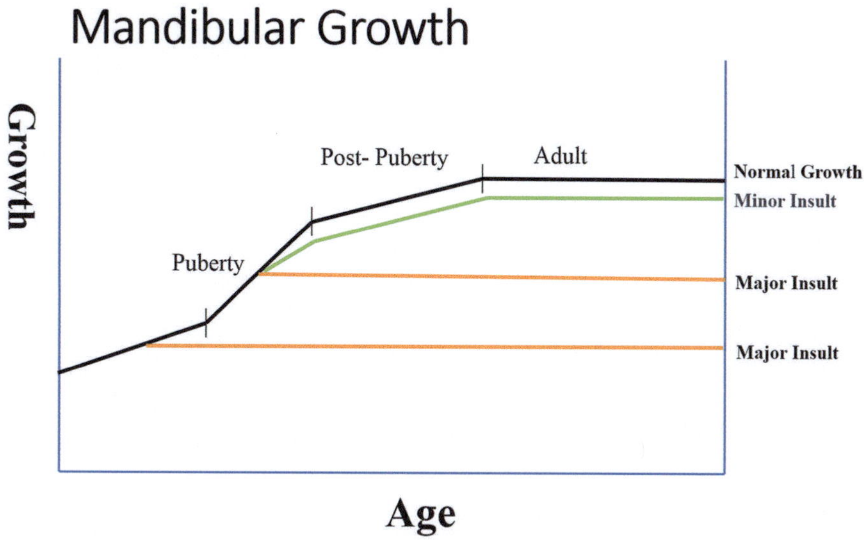

Fig. 1 Mandibular growth versus age. This graphic illustrates normal mandibular growth and the negative influence of minor and major TMJ insults on mandibular growth. The superior black line illustrates normal mandibular growth. The green line illustrates the influence of a minor insult, such as a disc displacement, on mandibular growth. The two orange lines illustrate that the degree of growth deficit is directly proportional to severity of the TMJ insult and inversely proportional to the age of the insult

mandible is larger than the contralateral half. The relative sizes of both halves of the mandible can be determined by comparison of the 3D image measurements of the anatomic components of the mandible. The anatomic components include the condylar process, ascending ramus, and body of the mandible. A pseudo-asymmetry may give the clinical appearance of an asymmetry, but both halves of the mandible are equal in size and the mandible is displaced or has an asymmetrical or warped shape. The next decision point in a true asymmetry is to determine if one side is too large or the contralateral size is too small. A mandible with a side too small is more common than those that are too large. Each condition leading to a mandibular asymmetry has unique features that can be identified through specific and detailed image analysis.

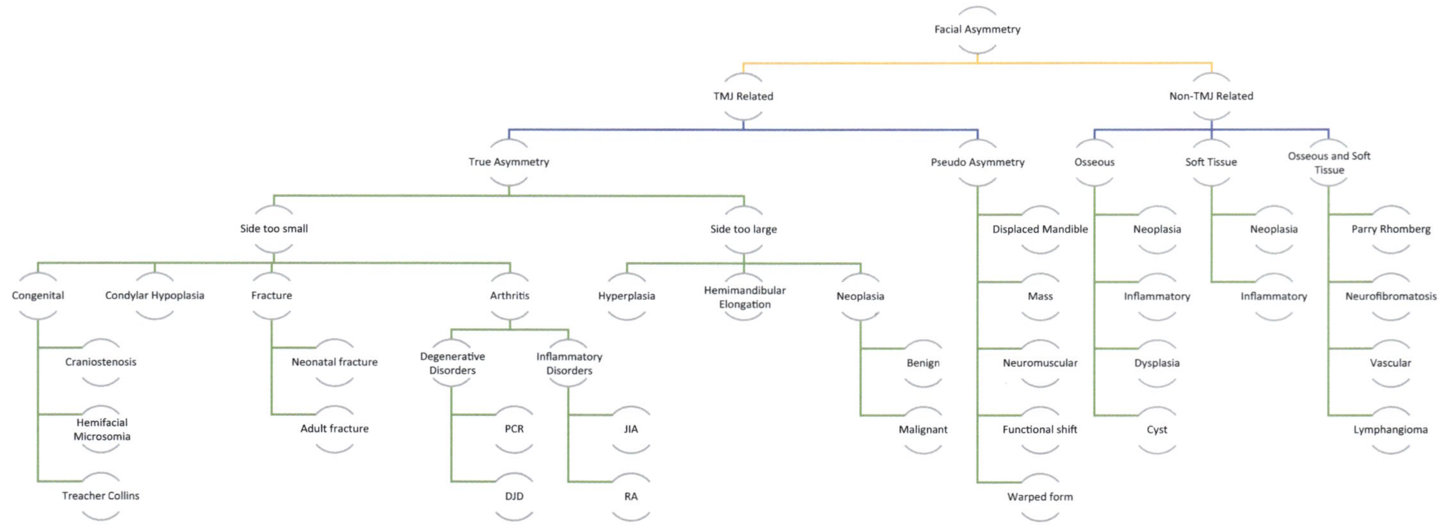

Fig. 2 Facial asymmetry decision tree. A flowchart of representative sources of facial asymmetry. The flowchart can be considered a differential diagnosis but organized into a decision tree. This tree represents decision points to arrive at a working diagnosis. Facial asymmetries are sorted by site of origin into those related to the temporomandibular joint and those not related to the TMJ. In all cases, it is important to localize and characterize the asymmetry. TMJ-related facial asymmetries are not uncommon and can initially be categorized into true asymmetries versus pseudo-asymmetry. A true asymmetry is one where one half of the mandible is larger than the opposite side. The bilateral component parts of the mandible can be measured to determine if a true asymmetry exists. If a true asymmetry exists, then the next decision point is to determine if one side is too large or the opposite side is too small. This decision can best be accomplished by determining the size and shape of the condyle and determining if the lateral development of the mandible is deficient. To further the diagnostic process, it is important to determine the etiology of the mandibular asymmetry and determine if the cause of the asymmetry is active

Imaging Strategies for Facial Asymmetry

The gold standard for all imaging is the accuracy and precision to reveal the anatomic truth. Multiple 2D and 3D static and dynamic diagnostic imaging methods have been developed, each with their own benchmark on a continuum to reveal the anatomic truth. Many of the diagnostic challenges that routinely present in clinical practice can benefit from imaging investigations. The art of imaging is choosing the appropriate imaging tool and optimizing that tool in order to fulfill the imaging objectives. The imaging objectives for facial asymmetry include 3D anatomic characterization and a determination of the etiology and activity state of the facial asymmetry. Multi-detector CT (MDCT) and MRI with or without contrast are recommended for conditions involving soft tissues, while MDCT or CBCT is recommended for the conditions involving the maxillofacial skeleton. Determining TMJ disc position is solely in the domain of MRI imaging. The wide view of a CBCT is ideal for imaging the maxillofacial skeleton to identify or rule out the presence and extent of a skeletal asymmetry. In the case of a skeletal asymmetry, a CBCT enables an anatomic component analysis to determine which skeletal elements are demonstrating deviant form and growth. The component analysis results are used to identify the etiology and activity status of the maxillofacial asymmetry. The first step in a component analysis is to reassign the Cartesian coordinate system generated by the image acquisition scanner to an anatomically based coordinate system. The reorientation of the scan volume is based on skull base landmarks and not the skeletal components involved in the asymmetry.

Biomechanics of the TMJ and Jaws

The maxillofacial region is composed of several interconnected anatomic elements that include the jaws, teeth, muscles, and TMJs. Each of the elements can individually be considered a local environment, while all combined elements could be considered as a regional environment. Mathematical modeling shows functional interaction of these anatomic elements generates and distributes forces among the regional environment [13–15]. The generated forces create tissue stresses and strains. Stress, an engineering term, depicts force per unit area, while strain describes physical tissue deformation (change in length/original length) resulting from applied stress. Stress/strain distribution, gradients, cycle number, and rate may influence bone modeling and remodeling. Mechanotransduction is a mechanosensory system that can have stratified interactions at the molecular, cellular, tissue, and organ levels [16–18]. Mechanical forces are involved in tissue development and injury through regulation of cellular biochemistry. There are two mechanisms of bone formation that can be observed during morphogenesis of the jaws: (a) intramembranous bone formation, and, (b) endochondral bone formation. Both mechanisms involve mesenchymal cell differentiation into either osteoblasts or chondrocytes. The direct differentiation of mesenchymal cells into osteoblasts occurs subjacent to periosteum and is called membranous or intramembranous bone formation. The differentiation of mesenchymal cells into chondrocytes occurs within the articular cartilage and forms an analgen that is replaced by bone and this is called endochondral bone formation [19, 20]. The cartilage analgen develops by interstitial and appositional growth and is later replaced by invading osteoblasts from the subchondral bone that replace and ossify the hypertrophic cartilage. The TMJ is a growth site that is a key driver for facial growth. The TMJ is a loaded joint that is subjected to a combination of compression, tension, and shear forces. The stresses and strains in combination with hormones and growth factors produce a dynamic environment that can modulate tissue response, such as tissue differentiation, growth, development, remodeling, modeling, mechanical failure, and tissue repair. The tissue response may be a tool set each individual possesses to facilitate environmental adaptation. Endochondral bone formation occurs at bone surfaces covered by fibrocartilage which is along the anterosuperior surfaces of the condyles and along the posterior slope and crest of the articular eminence. Membranous bone formation occurs at bone surfaces that are covered by periosteum which is along the posterior aspect of the condyles. Condylar growth contributes to a change in size and counterclockwise displacement of the mandible. The conformation of the skeleton is an outer cortical shell that is distributed around cancellous bone. The bones are able to absorb and release energy. The geometry of cancellous bone is optimized through remodeling to manage bone weight, sustain axial loading, and efficiently move functional forces away from the joint surface to the outer cortical shell of the mandible. The bones can model and remodel. Modeling is a process of surface bone formation that is generally not coupled with or preceded by bone resorption. Remodeling is a bone replacement process that begins with resorption and that is subsequently replaced by bone formation. Another form of modeling allows bone to drift in space by adding bone at an outer surface coupled with bone resorption on the endosteal surface of the same cortex. It also involves resorption of the surface of the opposite outer cortex and bone formation on the opposite endosteal surface. Remodeling occurs within the cortical bone and along the surfaces of the trabecular bone. Remodeling allows for repair of bone damage but also provides bone with the ability to adapt to functional changes during loading. Individual variations in anatomic spatial geometry, neuromuscular actions, and the adaptive capacity may contribute to a range of morphological modeling or remodeling outcomes. The location of muscle attachments, muscle orientation, and size and recruitment patterns interact to create regional deformation of the mandible, including regional sagittal bending, transverse bending, and torsion of the mandible. The deformation of the mandible produces stress gradients that may induce subperiosteal osteoblasts with subsequent bone formation [11]. The bending and torsional deformational forces of the mandible can be countered by increasing the mandibular dimensions along the lines of the principle forces. For example, sagittal bending can be resisted by an increase in the vertical dimension of the mandible, transverse bending can be resisted by increased mediolateral dimension, and torsional deformation can be resisted by changing the mandible to a more circular shape. In part, the bone's functional success is associated with its ability to adapt its size, shape, geometry, and mass to accommodate for changing mechanical and metabolic demands. It has been determined through mathematical modeling that the forces experienced by the TMJs are similar despite a wide range of craniofacial form. The local and regional environmental phenotypes presented in this chapter are integrated from information gained by imaging observations, mathematical modeling, and speculation that the tissue responses are adaptive mechanisms to permit the necessary high performance of jaw functions including mastication, respiration, phonation, and deglutination while keeping the tissue stresses and strains within a range that is compatible with health. An underpinning assumption is that tissue stresses and strains can be modulated as necessary responses to changing functional environments by adapting the biomechanical geometry (external form and internal structure) of the jaws and jaw structures. The modulation of tissue stress and strain occurs locally (near the point of force application) and regionally (away from the force application). Tissues and structures have a functional stress and strain capacity, that is, they can maintain health when subjected to a range of stress or strain levels . A TMJ that exceeds its functional capacity or health threshold may degenerate, and this initiates a response aimed to reduce excessive stresses and strains to levels that will promote tissue repair. Tissues repair and assume a new morphology through a process called tissue adaptation. During this process of degeneration and repair, involved tissues have an evolving functional capacity ranging from a very low functional stress capacity to one that is capable of meeting all functional demands.

Imaging observations indicate that a destructive process that reduces condylar volume may be followed by an ipsilateral change in jaw form. When asymmetrical mandibles were mathematically tested comparing the long and short side functional stress, no significant differences were noted, thereby suggesting that the form changes were secondary to adaptation. A reduction in condylar size can occur through multiple unique conditions, including degenerative and inflammatory arthritides, trauma, or hypoplasia, all of which can be identified by interpreting axially corrected images of the TMJs. The regional changes associated with this diverse group of conditions have a common form (size and shape). Local and regional changes may work in concert to maintain high-performance standards of the jaws while maintaining tissue stresses and strains within a range that is compatible with tissue health.

Dynamic aspects of joint surfaces in relative motion (tribology) are important to maintain tissue health. The TMJ surfaces include fibrocartilaginous covering of the condyle and eminence and subchondral bone, and in between these are the disc and synovial fluid for shock absorption, load distribution, lubrication, and nutrition. The TMJ disc is fibrocartilaginous and it does not have a homogeneous composition but rather, its structure correlates with regional functional demands. The biconcave disc and elliptical shape fills the wedge-shaped incongruences between the condyle and opposing temporal bone. The disc is composed predominately of Type I collagen, proteoglycans, glycoproteins, and water. Type I collagen resists shear and tensile forces. To a lesser extent, Type II collagen resists compressive forces. The disc is repeatedly subjected to high dynamic and static (clenching and bruxing) forces. The disc is divided into three anteroposterior areas/zones: the anterior band, intermediate zone, and posterior band. The distribution and arrangement of the disc components are not uniform throughout the zones of the disc. These zones or anatomic regions have material property differences related to their composition. The single-cell biomechanics of each zone reflect a structural relationship to their functional demands. The articular cartilage and intervening disc provide near frictionless movement and load. Loss or displacement of the disc may subject the articular cartilage to excessive stress concentrations and predispose the articular surfaces to degeneration.

Regional Changes Associated with a Small Condyle

The mandibular condyle is an adaptive growth site that contributes to the sagittal, vertical, and lateral development of the mandible. An insult that damages the condylar growth site will limit growth of the ipsilateral half of the mandible. The vertical dimensions of the condylar process, ascending ramus, and body of the mandible are shorter than the normal side. The lateral development of the affected side of the mandible is less than the normal side. The osseous midline of the mandible is shifted to the side with the short vertical dimension. On the ipsilateral side, the occlusal plane is elevated, while the cranial base near the TMJ is depressed. The mandibular and occlusal planes are steeper than the unaffected side. The regional changes are similar in almost every patient with small condyles, thereby suggesting that this phenomenon may likely be the result of an adaptive response of the jaws to optimize biomechanics through a process of mechanobiology. The severity of the regional changes are often directly proportional to the severity of the etiologic condition and inversely proportional to the age of onset (Fig. 1). Positional changes, such as repositioning of mandibular molars posteromedially and steepening of the occlusal plane, may create a biomechanical advantage that serves to optimize the joint loads while preserving necessary jaw function.

Conditions Leading to Facial Asymmetry

The following discussion does not represent all of the possible etiologies for facial asymmetry. Some represent common causes, while others are discussed to illustrate concepts of asymmetries. This chapter divides facial asymmetries into those directly derived from a TMJ anomaly and those that are not related to the TMJ anomaly.

Facial Asymmetries: TMJ-Related

All of the condyles under this heading display regional changes associated with a small condyle as previously described.

Congenital One of the more commonly encountered congenital anomaly associated with asymmetries is hemifacial microsomia.

Hemifacial Microsomia (HFM) This condition is an anomaly of unknown etiology involving first and second branchial arch derivatives. It unilaterally affects the ear, face, mandible, teeth, muscles, cranial nerve VII, and orbit regions [21]. HFM is characterized by an underdevelopment of the mandibular condyle that can range from a small condyle to condylar aplasia along with underdevelopment of the ipsilateral half of the mandible. HFM can be classified into three types:

- Type I: Mild hypoplasia of the condyle, ramus, and body
- Type IIA: Small flat condyle, poorly developed or absent glenoid fossa, small abnormally shaped ramus, and condyle normally positioned in fossa
- Type IIB: Same as IIA with condyle positioned inferior, anterior, and medial to the glenoid fossa
- Type III: Failure to form the TMJ, small or absent ramus, and small mandibular body

HFM Imaging The condyle is small or absent and fossa development is proportional to condylar development and function. Ipsilateral ramus and body development is decreased proportional to condylar development. The occlusal plane is elevated on involved side. A smaller malar bone and zygomatic arch, mastoid process hypoplasia, and lateroinferiorly displacement of the orbit along with middle and external ear defects are commonly seen on the affected side (Fig. 3).

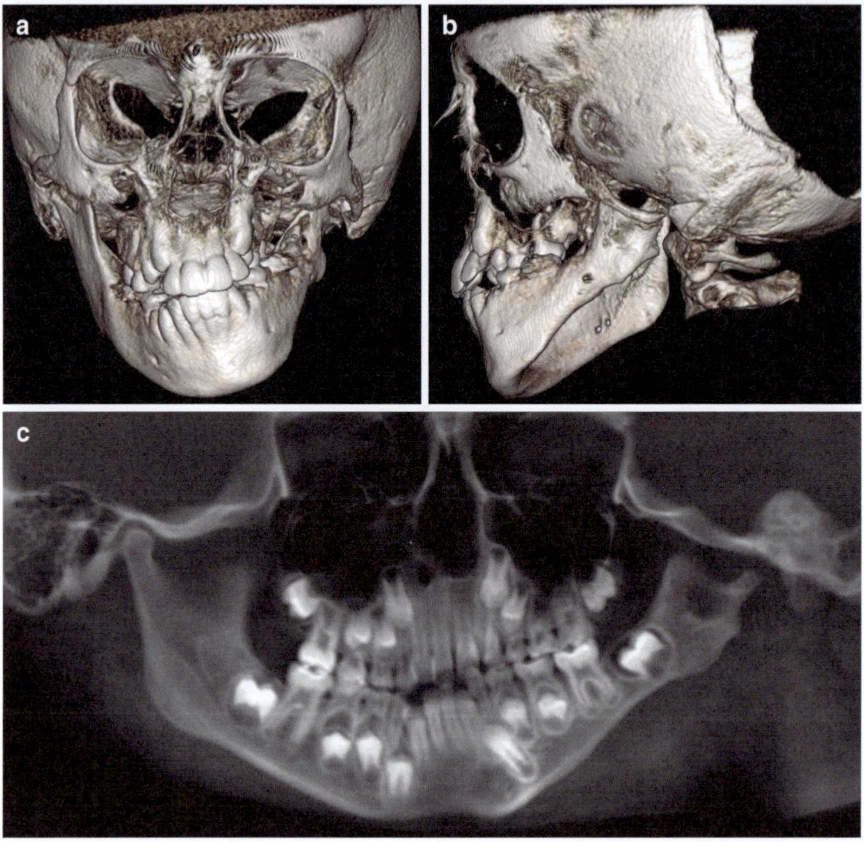

Fig. 3 Hemifacial Microsomia: (**a**) CBCT volume rendered coronal view showing a severe asymmetry in 7.5 year old female with left side hemifacial microsomia. The lateral development of the left half of the mandible is less than the right. The left angle of the mandible is elevated. The left posterior occlusal plane is elevated. The osseous midline of the mandible is shifted to the left. (**b**) Left lateral view shows the small left half of the mandible; short ramus, condylar process and body. There is a discontinuity in zygomatic arch. There is no external auditory canal. (**c**) CBCT reconstructed panoramic projection shows small left half of the mandible. Tooth # 18 is developing partially in the ramus. The left mastoid process is hypoplastic. The temporal bone anatomy is very dense. (**d**) Oblique sagittal view of the right TMJ show a normal TMJ. The osseous components of the right TMJ are smooth, rounded and without evidence of subchondral defects. The condyle fossa spatial relationships are within normal limits. (**e**) CBCT axially corrected oblique sagittal image of the left TMJ. The left condylar process is very small and has a posterior inclination. The left ramus and body have a short vertical dimension. The left glenoid fossa is very broad and without evidence of eminence development. There is no evidence of ear ossicles or ear canal. The mandibular plane is very steep and the gonial angle is obtuse. The joint space superior to the left condyle is very large

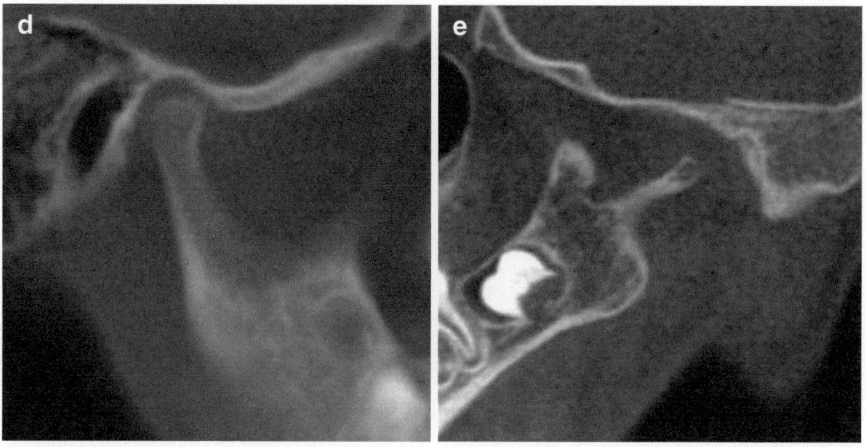

Fig. 3 (continued)

Developmental Causes of Asymmetry

Neonatal Trauma A subcondylar fracture occurring at or around the time of birth, often secondary to a difficult delivery [22].

Neonatal Trauma Imaging The proximal fragment displaces anteriorly, medially, and inferiorly. The distal end of the proximal segments overlaps the ramus and heals in that location. The distance from the condyle to the coronoid process is decreased and the angle formed by the two processes is acute. At the time of birth, the eminence is not developed and only develops if stimulated by functional forces from the articulating condyle. Without the condyle in normal contact with the temporal bone, no eminence develops and thus, the temporal portion of the TMJ is flat with a very shallow slope. The overlapping of the condylar process with the proximal end of the ramus and the acute angle between the coronoid and condylar processes creates the unique appearance that mimics scissors or shears. The joint insult is accompanied by reduced growth and development of the ipsilateral half of the mandible including short vertical dimensions of the ascending ramus and body of the mandible, decreased lateral development of the mandible, and an increased occlusal plane (Fig. 4).

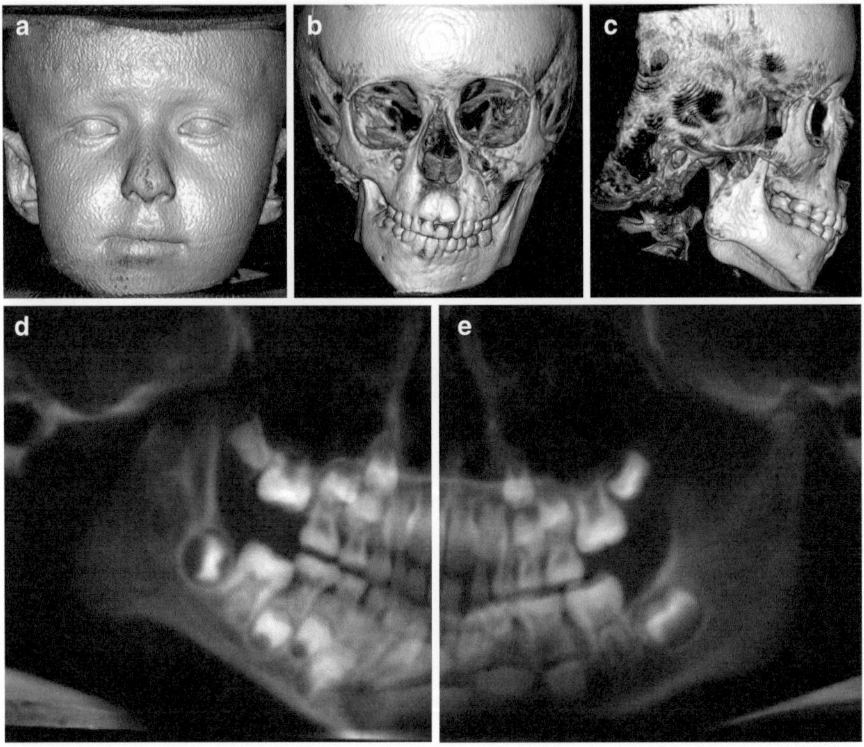

Fig. 4 Neonatal fracture. (**a**) CBCT frontal soft tissue volume rendered 3d view of 7 year old female face who had a right side subcondylar fracture during the birth delivery process shows that right lip commissure is elevated and depression of the soft tissues anterior to the right ear. (**b**) Frontal view of the skeleton shows the lateral development of the right half of the mandible is less than the left. The osseous midline of the mandible shifted to the right and the right occlusal plane is elevated. The right angle of the mandible is elevated. (**c**) Right lateral view of skeleton shows the AP and vertical dimensions of the right ramus are small. (**d**) CBCT right side panoramic reconstruction shows the overall size of the right half of the mandible is smaller than the left. The vertical dimension of the right condylar process is smaller than the left and is anteriorly displaced near the coronoid process. There is an acute angle formed between the right coronoid and condylar processes that creates a "shear or scissor" effect. The right antegonial notch is deeper than the left. The right second molar is forming in the anterior region of the ascending ramus. (**e**) CBCT left side panoramic reconstruction shows a normally developing left half of the mandible. (**f**) Axially corrected oblique sagittal view of the right TMJ shows no formation of the articular eminence and the condyle is displaced anterior to the articular portion of the temporal bone. The lack of an eminence indicates lack of functional loading that is responsible for eminence development. There is a cortex extending from the condyle to the follicle of # 31. This cortex was likely transported at the time of the fracture and caused anteroinferior displacement of the proximal segment. (**g**) Oblique sagittal view of the left TMJ shows that the osseous development of the left TMJ is normal. The left condyle is displaced anterior and inferior to the center of the fossa

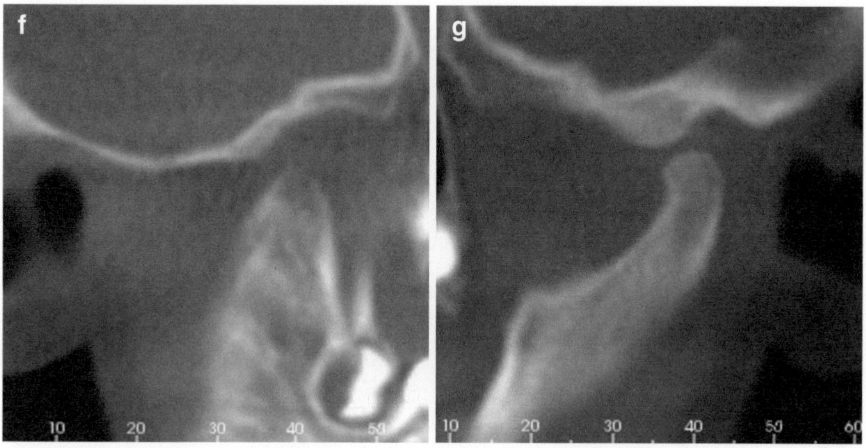

Fig. 4 (continued)

Inflammatory Disorders

Juvenile Idiopathic Arthritis (JIA) JIA is an autoimmune musculoskeletal inflammatory disease in children [23]. JIA affects 1–22 per 1000 children worldwide with higher female predominance than male. Polymorphism in the MIF and IL6 genes is associated with susceptibility to JIA. Three classification systems have been proposed for JIA with six subtypes that are based on clinical features occurring during the first 6 months of the disease: [1] oligoarticular (50–60%) [2]; polyarticular, JIA-positive or JIA-negative rheumatoid factor (30–50%) [3]; systemic (10–20%) [4]; juvenile psoriatic arthritis (2–15%) [5]; enthesitis-related arthritis (1–7%); and [6] Undifferentiated arthritis. JIA is more likely to involve large joints such as spine, knees, wrists, and ankles. The TMJ, craniovertebral junction, and spine are the primary sites of head and neck involvement. TMJ involvement is more likely in individuals with systemic disease, early age onset, and disease longevity.

JIA Imaging In the TMJs, JIA is most often bilateral with a symmetrical expression. The condyles show signs of erosions and flattening. The loss of volume can extend to the mandibular neck. The fossa can be shallow, broad, and flat. In early age onset cases, the articular eminence may not form. There may be secondary osteoarthritis with osteophyte formation. When changes are not bilaterally equal, JIA can cause facial asymmetry. JIA is characterized by bilateral short condylar processes, flat broad articular surfaces, and wide glenoid fossa. The anteroposterior dimensions of the mandible are small. The mandibular plane is steep, and there is a clockwise facial growth pattern tendency with a steep occlusal plane, and deep antegonial notches. The clockwise mandibular rotation may be associated with posteroinferior repositioning of the tongue and narrowing of the oropharyngeal airway dimensions. Autorotation of the mandible occurs around molar fulcrums, and as the condylar volume decreases, it moves the condyles in a more anterosuperior direction. The mandibular rotation may be associated with an increase in the anterior face height and anterior open bite. The coronoid processes may elongate and reposition superiorly as the condylar processes lose volume. MRI imaging using a T1 or proton density protocol will reveal the osseous anatomy as described above. T2-weighted protocols will reveal the presence of joint effusion, bone marrow edema, and disc position. A T1-weighted protocol with contrast will show joint space enhancement and may show signs of inflammation occurring prior to joint destruction (Fig. 5).

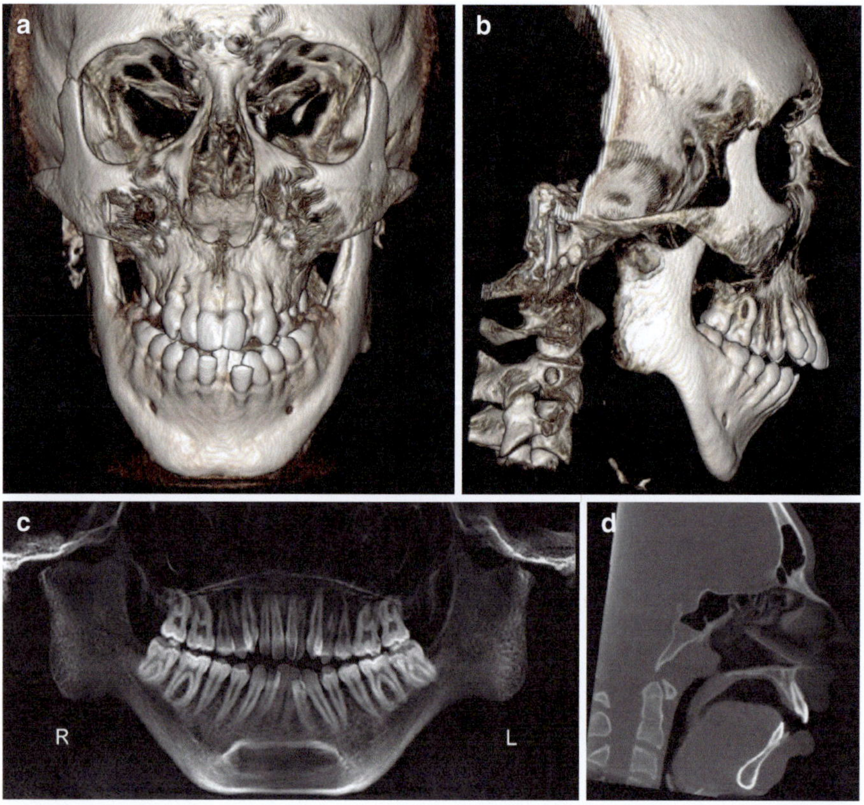

Fig. 5 Juvenile idiopathic arthritis. (**a**) CBCT volume-rendered frontal view of a 19-year-old patient with juvenile idiopathic arthritis (JIA) with the right side being slightly smaller than the left side. The osseous midline is shifted to the right. The transverse dimensions of the mandible are small with the right being the smallest. The maxilla has a small transverse dimension. There is a bilateral posterior crossbite and anterior open bite. (**b**) A lateral view shows an extremely steep mandibular plane and obtuse gonial angle. The vertical dimensions of the posterior portion of the mandible are steep and the anterior face height is large. The antegonial notch is steep and the hyoid bone is inferiorly positioned. (**c**) A CBCT panoramic reconstruction demonstrates the loss of condylar processes. The proximal ends of the mandible are articulating anteriorly on the temporal bone. Note the lack of eminence development indicating an early onset JIA. The coronoid processes are relatively large and superiorly repositioned. (**d**) A CBCT mid-sagittal section shows small airway. There is a large adenoid mass blocking posterior nasal choanae changing the mode of breathing to the mouth and lowering tongue posture. The vertical dimension of the anterior mandible is large but the labiolingual dimensions of the anterior alveolar process are small

Degenerative Disorders

Progressive Condylar Resorption (PCR) Progressive condylar resorption (PCR) also known as idiopathic condylar resorption is a localized non-inflammatory degenerative disorder of the TMJs that is characterized by lysis and repair of the articular fibrocartilage and the subjacent bone [24–31]. The incidence of this condition is unknown. PCR primarily affects females during the time of puberty, and therefore it is hypothesized that hormones and tissue response to functional biomechanics play an etiologic role. The natural history of PCR progresses through three distinct anatomic stages, and each has a clinical relevance when considering the therapeutic options and treatment timing: soft tissue phase, destructive phase, and reparative phase.

PCR Imaging

Soft tissue phase Soft tissue changes precede osseous changes. Early soft tissue change involves loss of proteoglycans. A nonreducing, displaced disc is often seen before the osseous destruction and loss of condylar volume.

Destructive Phase It is hypothesized that the sequence of events involving the osseous structures occur in the following order: (a) loss of the cortex along the anterosuperior surface of the condyles and (b) cavitation defects extending into the subchondral bone, resulting in a loss of condylar volume. During active phases, the TMJs may be particularly vulnerable to biomechanical forces. It is suspected that condylar resorption progresses until the compressive forces within the TMJ are reduced to a level compatible with tissue repair and health.

Reparative Phase The active phase is followed by condylar flattening and recortication. The flattening may form a congruent articulation with the opposing articular surface. Flattening and congruent articulations are thought to be functional adaptations to distribute loads over a larger stress-bearing area (Fig. 6). Because PCR occurs before growth is completed, asymmetry is commonly encountered when a unilateral joint is affected.

Condylar Hypoplasia Condylar hypoplasia occurs during the period of somatic growth and is characterized by a small condyle with a normal form (size and shape) [32]. A hypoplastic condyle is thought to occur secondary to a TMJ insult, such as a displaced disc or trauma.

Condylar Hypoplasia Imaging The condyle and the ipsilateral half of the mandible are relatively small. The small condyle has a normal shape without evidence of any destructive process. The vertical dimensions of the ipsilateral condylar process, ascending ramus, and body of the mandible are shorter than the contralateral side. The ipsilateral posterior occlusal plane may be elevated. The osseous midline of the mandible is shifted to the short side but the dental midlines are likely to be coincident. The lateral development of the ipsilateral half of the mandible will be reduced (Fig. 7).

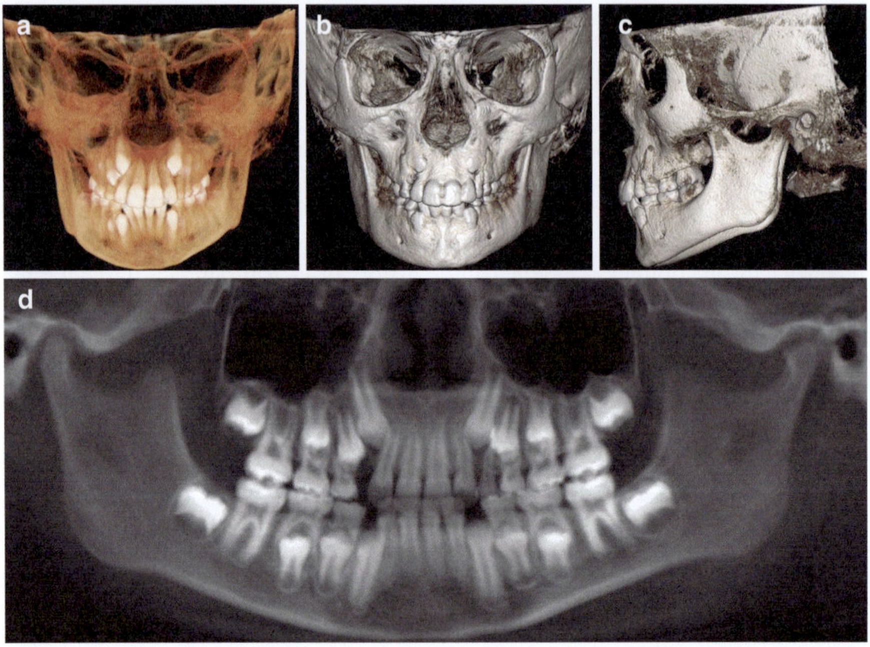

Fig. 6 Progressive Condylar Resorption (PCR). (**a** and **b**) Volume rendered 3d view of skeleton of an 8 year old female with PCR shows that the left side of mandible is smaller than the right. The lateral development of the left half of the mandible is slightly less than the right. The osseous midline of the mandible is shifted to the left but the dental midlines are co-incident. (**c**) Left lateral view shows that the left lower border of the mandible is elevated relative to the right. (**d**) CBCT reconstructed panoramic projection shows the vertical dimensions of the left condylar process, ascending ramus and body of the mandible are less than the right. The occlusal plane is slightly elevated on the left side. The left fossa is positioned inferior to the right on this oriented scan. (**e**) Axially corrected oblique sagittal and coronal views of the left TMJ show a loss of condylar height from its superior surface. The loss of height occurs through an erosive process. The anterosuperior of the left condyle is flat but relatively well defined. This TMJ in the repair phase of PCR. The superior joint space is wide suggesting the condyle is not seated therefore the occlusion may be orthopedically unstable. (**f**) Oblique sagittal views show that osseous components of the right TMJ are smooth, rounded and without evidence of subchondral defects

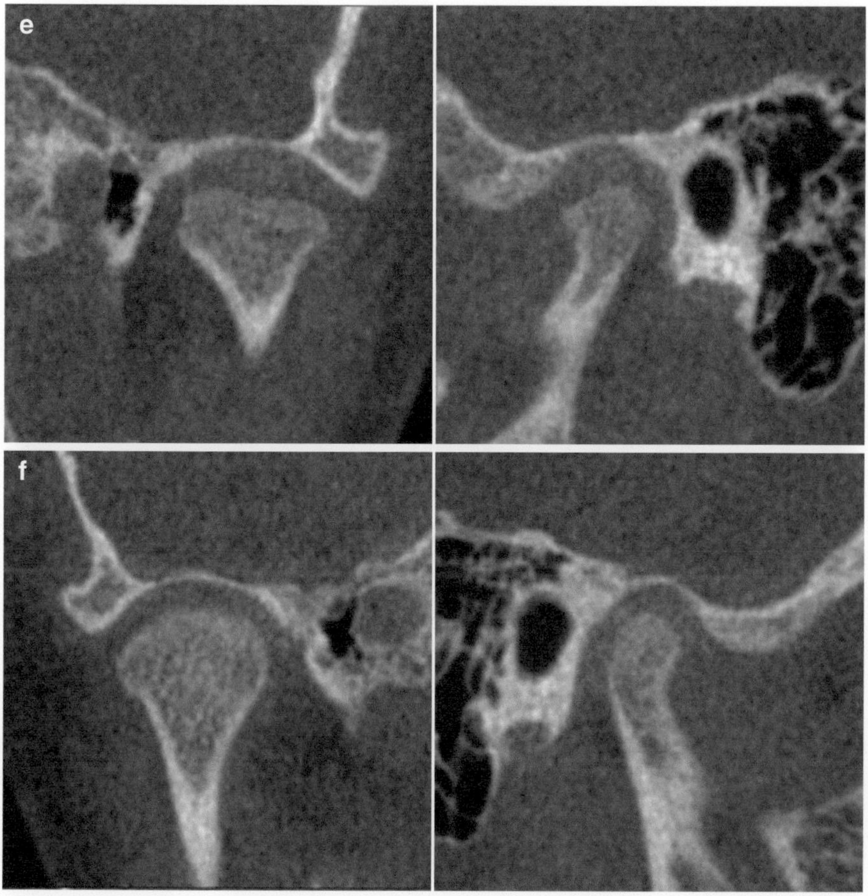

Fig. 6 (continued)

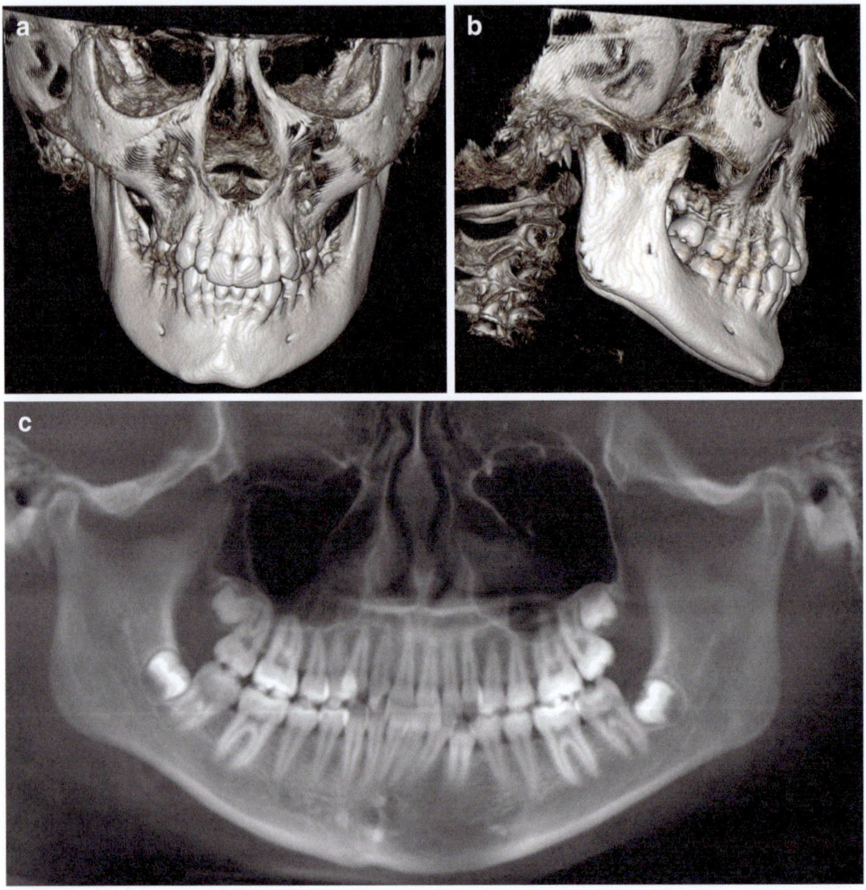

Fig. 7 Condylar hypoplasia. (**a**) Volume rendered 3d view of skeleton of a 15 year old female with a right side condylar hypoplasia shows that the right side of the mandible is smaller than the left. The lateral development of the right half of the mandible is less than the left. The osseous midline of the mandible is shifted to the right but the dental midlines are co-incident while right root apices are tilted to the short side. The occlusal plane is elevated on the right side. (**b**) Lateral view of skull. The right side lower border of the mandible is elevated compared to the left. (**c**) CBCT reconstructed panoramic view show the vertical dimensions of the right condylar process and ascending ramus are less than the left. There is a right side subdivision class II molar relationship. (**d**) Axially corrected oblique sagittal and coronal views of the right show that the right condyle has a normal shape but is slightly smaller than the left side. The superior joint space in the right TMJ is slightly less than the left. (**e**) Left TMJ images show that the osseous components have a normal size, shape, quality and spatial relationships. (**f**) Coronal view of TMJs show that the right TMJ fossa is positioned inferior to the contralateral side on this oriented scan

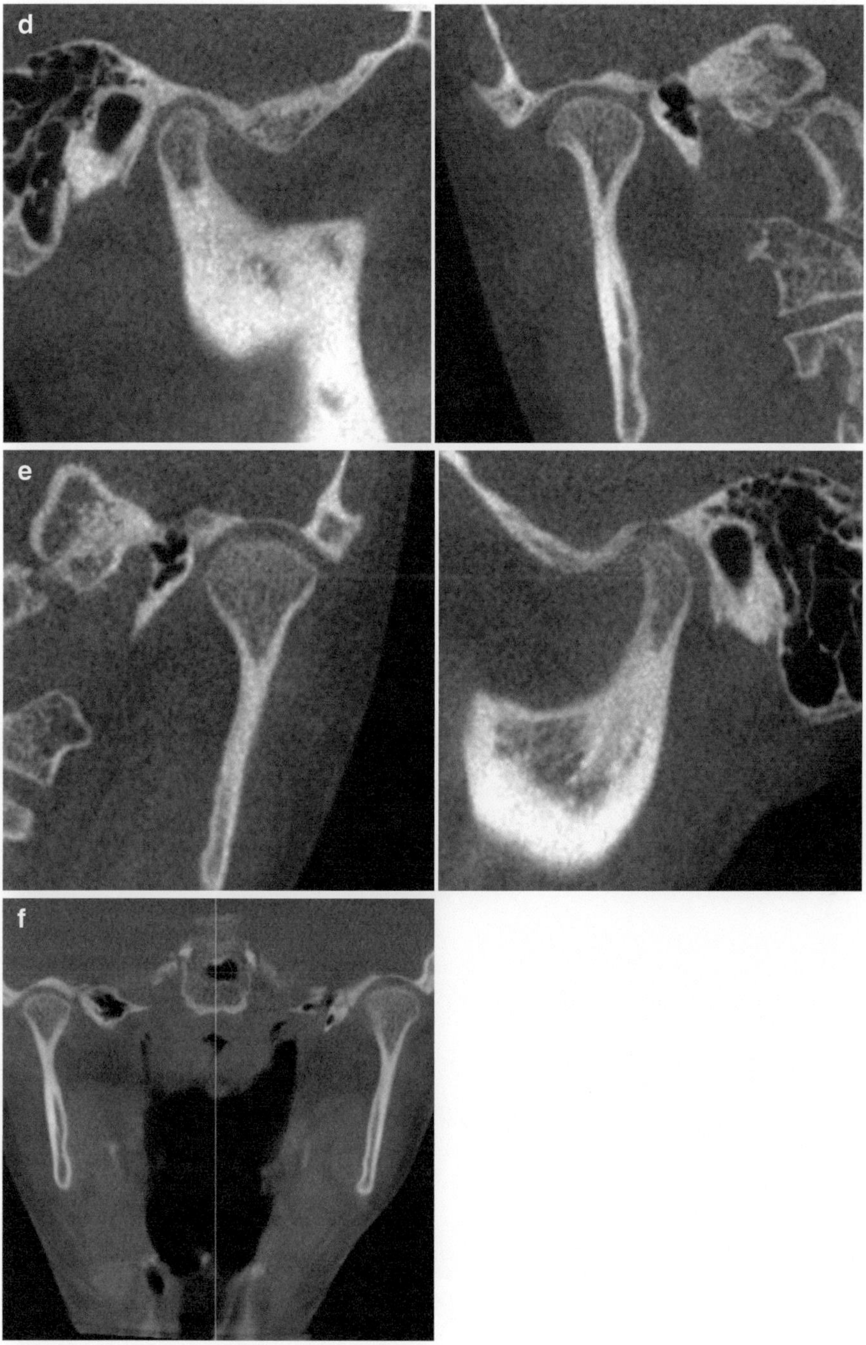

Fig. 7 (continued)

Acquired Causes of Asymmetry

Trauma An adult with a misaligned healed midface or mandibular fracture can result in a facial asymmetry [21] (Fig. 8).

Degenerative Joint Disease (DJD) DJD is a localized non-inflammatory disorder of synovial joints characterized by the destruction and repair of the articular fibrocartilage and underlying subchondral bone [32–35]. This condition is very similar to PCR, except that the age of onset is not at puberty but most commonly after the completion of somatic growth. DJD has been defined by Moffett as "the pathologic destruction of the articular tissues and bone that occurs whenever articular remodeling does not maintain equilibrium between form and function." This implies that TMJ has an adaptive capacity that requires function to maintain health but the func-

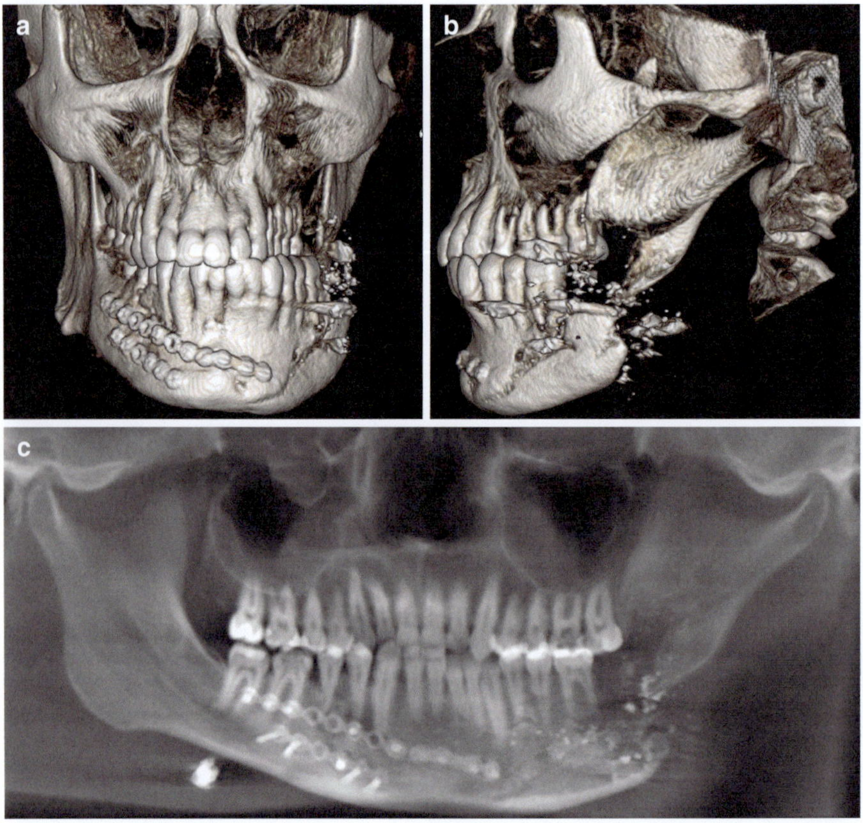

Fig. 8 Fracture GSW. (**a**) CBCT volume-rendered frontal soft tissue view showing a skeletal asymmetry with the left side nonhealing comminuted mandibular fracture secondary to a gunshot wound. Note that the left ramus is depressed medially. (**b**) Lateral view of the same patient shows anterosuperior displacement of the proximal fragment. (**c**) CBCT panoramic reconstruction shows proximal segment displacement in vector aligned with medial pterygoid muscle

tional demands need to fall within range that is compatible with tissue health. Excessive functional joint loading or trauma may contribute to the initiation and perpetuation of DJD. Similar to PCR, DJD progresses through the same three stages, namely, soft tissue, destructive, and reparative phases. The progression through the repair phase may be an adaptive mechanism that has a net effect of reducing stress and strain to a level that is commensurate with that is found in healthy tissues.

DJD Imaging Adult DJD is more likely than PCR to form osteophyte and subchondral bone cyst. Similar to PCR, soft tissue changes and disc displacement precede the osseous destructive phase.

Reparative Phase The active phase of DJD is followed by condylar flattening and recortication. The flattening may form a congruent articulation with the opposing articular surface. Flattening and congruent articulations are thought to be functional adaptations to distribute loads over a larger stress-bearing area. The later stage changes associated with DJD include osteophyte and subchondral cyst formation. An osteophyte is generally dense bone, develops in a low stress site, and forms a congruent articulation that increases the contact area between the opposing articular surfaces. Osteophyte formation most often occurs from the anterior surface of the condyle but other surfaces may also produce an osteophyte. A subchondral bone cyst is most often thought to form at the site of an erosive breach in the superior cortex. The hydraulic intrusion of synovial fluid into the subchondral cancellous bone will create a bone cavitation defect that will ultimately fill with connective tissue. If the cavitation phase is active, the margins of the defect will not be corticated, while in the repaired phase, the margins of the defect except for the connection to the articular surface will be corticated (Figs. 9 and 10).

Mandibular Asymmetries Associated with Condylar Enlargement

Large Condylar Process Either the entire condylar process or select portions may enlarge. The condylar process enlargement may be accompanied by enlargement of the ipsilateral half of the mandible. A condyle or mandible can be enlarged by both benign and malignant conditions. Examples of a large condylar process are osteochondroma, condylar hyperplasia, and hemimandibular elongation.

Osteochondroma An osteochondroma (OC) is a benign slow growth cartilage capped exophytic osseous lesion arising from areas where the cartilage exists [36]. An OC mostly occurs after completion of somatic growth but has been observed in growing individuals. The most common sites of occurrence are the anterior or superior surface of the condyle and rarely occur in the eminence and coronoid processes. It is not clear if an OC is a tumor or a hamartoma.

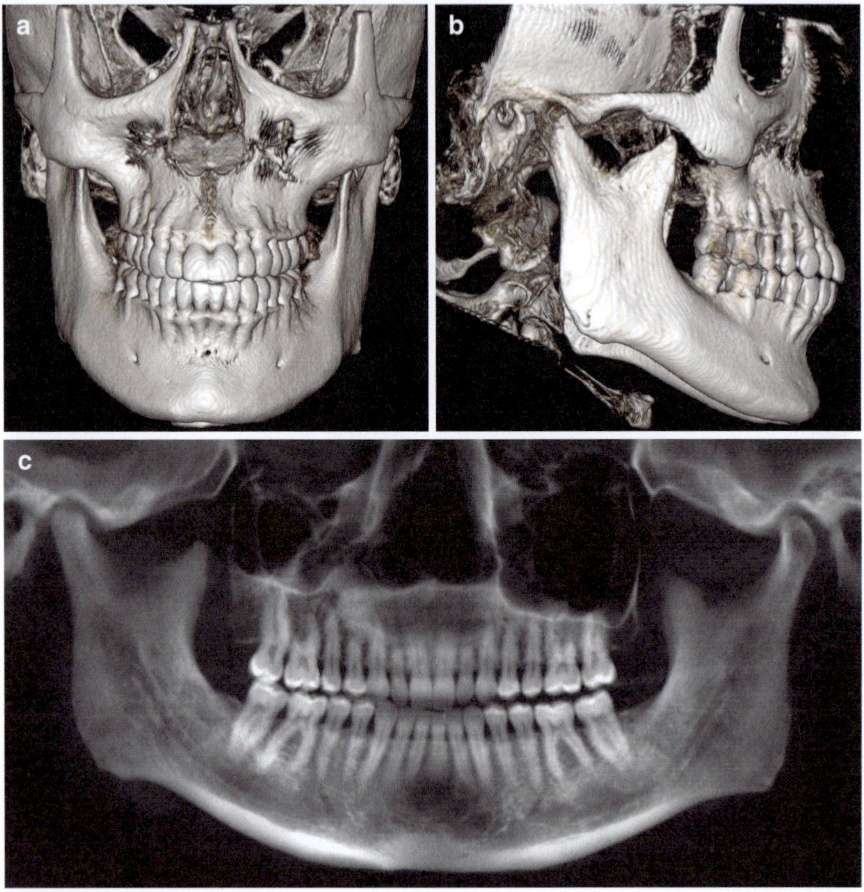

Fig. 9 Degenerative Joint Disease (DJD). (**a**) CBCT Volume rendered 3d view of skeleton of 39 year old female in the destructive or active phase of right TMJ DJD. The right angle of the mandible is elevated. (**b**) Right lateral view shows that the right lower border of the mandible is elevated relative to the left. (**c**) CBCT reconstructed panoramic projection shows the vertical dimensions of the right condyle is less than the left side. The right and left ascending rami and body of the mandible are equal size. There is an open bite with the only opposing tooth contact occurring between the right side molar teeth. (**d**) Axially corrected oblique sagittal and coronal views of the right TMJ show a loss of condylar height from its anterosuperior surface. This is considered to be in the destructive phase of DJD and this TMJ in vulnerable to biomechanical forces. The superior joint space is thin suggesting the a thinning or displacement of the interposing soft tissues and the condyle superiorly seated within the fossa following loss of condylar volume and creating a premature right side occlusion and a left side open bite. (**e**) Oblique sagittal views show that osseous components of the left TMJ are smooth, rounded, corticated and without evidence of subchondral defects. The left side condyle fossa spatial relationships are within normal limits

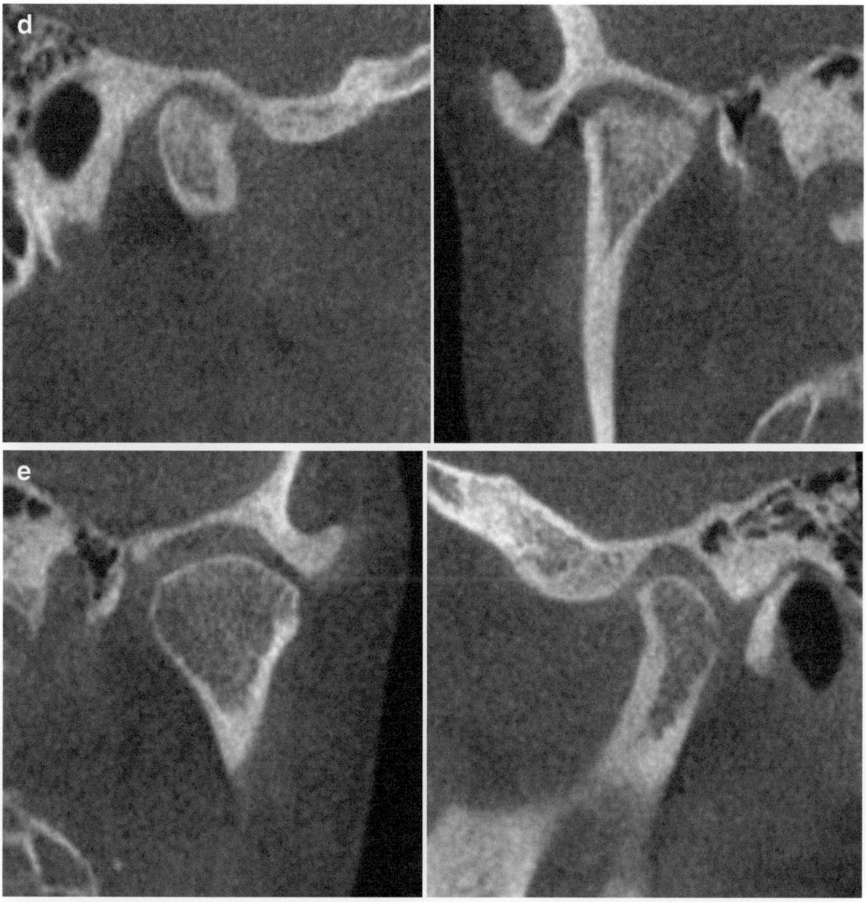

Fig. 9 (continued)

OC Imaging An exophytic enlargement localized to articular cartilage sites of the TMJ. Enlargement is limited to the tumor, but if it occurs in a growing individual, then it may also enlarge the ipsilateral ramus. In adults, the enlargement is confined to the lesion and not the rest of the mandible. An OC may continue to enlarge over time. The growth of this lesion, although originating on the condyle, may not always conform to the available space and therefore, may displace the mandible, creating a mandibular asymmetry and altering occlusion. A condylar OC can displace the mandible in a horizontal and/or vertical direction depending on the site of origin. A horizontal shift may create a contralateral posterior crossbite. An OC on the coronoid process often interferes with condylar motion.

The main differential diagnosis for an osteochondroma includes an osteophyte, osteoma, and condylar hyperplasia. The appearance of an osteoma and OC is very similar since the cartilage cap cannot be visualized on an image, and therefore anatomic knowledge of the cartilage versus periosteal surface sites is used to discriminate OC from an osteoma. A small OC originating from the anterior surface of the condyle mimics an osteophyte. An osteophyte is always associated with other signs of degenerative joint disease and will not displace the condyle (Figs. 11).

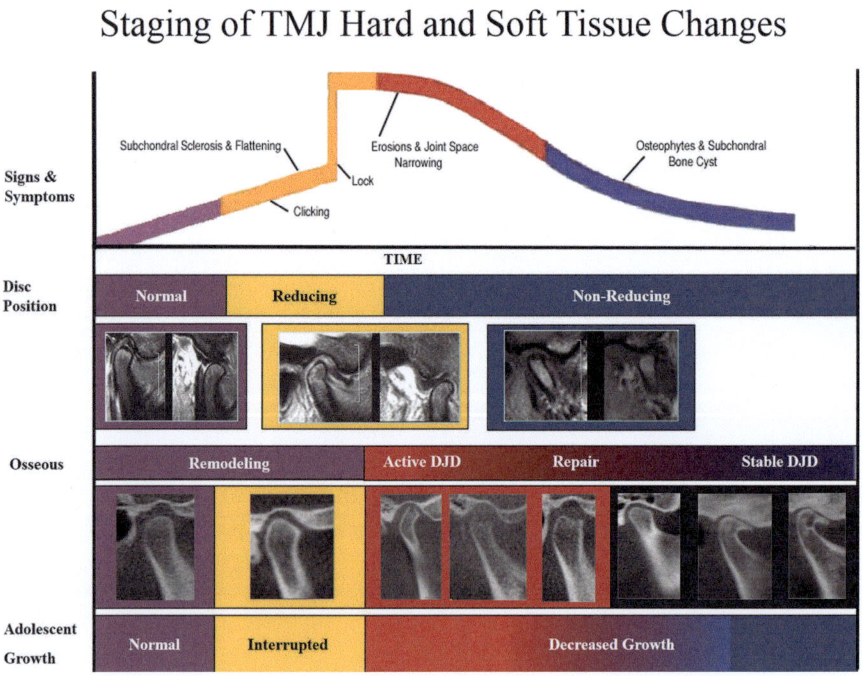

Fig. 10 DJD continuum graphic illustrator constructing. This graphic illustrates the hard and soft tissue changes occurring over time beginning with normal TMJ anatomy and terminating with end-stage degenerative joint disease. Soft tissue changes occur first with a precipitous increase in signs and symptoms occurring at the time of a nonreducing disc displacement. When the osseous anatomy radiographically expresses signs of degenerative joint disease, then it occurs after a nonreducing anteriorly displaced disc. The DJD progresses through several stages beginning with loss of a superior cortex and cavitation of the subchondral bone through an erosive process and resulting in a loss of condylar volume. The following stages progress through repair and terminate in a stable form. The repair process includes flattening and cortication of the articular surface. The clinical signs and symptoms tend to decrease over time as the osseous changes progress toward end-stage DJD. When these same degenerative changes occur during active period of growth and development, then regional growth deficits primarily involving the mandible will occur

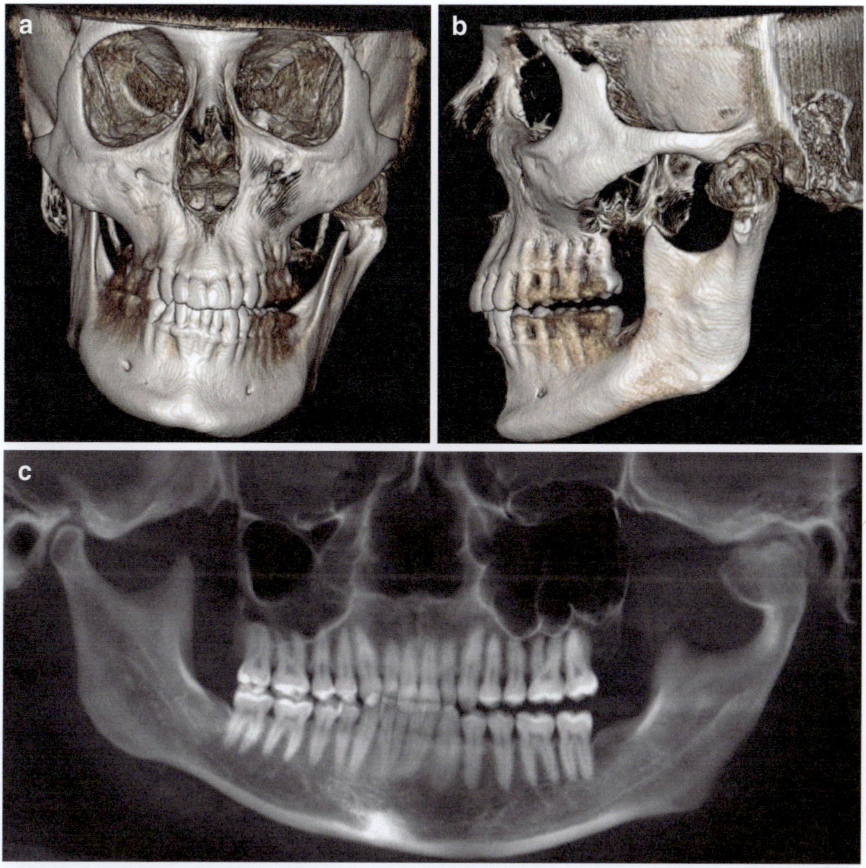

Fig. 11 Osteochondroma. (**a**) CBCT frontal volume rendering shows the left side being larger than the right. Note that the left ramus is displaced medio-inferiorly and not bowed laterally as seen in condylar hyperplasia. There is a mass noted along the superior surface of the displaced condyle. The osseous midline of the mandible is shifted to the right. (**b**) Volume rendered lateral view shows a large mass attached to the superior surface of the condyle and displacing the condyle. There is an ipsilateral open bite. (**c**) CBCT reconstructed panoramic projection and a large mass like structure extending from the anterosuperior surface of the left condyle. Note that aside from the osteochondroma extending from the left condyle the remainder of the left half of the mandible is of similar size as the right. (**d**) Oblique sagittal and coronal views of the left condyle. Note that the osteochondroma is extending from the articular cartilage portion of the condyle and that the native condylar cortex can be visualized. The outer margin of the osteochondroma has a cortex. (**e**) Oblique sagittal and coronal views of the right TMJ and is radiographically normal

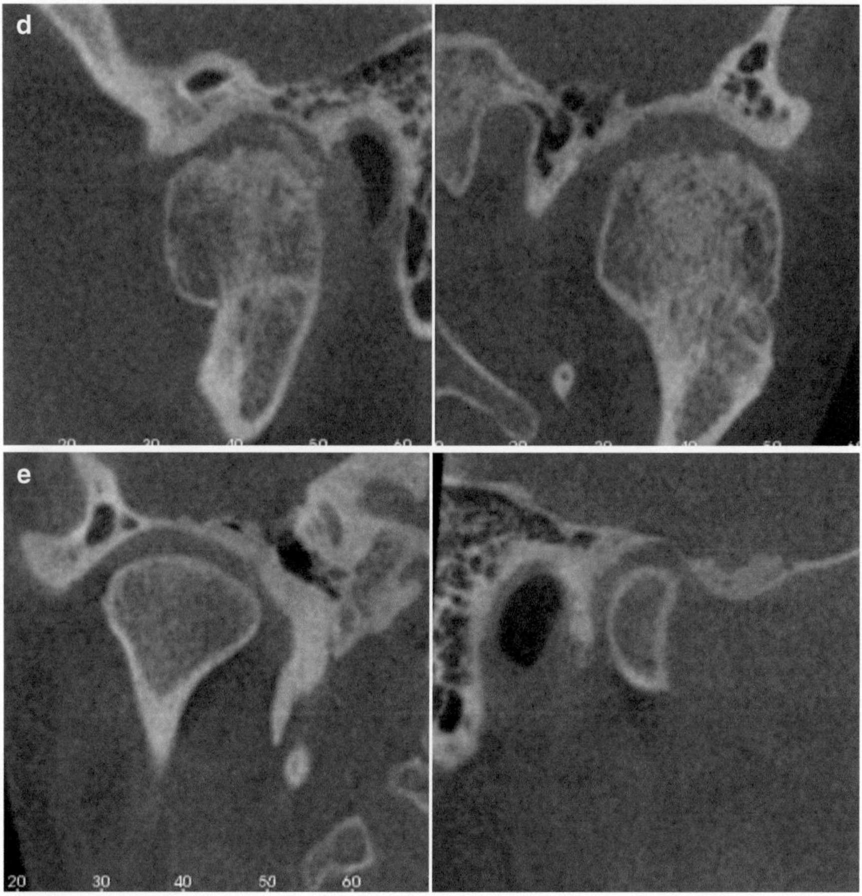

Fig. 11 (continued)

Osteoma

An osteoma is a benign slow-growing cancellous or compact bone-forming tumor arising from periosteal surfaces (intramembranous bone) typically in the craniofacial region [37]. Osteoma of the paranasal sinus region is the most common site, while the osteoma of the TMJ is rare. An osteoma is an acquired anomaly most commonly identified in the fourth decade, but can occur in other decades, both in males and females. Osteoma is generally asymptomatic until it enlarges sufficiently to interfere with mandibular function. An enlarging osteoma of the TMJ may displace the condyle/mandible, thus creating an ipsilateral posterior open bite (Fig. 12).

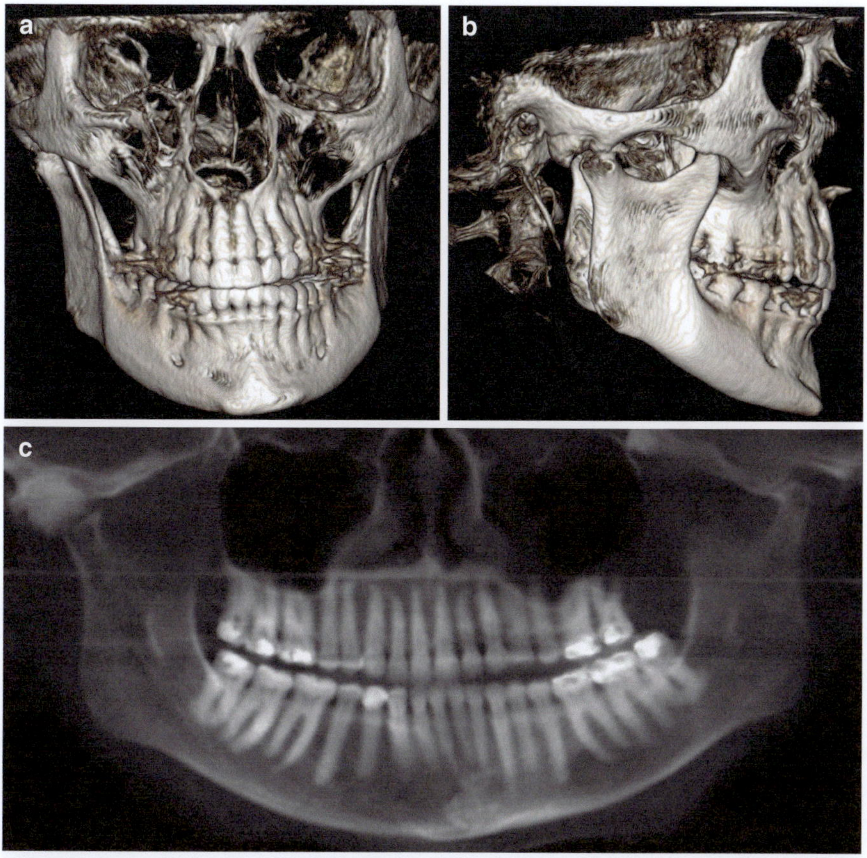

Fig. 12 Osteoma. (**a**) CBCT Volume rendered frontal view showing a mandibular asymmetry. The osseous and dental midlines are shifted to the left. (**b**) A lateral view shows that the right half of the mandible is anteriorly displaced as evidenced by the anterior position of the posterior border of the right ramus relative to the left ramus. Note that the lower borders of the mandible superimpose. (**c**) A CBCT panoramic reconstruction demonstrates a high density mass posterior to the right condyle. (**d**) Axially corrected oblique sagittal and coronal images of the right TMJ. An opaque mass with an attenuation value of dense cortical bone is extending from the posterosuperior regions of the right glenoid fossa. The proximal surface of the mass is located in the periosteal region of the glenoid fossa. There is a degenerative loss of volume from the condyle with a formation of an irregular but congruent articulation with the osteoma. (**e**) Left TMJ show a small condyle resulting from degenerative joint disease. The condyle is anteroinferiorly positioned within the glenoid fossa

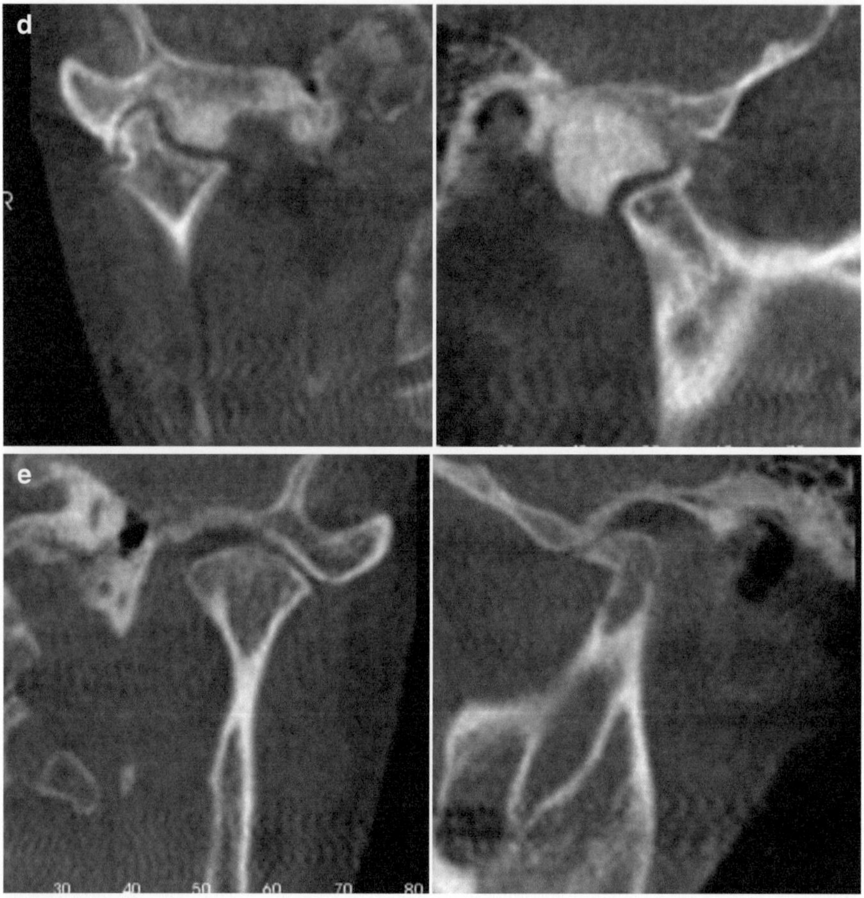

Fig. 12 (continued)

Condylar Hyperplasia

Condylar hyperplasia (CH) is a unilateral phenomenon characterized by vertical ipsilateral involvement of the mandible [38, 39]. CH has been reported to be active between the ages of 10 and 30 with a predominance between the ages of 15 and 19. This is a self-limiting condition and therefore not considered neoplastic. Hyperplasia refers to an increase in the number of cells leading to excessive growth. The condyle is a growth site and enlarges through endochondral bone formation. In the presence of CH, the growth rate is accelerated and growth duration extends beyond normal somatic growth. Two imaging strategies that are utilized to determine the activity status of CH are a nuclear scintigraphy bone scan or comparison of anatomic size on serial 3D imaging exams. The preferred bone scan method is single-photon emission tomography (SPECT) comparing uptake ratios to a control site.

CH Imaging The condyle and neck are elongated and may have an increased circumference. The bone within the enlarged condyle will be normal, but because of the biomechanical stresses and strains associated with function, modeling or remodeling may alter the shape and structure of the articular portions of the condyle and opposing fossa/eminence.

Since the fossa functionally develops and is nearly complete by the age of 12, a condyle fossa size and shape mismatch may occur with condylar hyperplasia. The vertical dimensions of the ipsilateral ramus and body may be increased. The concavity along the posterior border of the ramus and the inferior border of the mandible decreases or becomes convex. The combination of a convex posterior and lower border gives the appearance of a "rocking chair" shape. The ramus may become convex in a transverse direction. The mandibular canal will have a vertical relationship to the lower border of the mandible that is similar to the contralateral side. The mandibular occlusal plane will be depressed on the ipsilateral side with or without an open bite. The osseous midline of the mandible will be shifted to the contralateral side. The dental midlines may or may not be coincident but the mandibular incisor root apices may angle toward the contralateral side (Fig. 13).

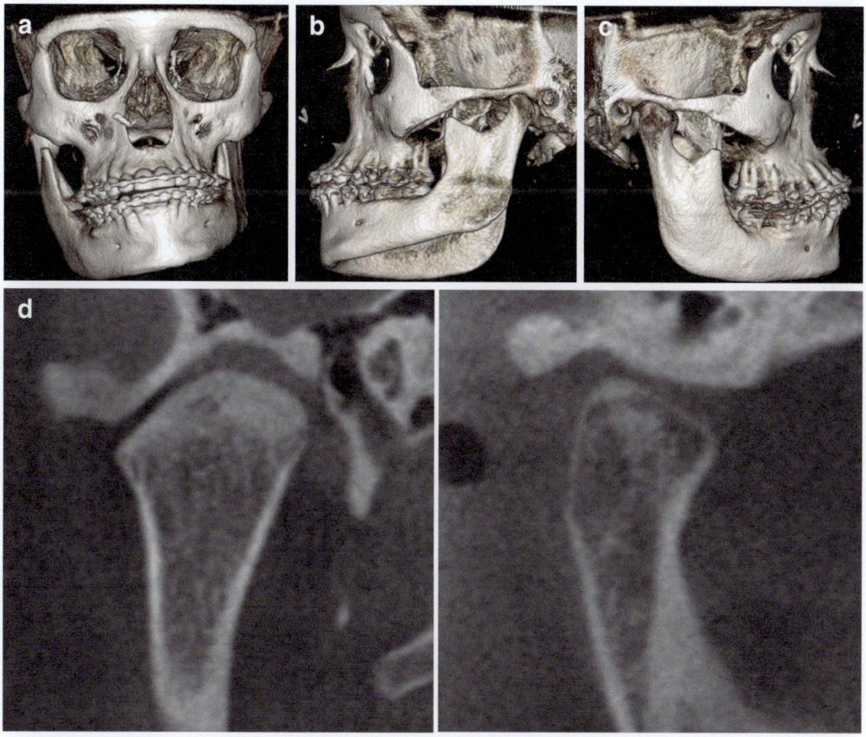

Fig. 13 Condylar hyperplasia. (**a**) Volume-rendered 3D view of skeleton shows that the right side is larger than the left. The lateral bowing of the right ramus indicates that the right side is too large. The occlusal plane is depressed on the right side. The osseous midline of the mandible is shifted to the left side. There is a right side posterior open bite. (**b**) The left lateral volume-rendered view shows the magnitude of the size discrepancy between the right and left halves of the mandible. Note that the discrepancy is vertical and not in an anteroposterior dimension. (**c**) Right lateral volume-rendered view shows convex shape of the lower border of the mandible and the reduction in convexity of the posterior border of the ramus creating a "rocking chair shape." (**d**) CBCT oblique sagittal and coronal views of the right TMJ show that the right condyle is relatively large when compared to dimensions of the ipsilateral fossa and the contralateral condyle. Note that the condyle is globally enlarged and surrounded by a normal but remodeled to a flattened superior and subchondral sclerosis. (**e**) CBCT oblique sagittal and coronal views of the left TMJ. The condyle has a normal size and shape. (**f**) CBCT-reconstructed panoramic view of the mandible showing large right half of the mandible with a rocking chair shape of the posteroinferior margins

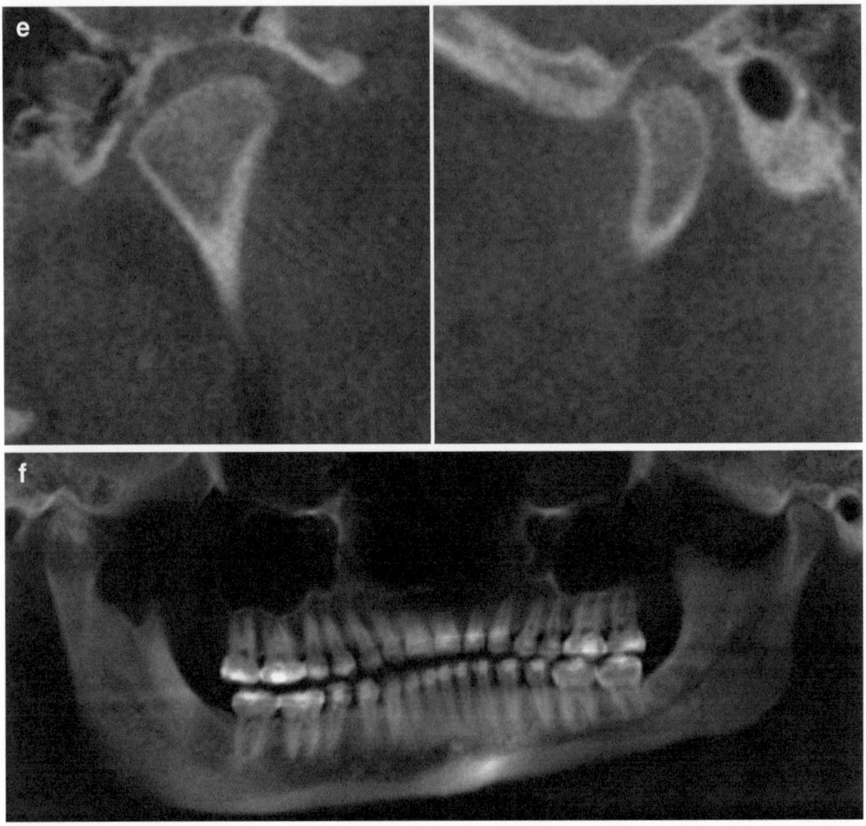

Fig. 13 (continued)

Hemimandibular Elongation (HME) The HME is primarily a unilateral elongation of the ipsilateral half of the mandible [40, 41]. Unlike condylar hyperplasia which extends beyond normal skeletal maturity timelines, HME is fully developed at cessation of somatic growth.

HME Imaging Vertical elongation of the ipsilateral condylar process (neck and condyle) without a significant change in condylar circumference or shape. Increased anteroposterior dimension of the ipsilateral half of the mandible is seen as equal to bilateral vertical dimensions of the rami and body of the mandible. The gonial angle on the ipsilateral side may be more obtuse than the contralateral side. The osseous midline of the mandible and the lower dental midline are shifted to the contralateral side. The anterior overjet ranges from a reduced overjet to an anterior crossbite. There is a class III molar relationship ipsilaterally with a tendency for a posterior crossbite on the contralateral side (Fig. 14).

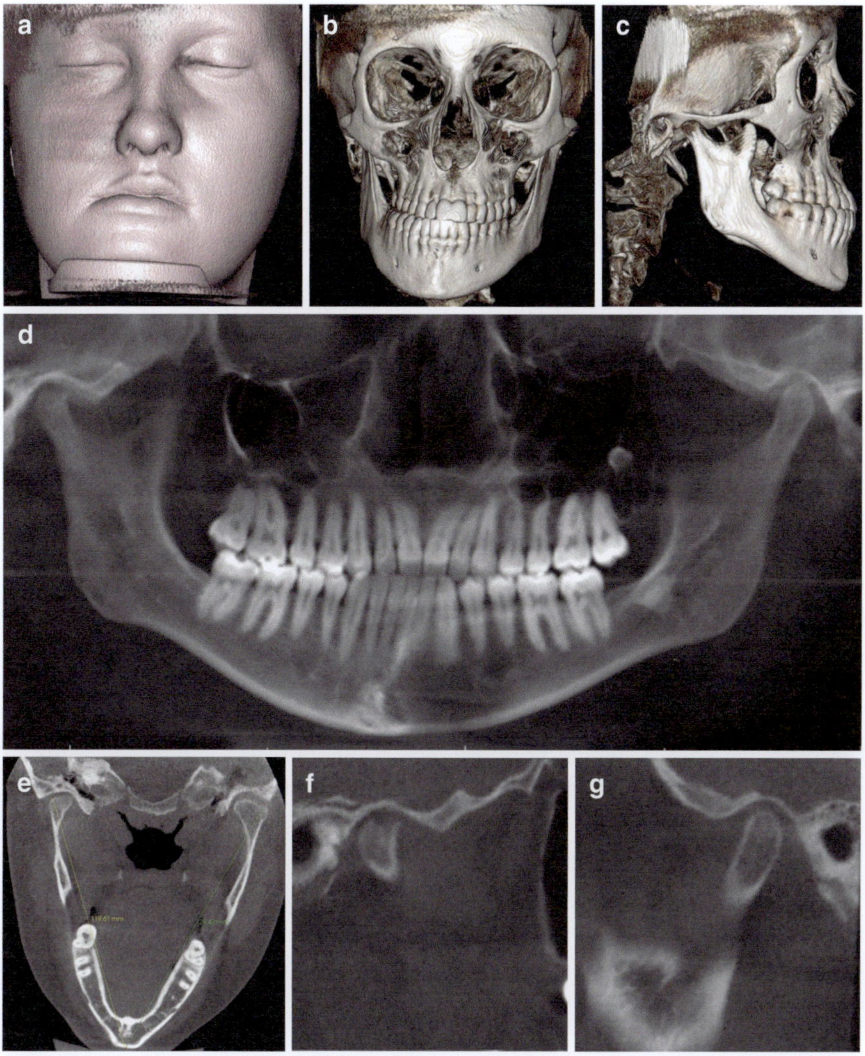

Fig. 14 Hemi-Mandibular Elongation. (**a**) CBCT volume rendered frontal soft tissue view showing a facial symmetry with the left side being larger than the right. (**b**) Frontal view of the skeleton show a displacement of the osseous and dental midlines to the right. There is a right side posterior cross bite and tendency toward a negative anterior overjet. (**c**) Lateral view showing left antegonial notch anterior to the right but no significant discrepancy in the vertical dimension of the lower border of the mandible. The right condylar process has a posterior inclination. (**d**) CBCT reconstructed panoramic projection shows the left condylar process is longer than the right but the vertical dimensions of the ascending rami and body are bilaterally equal. The left gonial angle is more obtuse than the right. There is a left side super-class III occlusion. The occlusal plane is horizontal. (**e**) Oblique axial view of the mandible shows that the anteroposterior dimensions of left half of the mandible are greater than the right. (**f**) Sagittal view of the right TMJ show a small right condyle with a relatively large active erosions extending into the superior surface. The erosion has resulted in a loss of condylar volume. The mandibular asymmetry may alter the mechanics of mandibular function and predispose the right TMJ to degeneration. (**g**) Axially corrected oblique sagittal view of the left condyle. The size, shape, quality and spatial relationships of the osseous components are within normal limits

Non-TMJ-Related Facial Asymmetries

Soft tissue All soft tissue types, including muscle, fat, neural, vascular, salivary, and lymphatic tissues, have the potential to be anomalous and can give rise to a facial asymmetry. Expanding lymphatic, neural, and vascular lesions can create a facial asymmetry from soft tissue distortion that causes a trophic effect on the adjacent skeleton. This trophic effect can enlarge (hypertrophy) or diminish (atrophy) bone size (Figs. 15 and 16).

Intraosseous Selected localized intraosseous lesions may create a focal expansion and therefore present as a facial asymmetry. Intraosseous lesion types to consider include cysts, benign and malignant tumors, and fibro-osseous lesions. Fibrous dysplasia will be discussed as a representative of an osseous condition leading to a facial asymmetry.

Fibrous Dysplasia (FD) This is a developmental condition that may enlarge the involved bone. There are monostotic (single site) and polyostotic (multiple bones) forms of FD. FD is not uncommon in the jaws but it rarely involves the TMJ. In this condition, normal bone is replaced with an admixture of fibrous connective and poorly formed cancellous bone and osteoid. The radiographic appearance of FD is the reflection of the composition and distribution of the bone and fibrous elements. Connective tissue forms low attenuation regions, while the bone has higher attenuation, thus creating bone pattern characteristics classically described as ground glass, orange peel, or thumb print. Fibrous dysplasia forms during the period of skeletal formation and has the unique ability to enlarge a bone by replacing all of the involved cancellous and cortical bone with dysplastic bone and then reforming an outer cortex (Fig. 17).

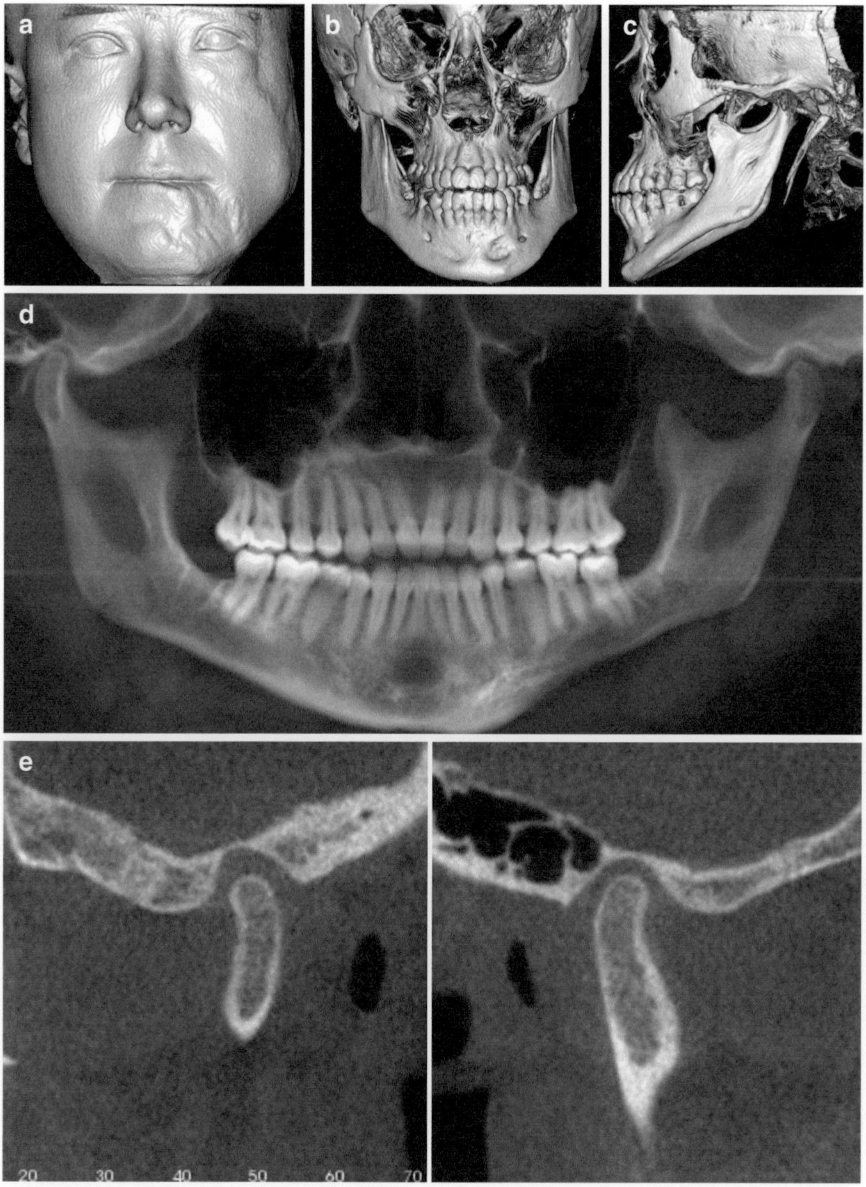

Fig. 15 Lymphangioma. (**a**) CBCT volume-rendered 3D view of the face of a patient with a lymphangioma shows the left half of the face is larger than the right with an irregular shape. Lymphangioma is responsible for the enlargement of the soft tissues but has an atrophic effect on the adjacent skeleton by reducing its size. (**b**) Frontal view of the skeleton shows the lateral development of the left half of the mandible is less than the right. The dental midline of the mandible is shifted to the left and there is an anterior open bite. Vertical dimension of the right body of the mandible is less than the left and lower border of the left side of the mandible is more concave than the right. (**c**) Left lateral view of skeleton illustrates size discrepancy between the two halves of the mandible. The left gonial angle is obtuse. (**d**) CBCT panoramic reconstruction shows the overall size of the left half of the mandible is smaller than the right. Note that the right and left condyles are symmetrical. (**e**) Right and left TMJ oblique sagittal views showing symmetrical condyles with normal growth and development

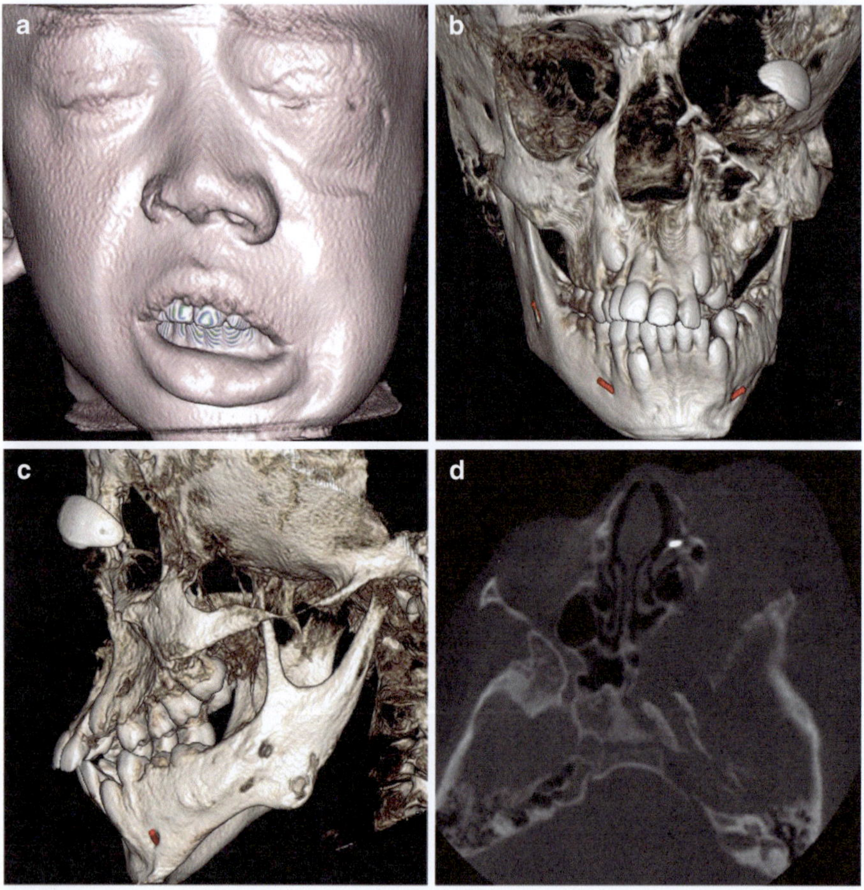

Fig. 16 Neurofibromatosis. (**a**) CBCT volume-rendered 3D view of the face of a patient with neurofibromatosis shows asymmetric face. The neurofibromatosis involves the soft tissues and has an atrophic effect on the adjacent skeleton. (**b**) Frontal view of the skeleton shows the lateral development of the left half of the mandible is less than the right. The osseous midline of the mandible shifted to the left and the left side occlusal plane is depressed. The right angle of the mandible is elevated. (**c**) Left lateral view of skeleton shows the AP and vertical dimensions of the left ramus are small. (**d**) CBCT axial section shows left side facial and orbital soft tissue enlargement. The left foramen rotundum, pterygopalatine fossa, and inferior orbital fissures are enlarged. The left side posterior ethmoid and sphenoid sinuses lack lateral development

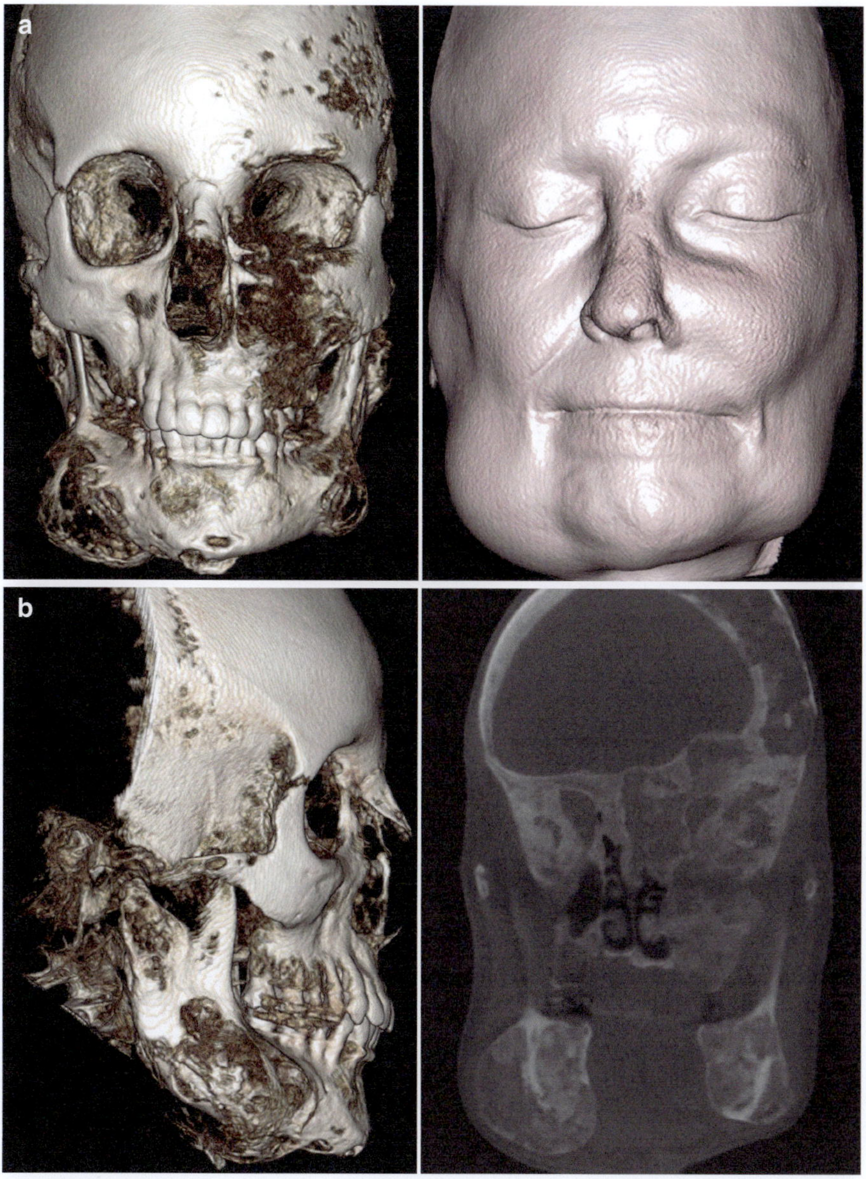

Fig. 17 Polyostotic Fibrous dysplasia. (**a**) Volume rendered frontal view of the asymmetrical facial soft tissues and the underlying skeleton. Note the asymmetrical enlargement of the mandible, left midface, orbit and frontal bone. (**b**) Volume rendering of right lateral skull view showing extensive enlargement of the mandible and right condylar process. Coronal sectional view showing bilateral involvement of the mandible, skull base, midface and left temporal and parietal bones. (**c**) Reconstructed panoramic projection shows asymmetrical enlargement of the mandible, TMJs, and left maxilla. (**d**) Oblique sagittal and coronal left and right side TMJs showing rare but extensive involvement of the TMJs

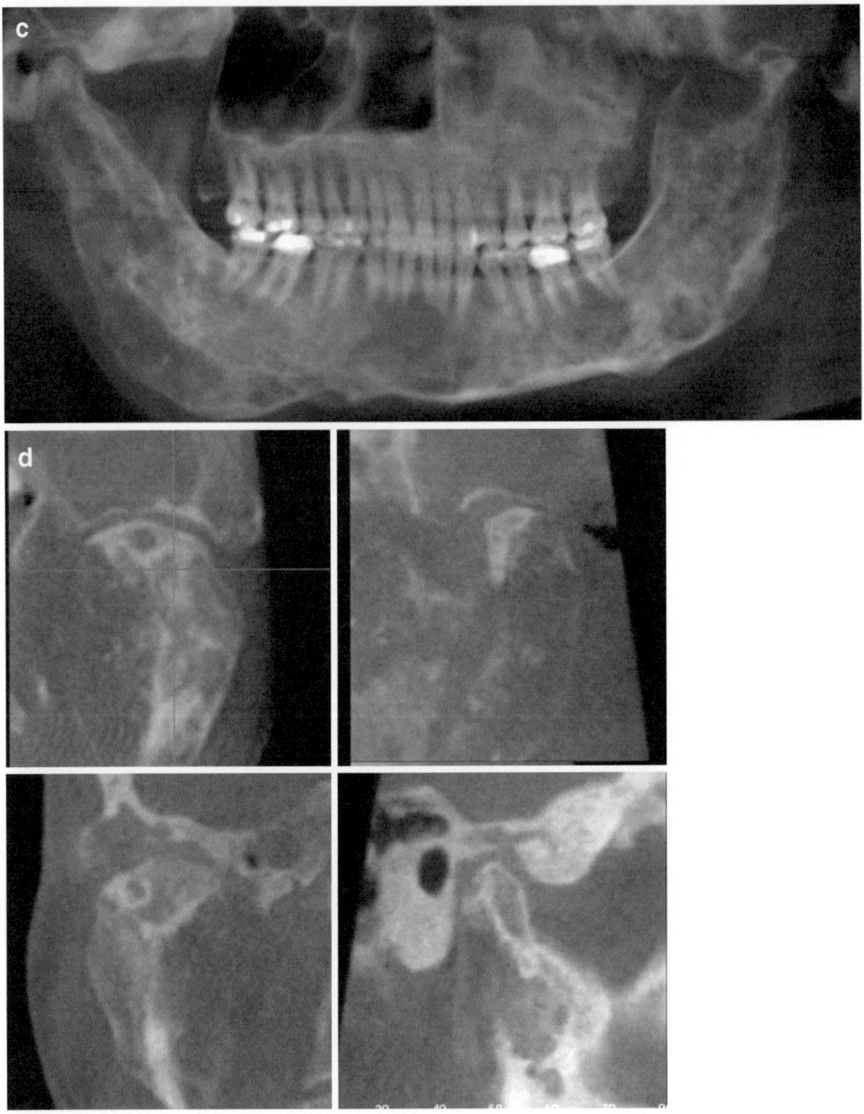

Fig. 17 (continued)

References

1. Sanders DA, Chankhoke TK, Uribe FA, Rigali PH, Nanda R. Quantification of skeletal asymmetries in normal adolescents: cone-beam computed tomography analysis. Prog Orthod. 2014;15:26.
2. Isberg A, Legrell PE. Facial asymmetry in adults following temporomandibular joint disc displacement with onset during growth. World J Orthod. 2000;1:164–72.
3. Nebbe B, Major PW. Prevalence of TMJ disc displacement in a pre-orthodontic adolescent sample. Angle Orthod. 2000;70:454–63.
4. Nebbe B, Major PW, Prasad NG. Adolescent female craniofacial morphology associated with advanced bilateral TMJ disc displacement. Eur J Orthod. 1998;20:701–12.
5. Nebbe B, Major PW, Prasad NG. Female adolescent facial pattern associated with TMJ disk displacement and reduction in disk length: part I. Am J Orthod Dentofac Orthop. 1999;116:168–76.
6. Trypkova B, Major P, Nebbe B, Prasad N. Craniofacial symmetry and temporomandibular joint internal derangement in female adolescents: a posteroanterior cephalometric study. Angle Orthod. 2000;70:81–8.
7. Bryndahl F, Eriksson L, Legrell PF, Isberg A, Bilateral TMJ disk displacement induces mandibular retrognathia, J Dent Res. 2006;85-12:1118–23.
8. Legrell PE, Reibel J, Nylander K, Horstedt P, Isberg K. Temporomandibular joint condyle changes after surgically induced non-reducing disk displacement in rabbits: a macroscopic study. Acta Odontol Scan. 1999;57:290–300.
9. Legrell PE, Isberg A. Mandibular length and midline asymmetry after experimentally induced temporomandibular joint disk displacement in rabbits. Am J Orthod Dentofac Orthop. 1999;115:247–25.
10. Kurita H, Ohtsuka A, Kobayashi H, Kurashina K. Alteration of the horizontal mandibular condylar size associated with temporomandibular joint internal derangement in adult females. Dentomaxillofac Radiol. 2002;31:373–8.
11. Legrell PE, Isberg A. Mandibular height asymmetry following experimentally induced temporomandibular joint disk displacement in rabbits. Oral Surg Oral Med Oral Pathol Oral Radiol Endod. 1998;86:280–5.
12. Bryndahl F, Legrell PE, Eriksson L, Isberg A. Bilateral TMJ disk displacement induces mandibular retrognathia. J Dent Res. 2006;85:1118–23.
13. Hatcher DC, Faulkner MG, Hay A. Development of mechanical and mathematic models to study temporomandibular joint loading. J Prosthet Dent. 1986;89:377.
14. Faulkner MG, Hatcher DC, Hay A. A three dimensional investigation of temporomandibular joint loading. J Biomech. 1987;20:997.
15. Koritoth TW, Hannam AG. Effect of bilateral asymmetric tooth clenching on load distribution at the mandibular condyles. J Pros Dent. 1990;64:62–73.
16. Sommerfeldt DW. Rubin CT biology of bone and how it orchestrates the form and the function of the skeleton. Eur Spine J. 2001;10:S86–95.
17. Carter DR, Beaupre GS. Skeletal Function and Form: Mechanobiology of Skeletal Development, Aging, and Regeneration. In: From and function, vol. 1-31. Cambridge University Press; 2007.
18. Carter DR, Beaupre GS. Skeletal function and form: mechanobiology of skeletal development, aging, and regeneration. In: Skeletal tissue histomorphology and mechanics, vol. 31-52. Cambridge University Press; 2007.
19. Mizoguchi I, Toriya N, Nakao Y. Growth of the mandible and biological characteristics of the mandibular condylar cartilage. Japanese Dental Sci Rev. 2013;49:139–50.
20. Pirttiniemi P, Peltomaki T, Muller L, Luder H. Abnormal mandibular growth and condylar cartilage. Eur J Orthod. 2009;31:1–11.
21. Hatcher D. Hemifacial microsomia. In: Tamimi D, Hatcher DC, editors. Specialty Imaging: temporomandibular joint. Salt Lake City (UT): Elsevier; 2016. p. 404–7.

22. Hatcher D, Petrikowski CG, Fracture TMJ. Adult and neonatal. In: Tamimi D, Hatcher DC, editors. Specialty imaging: temporomandibular joint. Salt Lake City (UT): Elsevier; 2016. p. 438–43.
23. Shah LM, Hatcher D. Juvenile idiopathic arthritis. In: Tamimi D, Hatcher DC, editors. Specialty imaging: temporomandibular joint. Salt Lake City (UT): Elsevier; 2016. p. 458–63.
24. Hatcher DC. Progressive condylar resorption: pathologic processes and imaging considerations. Semin Arthod. 2013;19:97–105.
25. Alsabban L, Amarista FJ, Mercuri LG, Perez D. Idiopathic condylar resorption: a survey and review of the literature. J Oral Maxillofac Surg. 2018 Jul;19
26. Arnett GW, Milam SB, Gottesman L. Progressive mandibular retrusions-idiopathic condylar retrusion-idiopathic condylar resorption. Part I- Am J Orthod Dentofacial Orthop. 1996;1(10):8–15.
27. Arnett GW, Milam SB, Gottesman L. Progressive mandibular retrusions-idiopathic condylar retrusion-idiopathic condylar resorption. Part II- Am J Orthod Dentofacial Orthop. 1996;1(10):17–27.
28. Posnick JC. Idiopathic condylar resorption: current clinical perspectives. J Oral Maxillofac Surg. 2007;65:1617–23.
29. Kristensen KD, Schmidt B, Stoustrup P, Pedersen TK. Idiopathic condylar resorptions: 3-dimensional condylar bony deformation, signs and symptoms. Am J Orthod Dentofac Orthop. 2017;152:214–23.
30. Kristensen KD, Schmidt B, Stoustrup P, Pedersen TK. Idiopathic condylar resorption: 3-dimensions condylar bone deformation, signs and symptoms. Am J Orthod Dentofac Orthop. 2017;152:214–23.
31. Kambylafkas P, Kyrkandides S, Tallents RH. Mandibular asymmetry in adult patients with unilateral degenerative joint disease. Angle Orthod. 2005;75(3):305–10.
32. Hatcher D, Koenig LJ, Petrikowski CG, Hypoplasia C, Editiors- Tamimi D, Hatcher DC. Specialty imaging: temporomandibular joint. Salt Lake City (UT): Elsevier; 2016. p. 414–7.
33. Milam SB. Pathogenesis of degenerative temporomandibular joint arthritides. Odontology. 2005;93:7–15.
34. Hatcher D. Degenerative Joint Disease. In: Tamimi D, Hatcher DC, editors. Specialty Imaging: temporomandibular joint. Salt Lake City (UT): Elsevier; 2016. p. 470–3.
35. Moffett BC. Definitions of temporomandibular joint derangements. In: Moffett BC, Westesson P, editors. Diagnosis of internal derangements of the Temporomandibular Joint. Proceedings of a Continuing Dental Education symposium, Seattle, February 17–18; 1984.
36. Hatcher D, Petrikowski CG. Osteochondroma. In: Tamimi D, Hatcher DC, editors. Specialty imaging: temporomandibular joint. Salt Lake City, UT: Elsevier; 2016. p. 540–5.
37. Koenig L, Harnsberger R. Osteoma. In: Tamimi D, Hatcher DC, editors. Specialty imaging: temporomandibular joint. Salt Lake City, UT: Elsevier; 2016. p. 548–51.
38. Hatcher D, Koenig LJ. Condylar hyperplasia. In: Tamimi D, Hatcher DC, editors. Specialty imaging: temporomandibular joint. Salt Lake City, UT: Elsevier; 2016. p. 418–23.
39. Xu M, Chan FC, Jin X, Xu J, Lu J, Zhang C, Teng L. Hemimandibular Hyperplasia: Classification and treatment Algorithm Revisited. J Craniofac Surg. 2014;25:355–8.
40. Posnick JC, Perez J, Chavda A. Hemimandibular elongation: is the corrected occlusion maintained long-term? does the mandible continue to grow? J Oral Maxillofac Surg. 2017;75(2):371–98.
41. Obwegeser HL, Melek MS. Hemimandibular hyperplasia-hemimandibular elongation J Maxillofac surg. 1986;14:183–208.

Orthodontic Considerations in the Management of Facial Asymmetries

Farhad B. Naini and Daljit S. Gill

Abstract

The purpose of this chapter is to describe the role of the orthodontist in the clinical management of patients with asymmetries affecting the middle and lower parts of the face. It will cover briefly the systematic clinical evaluation of bilateral symmetry for the bimaxillary complex and furthermore describe the analysis of two-dimensional and three-dimensional records. It will then cover in detail the five stages of orthodontic treatment required for the patient with dentofacial asymmetry undergoing orthognathic surgery, including the seven objectives of orthodontic preparation. The role of the orthodontist in the immediate preoperative appointment, potential intraoperative requirements and the immediate postoperative appointment will be discussed. Finally, postoperative orthodontics and retention regimes are described.

Keywords

Hybrid functional appliance · Preoperative orthodontics · Postoperative orthodontics · Post orthodontic retention · Facial asymmetry · Systematic facial evaluation

F. B. Naini (✉)
Kingston Hospital NHS Foundation Trust and Queen Mary's Hospital Sidcup,
King's College Hospital NHS Foundation Trust, London, UK

D. S. Gill
Great Ormond Street Hospital NHS Foundation Trust and UCLH Eastman Dental Hospital,
London, UK

P. Mehra, L. M. Wolford (eds.), *Management of Facial Asymmetry*,
https://doi.org/10.1007/978-3-030-44971-1_3

Introduction

The purpose of this chapter is to describe the role of the orthodontist in the clinical management of patients with asymmetries affecting the middle and lower parts of the face. Before embarking on the specific orthodontic considerations, it is worthwhile describing some of the more salient diagnostic features, which will be relevant to how the orthodontist prepares the positions of the teeth prior to surgery.

The clinical evaluation should begin with the frontal facial examination and go on to assess the face from different viewpoints and using various diagnostic records. Comprehensive diagnosis of craniofacial asymmetries has been described elsewhere [1, 2], but the most pertinent information related to jaw asymmetries is summarised in Table 1 (Figs. 1, 2, 3, 4, 5, 6, 7, 8, 9, 10, 11, 12, and 13). The patient should be in natural head position (NHP), though the clinician may need to make

Table 1 Systematic facial evaluation for bilateral symmetry of the maxilla, mandible and related structures

Clinical evaluation	
Frontal view	• Visually assess the approximate vertical distance of bilateral facial structures from a superior true horizontal line (Fig. 1) • Visually assess the approximate horizontal distance of bilateral facial structures from the facial midline • Mark midfacial structures with a skin pencil—e.g. soft tissue glabella, nasion, rhinion, pronasale, labrale superius, labrale inferius and pogonion. Assess their relative positions in relation to each other and the facial midline (Fig. 2) • Assess the relative inclination of horizontal reference lines to each other and to the true horizontal plane (Fig. 3): – Interpupillary line – Intercommissure line – Maxillary occlusal plane—Assess with a wooden tongue spatula or a dental mirror handle (Fig. 4); assess in incisor region, canines, premolar and molar regions. – Mandibular occlusal plane—Assess as for maxilla (Fig. 5) – Inferior chin plane • Assess the maxillary and mandibular occlusal planes with the transverse occlusal plane view, using an orthodontic cheek retractor or photographic cheek retractor (Fig. 6). The maxillary and mandibular occlusal planes may be assessed more clearly with the patient's teeth slightly apart • Assess maxillary incisor and canine exposure bilaterally in relation to the upper lip in repose and in animation (i.e. speech and smiling) • Assess vertical face height in the midline and bilaterally in the lateral aspect of the chin, inferior borders of the mandible and gonial angles • Is there a lateral deviation of the lower lip as well as the chin (signifying a horizontal mandibular asymmetry akin to hemimandibular elongation), or is the lower lip aligned with the upper lip?
Profile view	Assess contour of the inferior borders of the mandible

Table 1 (continued)

Submental view	• Assess the symmetry of the mandibular body and the base of the nose • Assess the horizontal position of the lower lip in relation to the upper lip and chin
Dynamic clinical evaluation	**Mandibular lateral displacement** Assess for a posterior crossbite (especially unilateral)—If a crossbite exists, check for a lateral displacement (functional shift) of the mandible, to ascertain whether *all or part* of the asymmetry is postural (Fig. 7). Clinically manipulate the mandible into occlusion by placing the knuckle of your curled index finger under the patient's chin and your thumb on the mental eminence. Ask the patient to relax, and to roll the tip of their tongue to the back of their throat, and then apply gentle pressure to move the mandible up and down, aiming to keep the condyles in their retruded position within the glenoid fossae. Look for an initial, premature dental contact; the patient may be better able to identify this area and point it out to you. Having established the premature contact, ask the patient to bite together and the displacement will become evident **Asymmetrical facial animation** An asymmetrical smile where the levator muscles of one side cause greater elevation of the upper lip than the contralateral side—This may be mistaken for a transverse cant of the maxillary occlusal plane
Maxillary dental midline	Should be aligned to the mid-philtrum of the upper lip Assess: • Midline deviation (bodily) to the left or right in mm • Mesiodistal angulation of incisors, and relation to maxillary occlusal plane (i.e. will the incisor angulation self-correct on correcting the jaw asymmetry?) (Fig. 8)
Mandibular dental midline	Assess in relation to: • Maxillary dental midline • Body of the mandible • Chin proper—i.e. is the dental midline coincident with the midpoint of the chin? Assess: • Midline deviation (bodily) to the left or right • Mesiodistal angulation of incisors, and relation to transverse occlusal plane cant (i.e. will the incisor angulation self-correct on correcting the jaw asymmetry?)
Radiographic-cephalometric evaluation	
Posteroanterior (PA) cephalometric radiograph	Assess the relative orientation of vertical reference lines drawn parallel to the midsagittal plane, through any pair of bilateral landmarks, to help identify transverse skeletal asymmetries (Fig. 9) Horizontal reference lines may be used to assess vertical dentoskeletal asymmetries (Fig. 10) Triangular analysis—This may be used to compare the left and right sides of the facial skeleton (Fig. 11) *Note:* These methods of analysis may now be used routinely with 3D images, such as CT scans

(continued)

Table 1 (continued)

Lateral cephalometric radiograph	Assess lack of superimposition of bilateral structures; in particular significant vertical differences between two separate inferior mandibular borders may indicate evidence of mandibular asymmetry, such as hemimandibular hyperplasia
Panoramic rotational tomography (OPT)	Assess the morphology and relative height of the mandibular condyle, ramus and body bilaterally (Fig. 12), visually and with comparative bilateral measurements Assess for degenerative changes to the condylar heads, such as from condylar resorption
Three-dimensional evaluation	
Dental study models	Assess the maxillary and mandibular arch forms separately in occlusal view—A transparent ruled grid may be oriented in the midline over the mid-palatal raphe, allowing direct observation of arch form This may be useful for monitoring occlusal changes in a growing patient
Facial soft tissue scans	May be useful for monitoring asymmetrical growth by superimposition of serial scans—This technology requires further development
Computed tomography (CT)/ CBCT	Useful for more severe asymmetries, particularly panfacial/craniofacial Relationship of horizontal and vertical reference planes may be compared (similar to PA cephalometric analysis), and comparison of the relative positions of trigeminal foramina (Fig. 13) [1] Stereolithographic models
Stereolithographic models	Fabricated from CT/CBCT data; these may be useful in diagnosis and planning the surgical correction of complex asymmetries

(Modified from: Naini FB, Gill DS (eds). Orthognathic Surgery: Principles, Planning and Practice. Oxford: Wiley-Blackwell, 2017; reprinted with permission.)

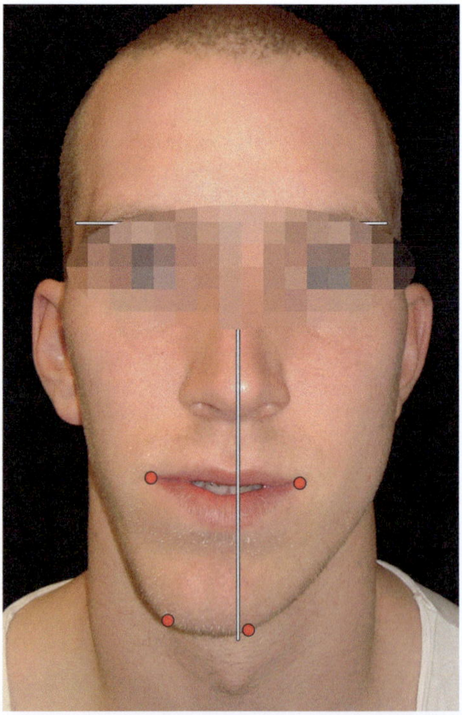

Fig. 1 Visually assess the approximate vertical distance of bilateral facial structures from a superior true horizontal line, and the approximate horizontal distance of bilateral facial structures from the facial midline. (From: Naini FB, Gill DS (eds). Orthognathic Surgery: Principles, Planning and Practice. Oxford: Wiley-Blackwell, 2017; used with permission)

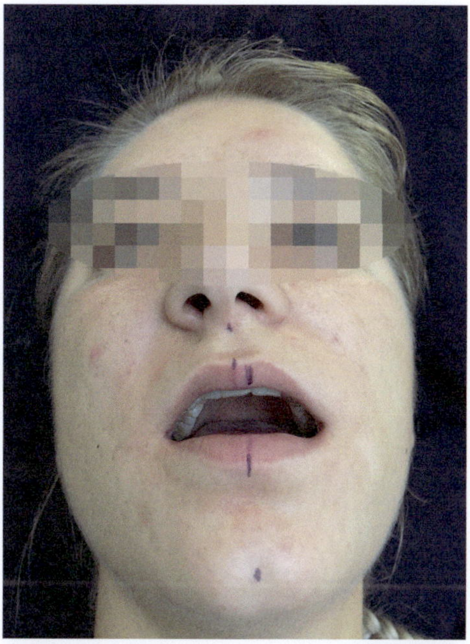

Fig. 2 Midfacial structures may be marked with a skin pencil, in order to assess their relative positions in relation to each other and the facial midline. In this patient, the position of the maxillary dental midline has also been drawn on the upper lip, demonstrating the deviation from the mid-philtrum of the upper lip

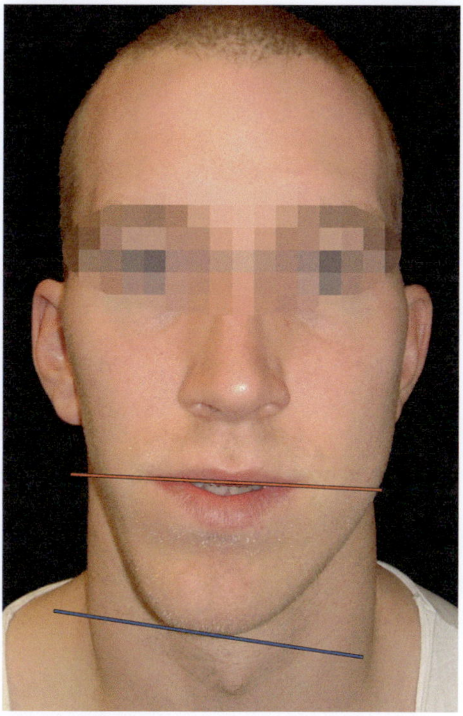

Fig. 3 The relative inclination of horizontal reference lines, such as the interpupillary line, intercommissure line and inferior chin plane may be compared to each other and the true horizontal plane. (From: Naini FB, Gill DS (eds). Orthognathic Surgery: Principles, Planning and Practice. Oxford: Wiley-Blackwell, 2017; used with permission)

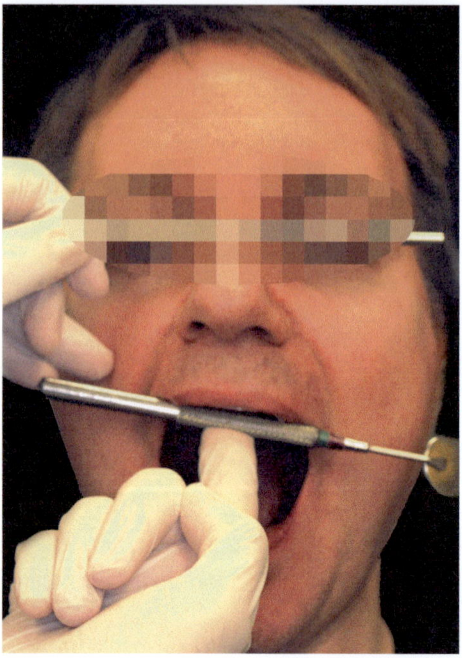

Fig. 4 The transverse inclination of the maxillary occlusal plane may be assessed with a wooden tongue spatula or a dental mirror handle. (From: Naini FB, Gill DS (eds). Orthognathic Surgery: Principles, Planning and Practice. Oxford: Wiley-Blackwell, 2017; used with permission)

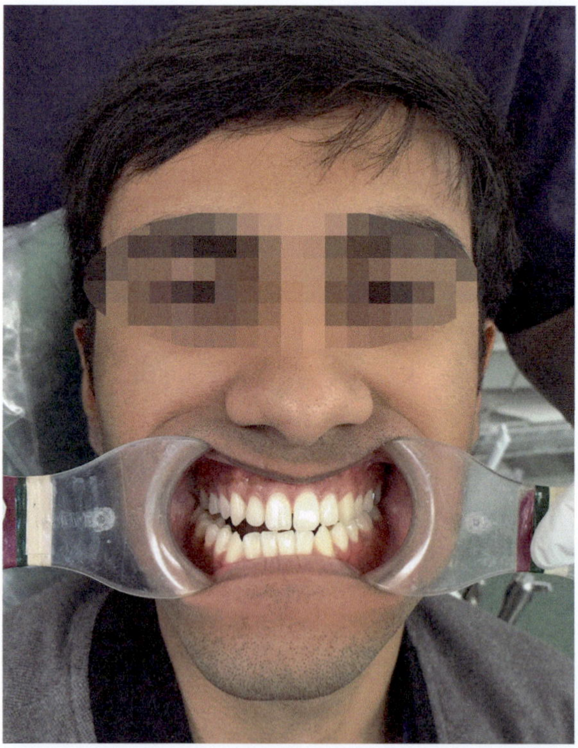

Fig. 5 In this patient, the maxillary occlusal plane is level, but the mandibular occlusal plane is canted down on the patient's right side

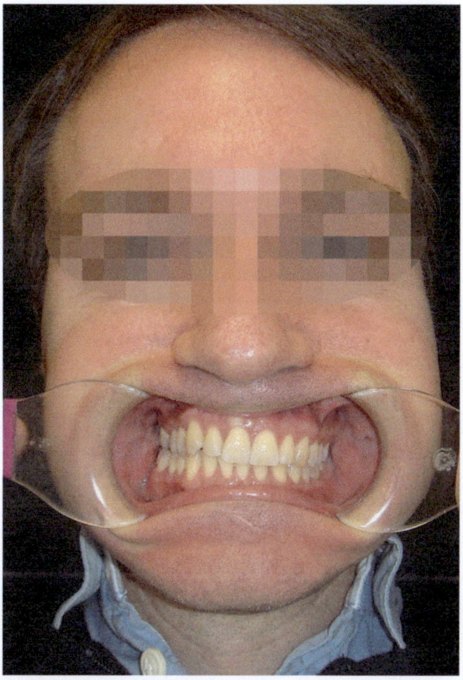

Fig. 6 Transverse occlusal plane view using a photographic cheek retractor. (From: Naini FB, Gill DS (eds). Orthognathic Surgery: Principles, Planning and Practice. Oxford: Wiley-Blackwell, 2017; used with permission)

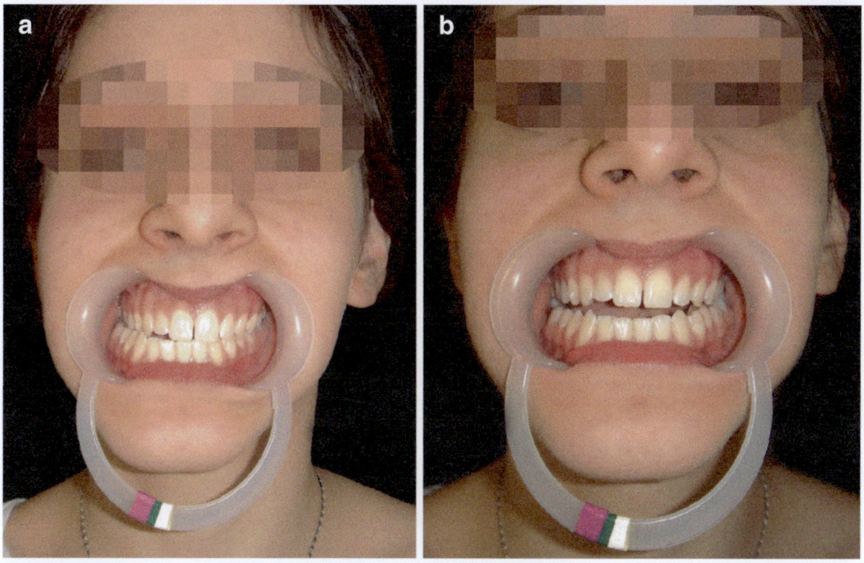

Fig. 7 Patient with mandibular asymmetry demonstrating (**a**) dental occlusion in centric occlusion, but the patient is also displaced to her right, which is evident in (**b**) demonstrating the undisplaced position of the mandible. (From: Naini FB, Gill DS (eds). Orthognathic Surgery: Principles, Planning and Practice. Oxford: Wiley-Blackwell, 2017; used with permission)

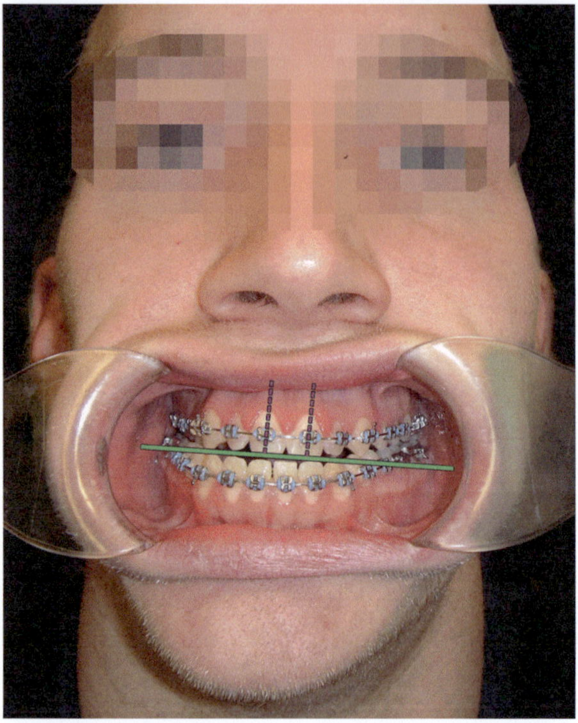

Fig. 8 The mesiodistal angulation of the maxillary incisors should be assessed in relation to the maxillary occlusal plane. The question is whether the incisor angulation will self-correct on correcting the jaw asymmetry or whether preoperative orthodontic preparation of the incisor angulations is required. (From: Naini FB, Gill DS (eds). Orthognathic Surgery: Principles, Planning and Practice. Oxford: Wiley-Blackwell, 2017; used with permission)

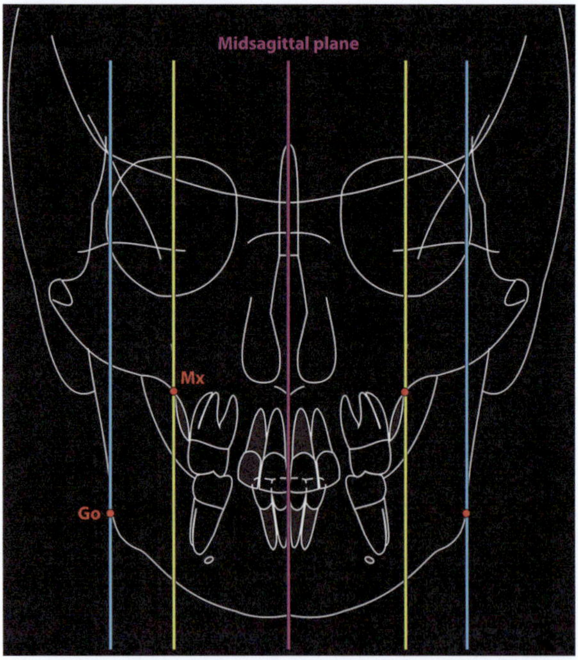

Fig. 9 Vertical reference lines may be drawn parallel to the midsagittal plane through any pair of bilateral landmarks to help identify transverse skeletal asymmetries. Mx, maxillare; Go, gonion. (From: Naini FB. Facial Aesthetics: Concepts and Clinical Diagnosis. Oxford: Wiley-Blackwell, 2011; used with permission)

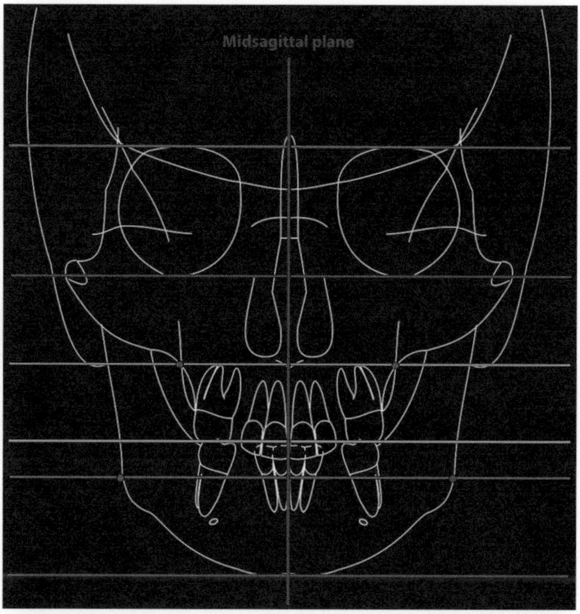

Fig. 10 Horizontal reference lines may be used to illustrate vertical dentoskeletal discrepancies. (From: Naini FB. Facial Aesthetics: Concepts and Clinical Diagnosis. Oxford: Wiley-Blackwell, 2011; used with permission)

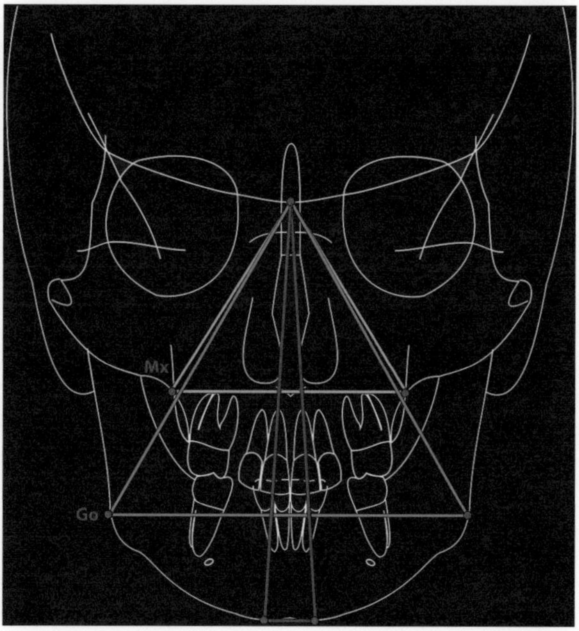

Fig. 11 'Triangular analysis' demonstrating the maxillary, mandibular and chin triangles. Comparison of the left and right legs of the triangles demonstrates transverse canting in relation to the cranial base. Comparison of the left and right halves of the bases of the triangles will indicate asymmetry and left-right difference in size (assuming no rotation of the patient's head around the vertical axis). (From: Naini FB. Facial Aesthetics: Concepts and Clinical Diagnosis. Oxford: Wiley-Blackwell, 2011; used with permission)

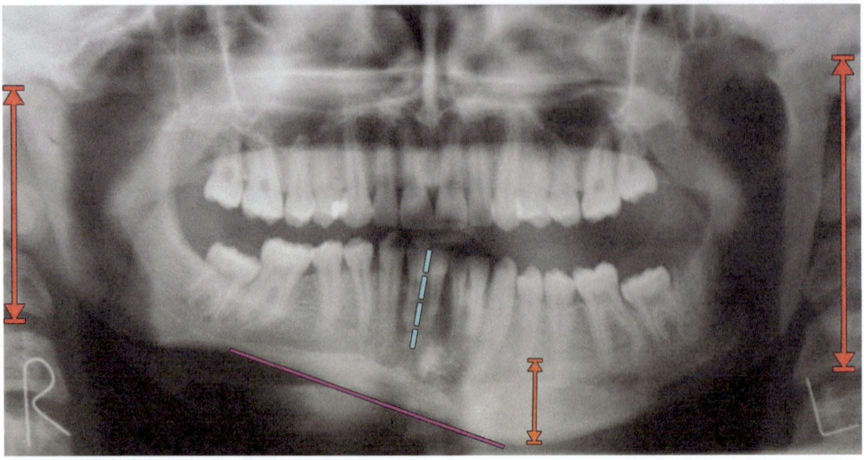

Fig. 12 Orthopantomograph (OPT) of a patient with left-sided hemimandibular hyperplasia, demonstrating excessive vertical growth of the left mandibular condyle and ramus, bowing of the left inferior border, increased bone height in the body of the mandible on the affected side, a transverse cant of the inferior chin plane and angulation of the mandibular incisors and dental midline to the affected side. (From: Naini FB, Gill DS (eds). Orthognathic Surgery: Principles, Planning and Practice. Oxford: Wiley-Blackwell, 2017; used with permission)

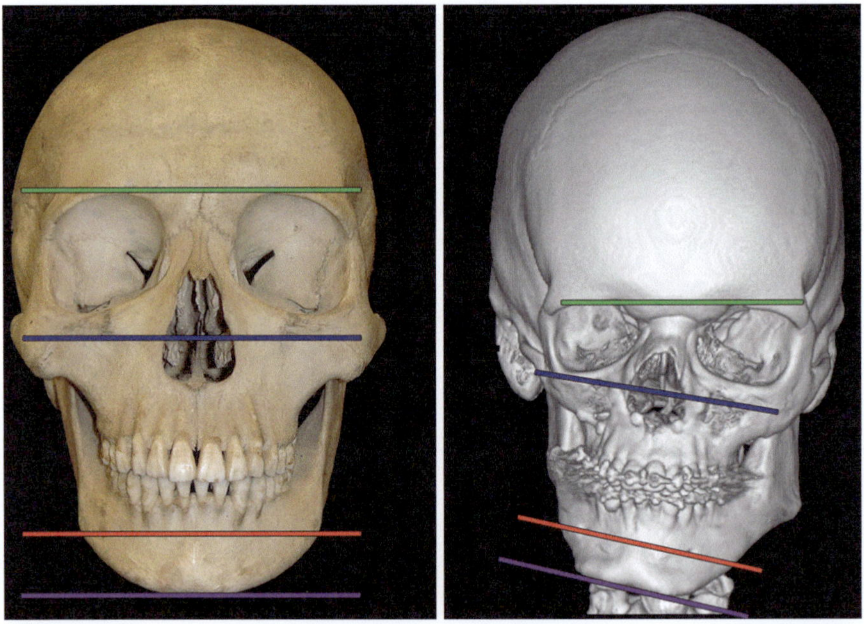

Fig. 13 Horizontal reference planes drawn through bilateral structures will be nearly parallel in the symmetrical skull. The relative orientation of these horizontal planes will demonstrate vertical asymmetry. This figure illustrates horizontal planes through the supraorbital, infraorbital and mental foramina and the inferior chin plane. (From: Naini FB. Facial Aesthetics: Concepts and Clinical Diagnosis. Oxford: Wiley-Blackwell, 2011; used with permission)

minor manual adjustments to the patient's head position, as patients may have developed a *compensatory head posture*, possibly to minimise the aesthetic impact of their facial asymmetry, often tilting their heads to the right or the left, around the sagittal axis [1].

Preliminary Considerations

In cases where a mandibular asymmetry or deficiency is identified at a young age, growth modification may be attempted by the orthodontist. Hybrid functional appliances are specifically tailored to address certain growth processes and development by combining several components, which may act by the following mechanisms: eruption (unilateral posterior bite planes to allow differential eruption of teeth to level a transversely canted maxillary occlusal plane), linguofacial muscle balance (unilateral shields or screens to allow unilateral expansion) and mandibular repositioning (construction bites or jaw registrations). It has been suggested that these appliances cause selective dentoalveolar eruption and, to a lesser extent, encourage a degree of normal mandibular growth to occur to compensate for asymmetrical deficiencies in growing patients. However, evidence for this is lacking. In general, it should be borne in mind that where a significant skeletal asymmetry exists, surgery will most likely eventually be required.

Treatment time for the patient undergoing orthognathic surgery is usually prolonged, and treatment of asymmetries is often more complicated than other dentofacial deformities. It is worth noting that attempts by the orthodontist to cut corners in order to reduce treatment time, or by the surgeon to undertake surgery without adequate preoperative orthodontic preparation, will inevitably lead to problems, for the patient and the clinicians. Poorly planned or executed orthodontics can make the required surgery very difficult or potentially impossible. Clearly, time should not be wasted by the orthodontist in the preparatory phase of preoperative orthodontics, but accuracy in placing the teeth of both arches into the desired positions far outweighs the speed of treatment and may well reduce the overall treatment time by reducing the length of postoperative orthodontics. It is imperative that the patient's oral health and hygiene be optimal before embarking on orthodontic treatment.

There are essentially five stages of orthodontic treatment required for the patient undergoing orthognathic surgery, which are:

1. Preoperative orthodontics
2. Immediate preoperative appointment
3. Intraoperative orthodontic requirements
4. Immediate postoperative appointment
5. Postoperative orthodontics

Preoperative Orthodontics

The amount of preparatory orthodontic treatment required for the orthognathic patient is quite variable. It depends on the complexity of tooth movements required and the type of surgery being planned. For example, dental extractions and subsequent space closure are likely to be more time-consuming than non-extraction treatment. Dental midline corrections often can be rather time-consuming, whereas a dental midline deviation planned to be corrected with rotation of the respective jaw requires less preoperative orthodontic preparation. Inevitably, this preparatory phase is the most prolonged phase of treatment. Nevertheless, attempts to rush this stage will lead to potentially avoidable problems at the time of surgery. The time quoted to patients should be realistic, but never underestimated, as patients will remember this information.

The type of appliance used is essentially down to the preference of the orthodontist, though usually some form of preadjusted edgewise appliance is likely to be employed. The fixed orthodontic appliance is not only employed to achieve the desired tooth movements before and after surgery but is also used by the surgeon to stabilise the jaws intraoperatively with intermaxillary fixation (IMF). The former standard edgewise appliance employed relatively similar brackets on the teeth and thereby required the orthodontist to place bends in the archwire to individually position each tooth in terms of their relative horizontal 'in-out' positions, their crown angulation (mesiodistal crown 'tip') and their crown inclination (buccolingual crown 'torque'). This prepared archwire then engaged the brackets in an 'edgewise' manner, hence the name. In the mid-1970s, Andrews introduced the 'straight-wire appliance' [3, 4], which modified the standard edgewise system such that the information for the in-out position of each tooth, its crown tip and crown torque was incorporated into the respective bracket for each individual tooth, i.e. the details of the *final* tooth position are incorporated in each 'preadjusted' bracket. This was achieved by varying the thickness of each bracket base (for the in-out position of the respective tooth), and by varying the angulation of each bracket slot relative to the long axis of each tooth in the mesiodistal plane (for the crown angulation) and contouring the base of the bracket occlusogingivally (for the crown inclination). Therefore, when the teeth are in their correct three-dimensional positions, there is a level bracket slot line-up, i.e. the bracket slots in each arch are at the same height, and there are no offset bends in the archwire. These preadjusted bracket systems have reduced the requirement for wire bending dramatically. Nevertheless, accurate tooth positioning in preparation for surgery and effective postoperative finishing and detailing of tooth positions will almost always require some degree of wire bending (Table 2) (Fig. 14). Much of the artistic flair in orthodontic finishing still emanates from the orthodontist's ability to bend wire.

In this context, the bracket slot size refers to the dimensions of the horizontal channel within a bracket that receives the orthodontic archwire. The most commonly used bracket slot sizes are the 0.018 × 0.025-inch (0.46 × 0.64 mm) and the larger 0.022 × 0.028-inch (0.56 × 0.7 mm). The type used is dependent on the preference of the orthodontist, but the 0.022 × 0.028-inch bracket slot does allow the use

Table 2 Classification of orthodontic archwire bends (after Tweed)

Type of bend	Archwire type required	Tooth movement generated
First-order bend (also termed 'in-out' or horizontal 'offset' bends; vertical step bends that do not alter the tooth's angulation are also in this category) (Fig. 14a and b)[a]	Round or rectangular stainless steel	Buccolingual offset of a tooth crown in the horizontal plane; or vertical translation of a crown *without* a change in angulation
Second-order bend (also termed 'tip bends' or 'angulation bends') (Fig. 14c)	Round or rectangular stainless steel	Mesiodistal angulation of the tooth crown and/or root
Third-order bend (also termed 'torquing bends' or 'inclination bends') (Fig. 14d)	Rectangular stainless steel or TMA (titanium-molybdenum alloy)	Buccolingual crown and/or root inclination

[a]Clinicians should be aware that the Tweed system, described by the pioneering American orthodontist Charles H. Tweed (1895–1970), describes first-order bends as horizontal adjustments only, and second-order bends for any vertical adjustment, i.e. vertical bodily extrusion or intrusion bends are classified as second-order according to Tweed

(Modified from: Naini FB, Gill DS (eds). Orthognathic Surgery: Principles, Planning and Practice. Oxford: Wiley-Blackwell, 2017; reprinted with permission.)

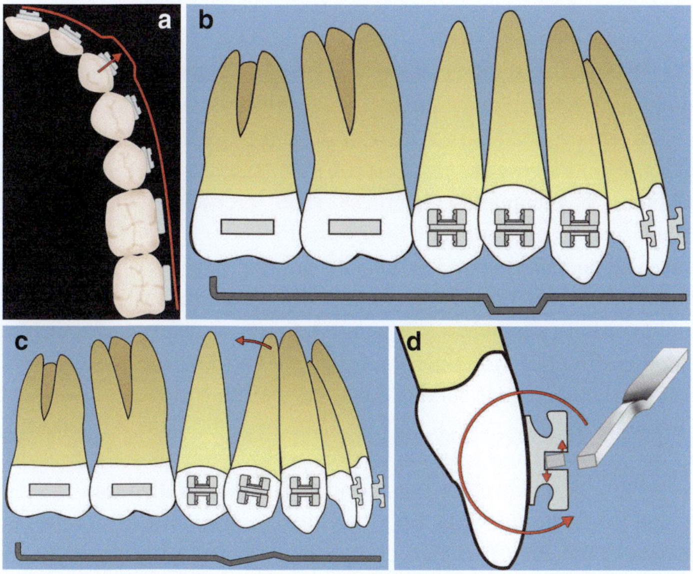

Fig. 14 (**a**) First-order bend to buccally offset a maxillary canine tooth. (**b**) First-order bend to vertically extrude a maxillary first premolar. (**c**) Second-order bend to correct the angulation of a maxillary first premolar. (**d**) Third-order bend to apply palatal root torque to a maxillary central incisor. (From: Naini FB, Gill DS (eds). Orthognathic Surgery: Principles, Planning and Practice. Oxford: Wiley-Blackwell, 2017; used with permission)

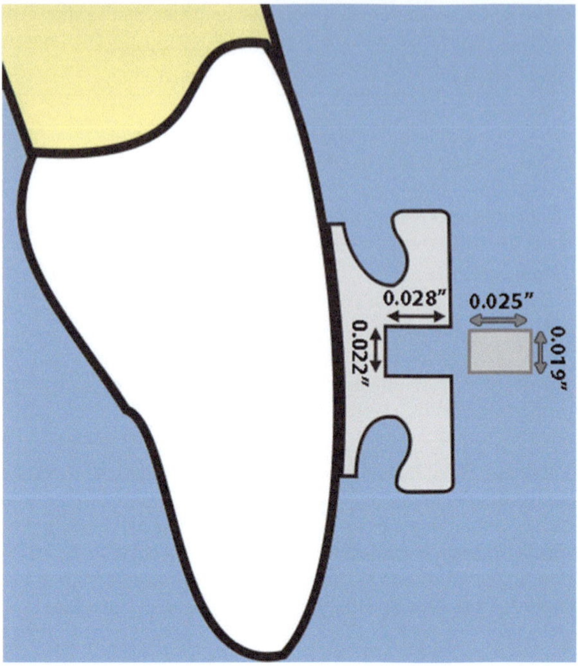

Fig. 15 Bracket slot dimensions and rectangular archwire dimensions in cross-section. A 0.022 × 0.028-inch bracket slot is shown, with a 0.019 × 0.025-inch rectangular archwire. (From: Naini FB, Gill DS (eds). Orthognathic Surgery: Principles, Planning and Practice. Oxford: Wiley-Blackwell, 2017; used with permission)

of heavier stainless steel archwires, which make dental arch levelling potentially easier (Fig. 15). To avoid long-winded terms in clinical practice, user-friendly abbreviations may be used at the chair side. The 0.018 × 0.025-inch bracket slot size is abbreviated and pronounced an '18-slot', and the 0.022 × 0.028-inch bracket slot a '22-slot'. A round archwire, e.g. a 0.018-inch stainless steel, is pronounced '18-steel', whereas a rectangular stainless steel archwire with the dimensions 0.019 × 0.025-inch is pronounced '19–25-steel'.

In modern orthodontics, bonded brackets are the norm for all the teeth, although molar bands are occasionally used, particularly when transpalatal arches or tooth-borne rapid maxillary expanders are required. Some surgeons prefer the molar teeth to be banded, particularly the final tooth in each arch, which is usually the second molar. The reasoning is that should this tooth be bonded rather than banded, and thereby debond during surgery, it may be a potential problem. Alternatively, it may be argued that a loose band may not be noticed for some time. If the final tooth in the dental arch is bonded rather than banded, it is imperative that the archwire is cinched distal to this tooth. Molar bands are also required if a band tube needs to be converted into a bracket. This is accomplished by removing the buccal cap of a convertible tube on the first molar band, thereby transforming the tube into a bracket. More recently, self-ligating molar tubes have been introduced, which may be used instead of a convertible tube. A second, or auxiliary, archwire tube can be incorporated into a molar bond or band. This is useful in cases requiring segmental surgery, if an auxiliary wire needs to be constructed for placement into the auxiliary tubes to stabilise the segments immediately after segmental repositioning. The use of lingual and palatal cleats on molar bands for attachment of elastics may be required in either the preoperative or postoperative phases; however, where bonded molar tubes have been used rather than molar bands, lingual or palatal buttons may be bonded directly onto the teeth if required. The canine brackets, and ideally the premolar brackets, would have integrated hooks, facilitating elastic wear as required, particularly postoperatively. A specific bonding problem may occur in patients with unilateral TMJ ankylosis and resultant asymmetry, as there is often very little space between the buccal surface of the posterior dentition and the inside of the cheek. A similar problem may occur in patients with craniofacial microsomia, where the affected cheek may be very tight against the molar teeth, possibly due to lack of tissue or scarring from previous surgery, such as macrostomia repair. This lack of space can make placement of brackets very difficult, and bands may be somewhat easier to place.

Labial orthodontic appliances are superior to lingual appliances in orthognathic patients for a number of reasons. Firstly, lingual appliances cannot be used by the surgeon intraoperatively for application of temporary intermaxillary fixation, and some form of labial attachment will be required, e.g. buttons or brackets bonded onto the labial aspects of the teeth, or temporary anchorage devices (e.g. microscrews) in the labial alveolar bone. Secondly, if a lingual bracket debonds during or immediately after surgery, it is very difficult to rebond in the immediate postoperative period, as the patient has discomfort, an inevitable degree of trismus leading to limited mouth opening, and often a mouth laden with blood-stained saliva. Thirdly, the same factors may potentially make it more difficult for the patient to keep the teeth and appliances clean if the brackets are lingual. Finally, an upper lingual appliance may also interfere with complete overbite correction in anterior open bite (AOB) cases. Some patients may demand labial 'aesthetic' brackets, in which case informed consent is essential. However, routine stainless steel brackets and bands/tubes are superior to aesthetic labial brackets in patients undergoing orthognathic surgery, as aesthetic brackets have a greater susceptibility to fracture, which is a particular problem intraoperatively, they can lead to serious tooth wear from abrasion with the enamel of teeth in the opposing arch, and they may impede or reduce tooth movement due to problems of increased friction.

Objectives of Preoperative Orthodontics

The overall purpose of preoperative orthodontic treatment is to place the teeth into the correct position for their respective jaw, so that on repositioning the jaws, the surgeon may attain the desired skeletal movements *and* obtain the best possible dental occlusion. *The preparatory orthodontic tooth movements should be determined in relation to the proposed surgical movements of the jaws.* The intended tooth movements may be described in relation to the six objectives of preparatory preoperative orthodontic treatment [2]:

- Alignment
- Levelling
- Decompensation
- Incisor inclination preparation
- Arch coordination
- Elimination of occlusal interferences

There is a seventh objective if segmental surgery is required:

- Creating interdental space for osteotomy cuts. This will be described under the 'Alignment' section below.

These objectives of orthodontic preparation are not always achieved in the same order. For example, decompensation may occur prior to arch levelling, or maxillary arch expansion to coordinate the arches may be required at the beginning of treatment. In certain circumstances, some of these phases occur together. They are described separately below for enhanced descriptive clarity.

Alignment

Alignment is usually, though not always, the first step in preoperative orthodontics (arch expansion is sometimes undertaken prior to alignment). Some arch levelling also begins at the same time as alignment, i.e. when the initial archwire is engaged into the brackets, the teeth will begin to level. However, for the purpose of clarity, levelling will be described separately in the next section. The purpose of alignment is to correctly angulate ('tip') the crowns of the teeth into the correct position for their respective jaw and to correct tooth rotations.

Time taken to accurately position the brackets is never wasted. The brackets must be bonded into the correct position for each tooth. Minor variations in bracket positioning may be required in some patients. In orthognathic patients, the coordination of the maxillary and mandibular labial segments, i.e. the canine-to-canine region, is paramount. Often, interference may occur between the tip of the mandibular canine and the mesio-palatal aspect of the maxillary canine, which prevents the intercuspation of the teeth. Therefore, it is advisable to bond the maxillary canine bracket approximately ½ to ¾ of a millimetre mesial to the long axis of the tooth, leading to slight mesio-labial rotation of the tooth, and better ultimate interdigitation of the labial segment. Bonding the maxillary second molars may lead to their extrusion, which will become a major interference in attempting arch coordination. If they must be bonded/banded, e.g. to derotate, then care should be taken to bonding the brackets somewhat occlusally. If a convertible tube is placed onto the first molar, steps can be added to an archwire to also minimise extrusion of the second molar.

If segmental surgery is planned, some interdental space is required, both between the crowns and roots of the teeth on either side of the planned osteotomy, to permit space for the surgical cuts without damaging the teeth. The crowns of the teeth on either side of the planned osteotomy may be separated using active coil spring, but

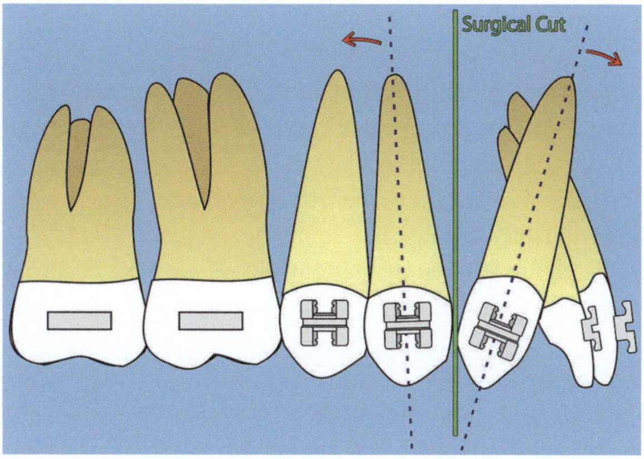

Fig. 16 Root divergence prior to segmental surgery. (From: Naini FB, Gill DS (eds). Orthognathic Surgery: Principles, Planning and Practice. Oxford: Wiley-Blackwell, 2017; used with permission)

root divergence may be achieved by either having the brackets in the correct positions and placing second-order bends in the archwire, or bonding the brackets at an angle to diverge the roots, and rebonding them in the correct position postoperatively (Fig. 16). If the surgical cut is planned distal to the canine teeth, contralateral canine brackets may be bonded, which reverses the tip in the brackets and angulates their roots mesially. Following surgery, the correct brackets may be bonded to correct the canine angulations.

For archwire selection, a thin, round archwire is ideal for initial alignment, producing little binding and friction, and permitting relatively free tipping of the tooth crowns. The forces should be as light as possible, whilst permitting tooth movement. Nickel-titanium alloy (NiTi) is the initial aligning archwire material of choice, having both shape memory (i.e. it returns to its original form following plastic deformation, e.g. being ligated to a malpositioned tooth) and superelasticity (i.e. a flat 'superelastic' plateau in the middle of the force-deflection curve, allowing appreciable distortion of the wire in order to engage brackets on considerably displaced teeth whilst maintaining acceptable force levels). Typical sequencing of archwires for an orthognathic patient is variable, depending on the desired goals of treatment. Assuming a 0.022 × 0.028-inch bracket slot, the preliminary archwire is usually a round 0.014-inch, followed by a 0.016-inch NiTi or 0.018-inch copper NiTi after one to two visits of religation. If sliding mechanics are required, e.g. to correct a dental midline shift, a working archwire of 0.018-inch stainless steel may be used, though a working wire should always be ligated into the brackets for at least a month, allowing levelling of the bracket slots, prior to any sliding mechanics being undertaken. This helps to make the archwire passive and thereby avoids binding of the brackets onto the archwire. The 0.018-inch stainless steel archwire is also very useful for correcting the inclination of incisor teeth, as the teeth rotate round the transverse axis. If such movements are not required, then an interim 0.019 × 0.025-inch NiTi archwire is used to help prepare for the ligation of the 0.019 × 0.025-inch stainless steel archwires, on which surgery is usually carried out. 0.019 × 0.025-inch stainless steel archwires are also useful for coordinating the dental arches and for levelling.

Levelling

Dental arch levelling refers to the stage of orthodontic treatment which aims to flatten (or almost flatten) the curve of Spee, by permitting the relative vertical movement of the teeth in each arch to bring their marginal ridges to lie approximately in the same horizontal plane. A relatively flat (i.e. 'level') curve of Spee is one of the prerequisites to a normal dental occlusion.

In the orthognathic patient, levelling may be undertaken at different stages of treatment, depending on the requirements of the respective case:

- Preoperatively—In the majority of patients, most or all the levelling may be undertaken prior to surgery.
- Intraoperatively—The preoperative phase is used to segmentally align 'segments' of each dental arch and the segments are subsequently surgically levelled.
- Postoperatively—Some or most of the levelling is undertaken following surgery, e.g. a three-point or tripod landing (interarch tooth contact at the incisors and terminal molars only) used to increase the lower anterior face height and reduce the incisor overbite (see below).

The decision on how to level in the maxillary arch is predominantly based on the final desired position of the maxillary incisors in relation to the upper lip and face. Once the desired postoperative position of the maxillary incisors has been planned, the decision on how to level the mandibular arch depends on the planned postoperative position of the mandibular incisors in relation to the maxillary incisors and the effect of this position on the lower anterior face height (LAFH). If no increase in LAFH is desired, the mandibular arch is levelled preoperatively by incisor intrusion. However, if an increase in LAFH is desired, the mandibular arch curve of Spee is either partially levelled if only a small increase in LAFH is desired, the curve is maintained if already present at the required depth, or the curve is accentuated if a significant increase in LAFH is desired, i.e. the degree of preoperative levelling depends on how much of an increase in LAFH is desired. As the mandible is advanced, the degree of anterior-inferior movement of the mandibular incisors will determine the increase in LAFH.

In the preoperative phase of treatment, the levelling of each individual dental arch may be total, partial or segmental. In addition, there is a space requirement for orthodontic levelling, with approximately 1 mm of space required to level a 3 mm depth curve of Spee [5].

Decompensation

The discrepancy between the jaws in all three planes of space has an indirect yet considerable influence on the dental-occlusal relationship as a result of dentoalveolar compensation. Dentoalveolar compensation describes the variations in the positions of the teeth, in the sagittal, vertical and transverse dimensions, that may

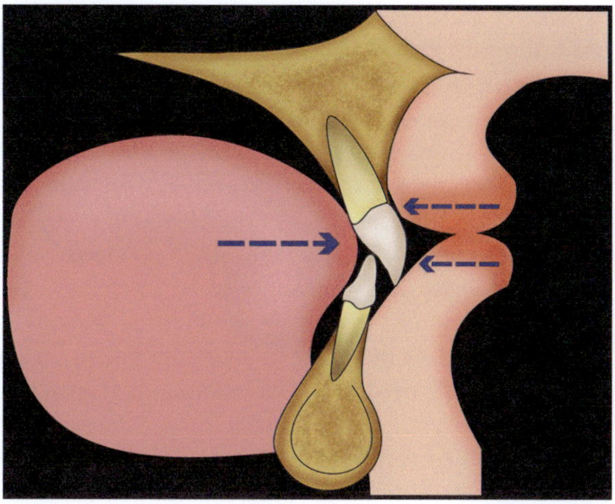

Fig. 17 The soft tissue envelope of the tongue and lips/cheeks; the teeth are in a position of soft tissue equilibrium between the opposing forces of the tongue and lips/cheeks. (From: Naini FB. Facial Aesthetics: Concepts and Clinical Diagnosis. Oxford: Wiley-Blackwell, 2011. Reprinted with permission)

compensate for variations in the skeletal pattern, i.e. it is nature's way of trying to get the teeth to meet when the jaws are growing away from one another [1]. In the normal situation, the erupting maxillary and mandibular teeth are guided towards each other by the surrounding soft tissue envelope of the tongue, lips and cheeks; hence, they erupt into a position of soft tissue equilibrium between the opposing forces of the tongue and lips/cheeks (Fig. 17). Therefore, in the presence of *sagittal* or *transverse* skeletal discrepancies, alterations in the inclination of the teeth *compensate* for the skeletal discrepancy. In such cases, the occlusal discrepancy will appear less severe than the underlying skeletal discrepancy. For example, in a patient with a severe Class III skeletal pattern, the dentoalveolar compensation involves proclination of the maxillary incisors and retroclination of the mandibular incisors. This compensatory mechanism may be unsuccessful either because the skeletal discrepancy is too severe or because the soft tissue pattern is unfavourable. For example, in a Class II skeletal discrepancy, if the soft tissues are unfavourable and the lower lip is unable to control the labial aspect of the maxillary incisors and instead falls behind them, it will lead to their proclination and thereby magnify rather than compensate for the skeletal discrepancy. In the *vertical* plane, the incisors will tend to overerupt to compensate for increasing lower anterior face height, unless a forward tongue position prevents their overeruption. If the face height is dramatically increased, the incisors may not be able to fully compensate and an anterior open bite (AOB) will ensue.

Orthodontic preparation for orthognathic surgery requires orthodontic decompensation of the dental arches in *all three planes of space*, i.e. the process of removing the dentoalveolar compensations that may be present in the sagittal, transverse and vertical planes, and re-establishing the correct position of the teeth with regard to their own skeletal base, thereby permitting adequate surgical correction of skeletal discrepancies. The primary objective of preparatory orthodontics in an asymmetry patient is to remove the dental compensations and *to make the dental-occlusal asymmetry match the skeletal asymmetry*, which will allow correction of the dental occlusion with the skeletal repositioning.

There is frequently a 'worsening' effect on the dental occlusion and facial appearance in this stage of preoperative orthodontics. Just as dentoalveolar compensation tends to mask the extent of the underlying skeletal discrepancy, *orthodontic decompensation unmasks the true extent of the underlying skeletal discrepancy*. For example, a patient with a Class III skeletal discrepancy will often have retroclined mandibular incisors and possibly some proclination of the maxillary incisors. As such, orthodontic decompensation results in retroclination of the maxillary incisors and proclination of the mandibular incisors, thereby increasing the reverse incisor overjet and making the lower lip more prominent. In asymmetry patients, the dental midlines usually need to be corrected to their respective jaw preoperatively, often making the overall dental midline and occlusal asymmetry discrepancy worse, which is then corrected with the skeletal repositioning. This is one aspect of treatment that may displease patients a great deal. Dental-occlusal function may also deteriorate during this stage of treatment. As such, it is extremely important that patients are made aware of this issue prior to embarking on treatment, and as part of informed consent.

Either Class II or Class III interarch elastics may be required in order to help incisor proclination/retroclination, but in the orthognathic asymmetry patient, these elastics may be employed in the opposite direction to conventional orthodontics, in order to slide the dental midlines towards their desired preoperative position.

Dental extractions, when required, will be so as to permit the maximum extent of decompensation achievable and thereby allow the desired extent of surgical movement of the jaws. In preparation for orthognathic surgery, dental extraction patterns are usually the opposite of those used in conventional orthodontics. In addition to preparing the dental midlines based on the type of surgery planned, the mesio-distal incisor angulations should be prepared when occlusal plane rotation around the sagittal axis is being planned. As such, the surgical repositioning of the respective jaw automatically corrects the incisor angulations. If maxillary surgery is not required, maxillary dental midline deviation correction may well require dental extractions to create space. This usually involves extraction of the first premolar on the side to which the dental midline is to be moved. However, all things being equal, it is better to avoid extractions in the maxillary arch only, as there is a tendency to narrowing of the arch width, making arch coordination more difficult. This is particularly true in Class III asymmetrical patients, where the maxilla may be rather small relative to the mandible. All extraction patterns should be planned after undertaking a comprehensive space analysis.

Incisor Inclination Preparation

The orthodontic treatment required to prepare the maxillary and mandibular incisor inclinations for surgery often occurs as part of incisor decompensation (see above). However, preoperative incisor inclination changes are not always, by definition, strictly speaking decompensation. For example, Class II patients with mandibular retrognathia often develop a lower lip trap, i.e. the lower lip gets caught behind the maxillary incisors and leads to their proclination. This is not a compensatory proclination, but the inclination of the maxillary incisors needs to be corrected prior to mandibular advancement surgery.

Incisor inclination preparation for orthognathic surgery depends on whether surgery is being planned for a jaw, and whether that surgery involves rotation of the jaw round the transverse axis. If surgery is not being planned, then the incisor inclination for that jaw should be corrected prior to surgery, e.g. proclined maxillary incisors should be corrected preoperatively when only mandibular advancement surgery is being planned. If surgery is being planned for either jaw, that will only entail sagittal bodily translation of the jaw, or if only vertical maxillary movement is required, then the incisor inclination for that jaw should again be corrected prior to surgery. However, if either jaw is being planned for surgery, that will involve the rotation of the jaw round the transverse axis, such as differential posterior impaction of the maxilla, or autorotation of the mandible, which thereby alters the inclination of the incisors, then the incisor inclination should be prepared preoperatively to take into account the change in incisor inclination that will occur as part of the surgical repositioning of the respective jaw [2].

Arch Coordination

Dental arch coordination refers to the aspects of orthodontic treatment which ensure that the maxillary and mandibular dental arches will fit well together in occlusion, with maxillary and mandibular arch forms that correspond to one another, and with normal incisor, canine and buccal segment overjet.

Of all the parameters that must be dealt with in orthodontic preparation, the coordination of the maxillary arch with the mandibular arch is often the most important, commonly the most challenging and usually the most likely to cause problems at the time of surgery and in the postoperative phase of treatment.

Ideally, the dental arches should be as well-coordinated as possible prior to surgery. However, in some patients, if the occlusion is so well-interdigitated as to make expansion difficult, particularly in low angle patients, glass ionomer cement blocks may be placed on the occlusal surface of the maxillary first molars to disclude the arches and permit easier expansion. Conversely, some of the posterior buccal segment expansion (perhaps 3–4 mm, i.e. no more than 2 mm per side) may be completed postoperatively. However, *the coordination of the canine-to-canine region of the maxilla to that of the mandible is the single most important preparatory requirement of preoperative orthodontics* [2]. Good preoperative coordination of this region is mandatory.

Judging the arch width of the opposing jaws for arch coordination is best accomplished by hand articulating the dental study models, which will demonstrate the requirement for arch expansion or contraction (Fig. 18a, b). In the asymmetrical patient, arch coordination may necessitate unilateral arch expansion and/or

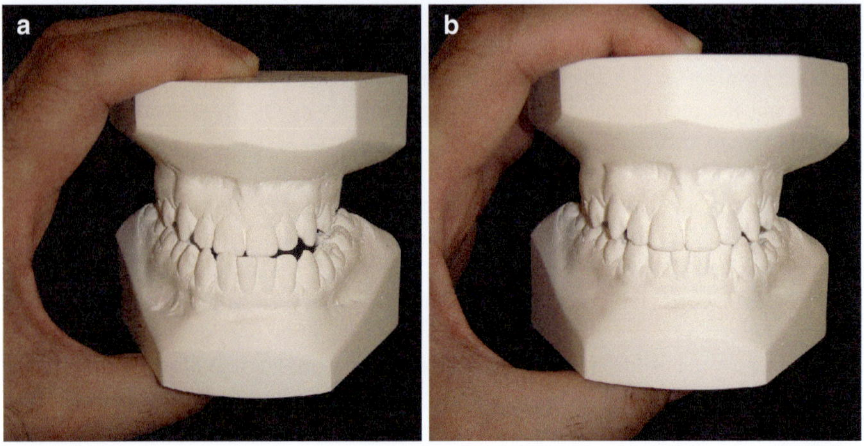

Fig. 18 (**a**) Pretreatment study models in pretreatment occlusion. (**b**) Hand articulated pretreatment study models in the approximate postoperative position of the skeletal bases. Hand articulating pretreatment study models in the approximate proposed postoperative position for the skeletal bases will provide an idea of the degree of arch coordination that will be required

contralateral arch contraction of the maxilla. This may be achieved using coordinated rectangular stainless steel archwires, and the use of cross-elastics may also be useful.

Additionally, the buccolingual inclination of the molar and premolar teeth relative to their respective skeletal base should be observed. In patients with transverse occlusal plane cants, the inclination of the buccal segments should be prepared such that surgical cant correction automatically corrects the buccal segment dental inclinations.

In asymmetry patients requiring orthognathic surgery, coordinated rectangular stainless steel archwires will eventually be required as the buccal root torque expression helps to limit buccal flaring, to elevate hanging palatal cusps and correct the inclination of the posterior teeth relative to their basal bone. If preoperative maxillary arch expansion is required, a number of methods are available, including expanded archwires, removable appliances with expansion screws, auxiliary archwires, quadhelices, rapid maxillary expansion and surgically assisted rapid palatal expansion (SARPE).

Elimination of Occlusal Interferences

Planning to prevent occlusal interferences begins before a single bracket is bonded. Additionally, during treatment the dental arches should be checked at every visit, in order to continue preventing the formation of potential interferences, and eliminating them when they occur.

It is vitally important to check the patient's individual dental arches and their occlusion with keen observation and with interim 'snap models' when required, in order to detect potential occlusal interferences. The two most common potential interferences in orthognathic patients are lack of coordination of the intercanine width, usually due to a narrow maxillary intercanine width, and extrusion of maxillary second molar teeth, which will prevent good dental interdigitation. In addition, excessive buccal flaring of maxillary molars, inadvertent premolar extrusion (usually due to incorrect bracket positioning), overeruption of preoperatively unopposed teeth, dental substitutions and prominent cusps may all lead to interferences, which should be identified and resolved prior to surgery.

Immediate Preoperative Appointment

This appointment should be ideally no more than 2–3 weeks prior to the date of the operation. The purpose of this appointment is to ensure that the brackets and bands are all secure, to ligate the brackets securely with stainless steel ligatures (Fig. 19), (except for self-ligating brackets, where ligatures are only required on a specific bracket if the orthodontist is concerned that the specific archwire engaging mechanism may not hold intraoperatively), and the placement of surgical hooks (unless integrated hooks are present).

Both the surgeon and orthodontist should check the preoperative model surgery. Patients with jaw asymmetries present a unique set of challenges for model surgery, and special considerations are required. *The most important principle to follow is that the direction and magnitude of the surgical movements must be decided clinically.* No attempt should be made to make alterations or adjustments when just viewing the articulator-mounted dental models. Three-dimensional virtual surgical planning (3D-VSP) can be very beneficial for complex asymmetries.

It is also important for the orthodontist to put aside enough time to discuss any final issues with the patient. Despite previous information provision, patients may still have some questions at this stage. Finally, patients will be understandably anxious at this close stage to the operation, and the orthodontist should reassure the patient that they will be in the safe hands of an experienced surgeon and anaesthetist.

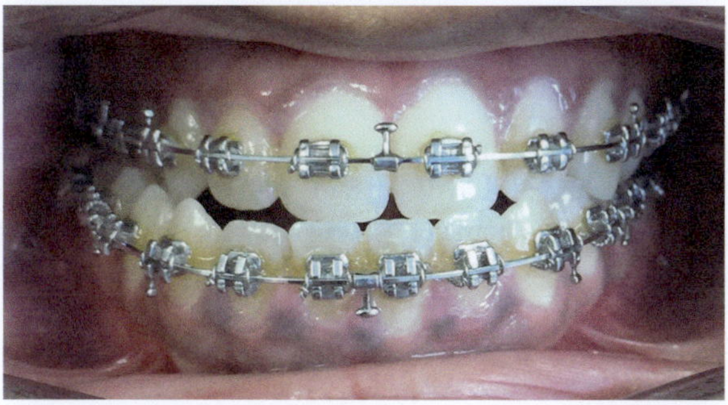

Fig. 19 Brackets are ligated with stainless steel ligatures, and surgical hooks are placed in preparation for surgery

Intraoperative Orthodontic Requirements

Surgical finesse is vital, and excessive surgical force in placement of intermaxillary fixation may debond brackets. Nevertheless, debonds do occur intraoperatively and can usually be ignored (hence the importance of reliable ligation) and repaired by the orthodontist postoperatively. However, if a band which is part of an RME appliance becomes loose, it may need to be repaired intraoperatively. Additionally, in segmental surgery, continuous archwires may need to be placed intraoperatively, or over-tied to the segmented archwires, once the jaw has been surgically segmented and repositioned. Therefore, the presence of an orthodontist may occasionally be required in the operating theatre.

A number of inaccuracies may occur during splint wafer construction, and, as such, the fact that a patient is occluding well into the surgical wafer is no guarantee that they will occlude well once the wafer has been removed. Wafers should be removed at the end of the operation, and the dental occlusion checked.

Immediate Postoperative Appointment

The patient should be seen by the orthodontist, together with the surgeon, on the day following surgery. It is important for patients to be mobilised as soon as possible following surgery. As such, it is better for patients to come from the ward to the maxillofacial department, walk and sit in the dental chair to be examined. At this stage, the vast majority of patients feel absolutely terrible. Though they should have been informed preoperatively, it is important to reiterate to the patient that the first few days are always the worst and that they will feel much better soon. Despite feeling dispirited, this encouraging information will hearten the patient and their parents/carer.

The main purpose of this appointment is *to check that the skeletal and dental-occlusal aims of the surgery have been achieved.* Despite the obvious facial soft tissue oedema, it is also important to check that potential untoward soft tissue changes have been minimal. Prior to clinical evaluation, the patient should be reassured by the clinician that they will be very gentle in their oral examination. Blood-stained saliva may be gently aspirated as far as possible, and any intermaxillary elastics placed intraoperatively may be removed. The patient's mandible may then be gently guided by light finger pressure in order to check the dental occlusion with the maxillary arch or into the wafer if it has not been removed.

Specific clinical parameters to be checked for asymmetry patients at this stage are the maxillary incisor exposure in repose (is the maxillary incisor display in relation to the upper lip correct and symmetrical?), the position of the maxillary dental midline (is this coincident with the mid-philtrum of the upper lip and facial midline?), the mandibular dental midline (is this coincident with the maxillary dental midline and chin?) and transverse canting (is the transverse maxillary occlusal plane level, have any preoperative transverse cants been corrected, and has any transverse canting been inadvertently introduced?). The patient is then sent for postoperative radiographs prior to returning for placement of intermaxillary guiding elastics as required. The radiographs are used to check postoperative condylar positions (e.g. do the condylar positions in the postoperative radiographs correspond to the positions on the preoperative radiographs?), the alignment of the bony borders in the surgical regions, and chin position after a genioplasty.

As already mentioned, some surgeons prefer to maintain the wafer initially, usually ligated to the maxillary fixed appliance. Either way, as soon as the wafer is removed in the postoperative period, the dental occlusion should be checked. At this stage, a mild deviation (no more than 2–3 mm) of the mandibular dental arch, either anteriorly or laterally, may result from altered proprioception in the immediate postoperative phase, from minor dental interferences not picked up preoperatively, or from oedema of the intraoral soft tissues, particularly in the retromolar regions. In these situations, light intermaxillary guiding elastics, also known as training elastics, may be placed to override the proprioceptive impulse of minor dental or soft tissue interference and gently guide the patient's teeth into occlusion. However, if a major discrepancy in the position of the jaws is observed, the patient will almost certainly need to return to the operating room for surgical adjustment as required. Attempting excessive intermaxillary elastic placement with heavy forces, almost akin to intermaxillary fixation, is inappropriate and should be avoided. If the jaws have been rigidly fixed in an incorrect position, no amount of elastic force will correct this position, and one is simply delaying the inevitable. Additionally, immediate return to surgery, though an unwelcome news for the patient, will be preferable to reoperating after a few weeks, both psychologically for the patient and for the clinician, as bone healing may occur very quickly in a young healthy adult, as any surgeon attempting to reoperate after a few weeks will testify.

Postoperative Orthodontics

Whether the surgical splint is removed early or not, active orthodontic treatment is usually delayed for 2 weeks, until the patient feels up to having treatment. During this time, the patient will usually be wearing light intermaxillary guiding elastics, which help to guide the patient into the planned dental occlusion. These should be worn full time, and the patient should be seen by the surgeon and orthodontist weekly for the first 2 weeks, for close observation of any changes to the dental occlusion. Some patients will have an obvious, well-interdigitated dental-occlusal result postoperatively. However, others may need closer observation, with variations in the intermaxillary elastic vectors made as required during this time (see below). Repairs to the orthodontic appliance should be made as soon as practically possible during this initial period. If a bracket has debonded or a band is loose, it should be repaired or removed.

If full-thickness stainless steel archwires had been placed prior to surgery, i.e. 0.0215 × 0.025-inch archwire in a 0.022 × 0.028 bracket slot, then these stabilising archwires will need to be replaced with working archwires. However, most orthognathic surgeons are happy to operate with a larger dimension stainless steel working archwire, e.g. 0.019 × 0.025-inch stainless steel archwire, so long as it has been placed for at least one visit and is considered passive, prior to the maxillofacial technologist's impressions (or 3D-VSP CT scan) in preparation for surgery. If a working archwire is already in place, there is no requirement to change it at this stage.

The type of working archwire required in either the maxillary or mandibular arch depends on the tooth movements desired. Often the most important initial movement is to guide the teeth vertically into a better dental occlusion. The orthodontist must decide on the teeth they would like to extrude, and in which arch. For example, if the maxillary arch is level, the 0.019 × 0.025-inch stainless steel archwire may be maintained in position. If there is a lateral open bite in the mandibular canine and premolar region, these teeth need to be extruded by elastic force; therefore, a flexible mandibular archwire is required. The dimensions and material of the flexible archwire depend on the other types of movement that may be required, e.g. torque control, but rectangular braided (multistrand) stainless steel, TMA (titanium-molybdenum alloy) or nickel-titanium (NiTi) is commonly used postoperatively.

The potential for slight variation in the actual postoperative dental-occlusal position compared with the planned position in asymmetry cases is greater than with orthognathic surgery in more straightforward sagittal and vertical discrepancies. As such, the postoperative orthodontics may need to compensate the dentition for an essentially minor skeletal malocclusion. Asymmetrical use of intermaxillary elastics may be required in some patients if the dental occlusion and midlines are not quite coincident, but were planned to be, i.e. Class II elastic on one side and Class III on the contralateral side (Fig. 20). An anterior cross elastic may also be required, which should usually only be worn at night. The elastic force should be kept light, in order to avoid unwanted vertical extrusion of teeth and potential transverse rotation of the occlusal plane. This is particularly pertinent where a unilateral maxillary

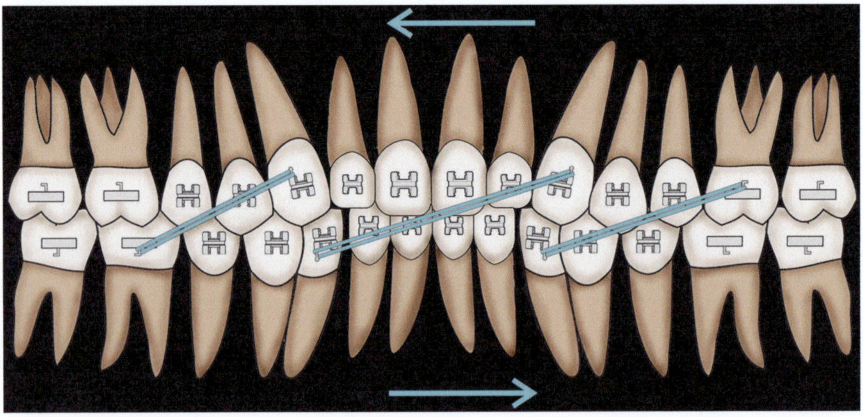

Fig. 20 Anterior diagonal elastic, with Class II and Class III elastic traction, which is a combination commonly used for dental midline correction. Archwires are not shown to improve clarity. (From: Naini FB, Gill DS (eds). Orthognathic Surgery: Principles, Planning and Practice. Oxford: Wiley-Blackwell, 2017; used with permission)

impaction has been undertaken to level the maxillary plane. Small posterior or lateral open bites may also be present, which will require light vertical elastics on flexible archwires, allowing dental extrusion.

The configurations and vectors of the working intermaxillary elastics depend on the type and direction of desired tooth movement. Incorrectly placed elastics will result in undesirable tooth movement; therefore, every effort must be made to ensure that patients do not incorrectly position them. A schematic drawing demonstrating exactly which teeth should engage the elastics may be provided to the patient as a reminder or they may take a photograph of the elastics positioned whilst still in the clinic. Vertical tooth movement in the buccal segments is usually facilitated with box elastics, maintaining a vertical vector as far as possible (Fig. 21). Vertical intermaxillary elastics, whether box type or triangular in configuration, aim at extrusion of selected teeth to improve the interdigitation of the dental arches. Box elastics are required to level a mandibular curve of Spee. If necessary, a Class II or Class III vector may be advisable on one or both sides, depending on the desired tooth movements.

Short intermaxillary elastics, either Class II or Class III, may be useful, providing the Class II or III vector but limiting the potential detrimental vertical eruption of the maxillary or mandibular molars from routine Class II or III intermaxillary elastics. These may also be placed in a triangular configuration (Fig. 22). Persistent dental midline deviations may require a Class II elastic vector on one side and Class III on the contralateral side. Sometimes an anterior diagonal elastic may also be

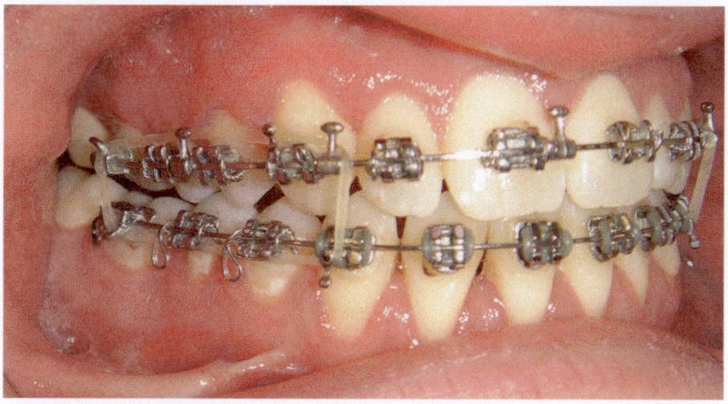

Fig. 21 Vertical tooth movement in the buccal segments may be facilitated with box elastics, maintaining a vertical vector as far as possible. The position of surgical hooks, integrated hooks on brackets and Kobayashi ligatures allows the orthodontist to vary the elastic vectors as required

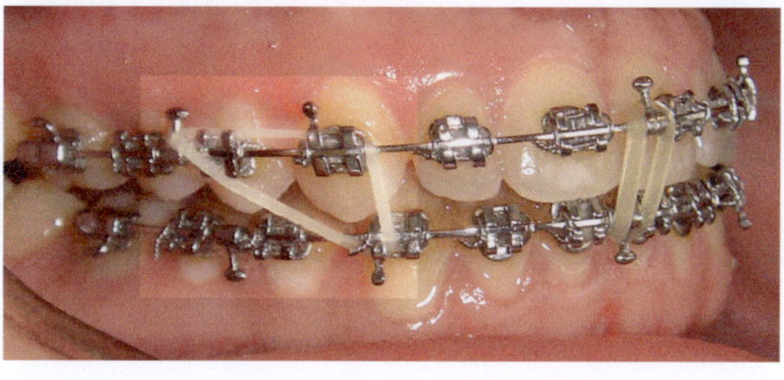

Fig. 22 Short triangular intermaxillary elastic with a Class III vector

added (usually just night times) (Fig. 20). In such situations, care must be taken not to cause transverse canting of the maxillary occlusal plane by extruding the teeth attached to these elastics; theoretically temporary anchorage devices may be used in one arch as a means of elastic attachment instead of the teeth, though in practice this is rarely required.

Occasionally, the exact planned surgical result may not have been attained. Where the discrepancy with the planned result is relatively minor, and the facial aesthetic improvements are acceptable, the orthodontist and surgeon may decide if the case can be 'salvaged' by orthodontic treatment alone. This often involves some form of compensatory tooth movement, particularly in relation to incisor inclinations. For example, if a Class II mandibular advancement has been slightly over-advanced, with an edge-to-edge type incisor relationship, Class III elastics may be used, perhaps in conjunction with a round steel archwire in the mandibular arch, to improve the incisor relationship. Alternatively, if a Class III case has a slightly edge-to-edge incisor relationship postoperatively, Class III elastics may be beneficial in improving this relationship. Whatever the circumstances, the clinicians need to be aware that miracles are not possible, and significant problems resulting from surgical shortcomings may need further surgical modification.

If segmental surgery has been undertaken, the roots of the teeth on either side of the planned segmental surgical cut will usually have been diverged in preparation for the surgery. Either repositioning of the brackets or second-order bends in the archwire will be required to achieve correct root angulation postoperatively. This is sometimes referred to as 'root paralleling', though the term is somewhat of a misnomer as the objective is correcting the angulations of the teeth, not necessarily making the roots parallel. Much of the active vertical orthodontic settling occurs with the intermaxillary working elastics. Intermaxillary elastic wear will be markedly reduced, if required at all, in the finishing stages of orthodontic treatment. Elastic wear should be completely stopped for at least 6 weeks prior to appliance removal, to ensure that a stable result has been achieved.

Minor variations in tooth crown morphology combined with minor variations in bracket position will mean that some tooth repositioning by 'artistic' wire bending is likely to be required in the finishing stages of treatment. Occasionally, first-order bends to vertically extrude specific teeth or second-order angulation bends for the incisor teeth may be required, as is labial or lingual root torque (third-order bends) for specific teeth (usually maxillary lateral incisors). The postoperative phase of orthodontic treatment typically takes anything from 3 to 6 months, depending mainly on the degree of postoperative tooth movement required.

Retention

Retention protocols and regimes vary from unit to unit. Retainers should ideally be made and fitted on the same day as appliance removal, or at least within 1–2 days. Retainer wear begins close to full time, except for eating and cleaning of the teeth and retainers. This first 3–4 months of close to full-time wear is to permit time for reorganisation of the periodontal ligament and supporting tissues [6, 7]. Wear may be reduced to evening and nights only after 3–4 months, and gradually onto nights only, which may be continued for between 12 and 24 months. Certain orthodontic tooth movements will require a longer period of full-time retention, e.g. derotation of teeth, and may even require bonded retention. Realistically, many patients reduce retainer wear gradually to every other night, and eventually down to a few nights per week, which should then be maintained on a long-term basis. However, for many patients, the degree of stability of their orthodontically repositioned teeth is difficult to know with any degree of certainty; as such, the orthodontists' advice is usually for patients to continue their night time retainer wear *indefinitely*.

Patients may be given some choice as to the type of removable retainer. Vacuum-formed, Essix type retainers have superior aesthetic qualities, but the patient's oral hygiene must be excellent; otherwise, problems may result. They are often not particularly sturdy and may crack, wear and have to be remade after some variable interval. They may also reduce settling of the teeth as they cover the occlusal surfaces.

When maxillary expansion has been undertaken, Hawley type retainers are preferable as the palatal acrylic helps to maintain the expansion and prevent transverse relapse. An alternative is a combined retainer, the Hawlix or 'aesthetic' retainer, which combines the anterior aesthetic advantage of the Essix retainer and the palatal acrylic of the Hawley retainer [8]. This retainer is particularly useful following treatment in cleft lip and palate patients in order to improve the aesthetics of anterior maxillary dentoalveolar cleft defects. Begg type retainers are ideal for patients requiring dental-occlusal settling.

If mild relapse is predicted, features may be built into the retainers to help provide 'active' retention. For example, placement of hooks on the Hawley retainers will allow intermaxillary elastics to be worn in Class II, Class III or anterior diagonal configurations, should the dental midlines begin to slip. Natural vertical settling continues when retainer wear is reduced to part time, particularly with retainers that do not employ occlusal coverage. This is why the dental occlusion sometimes looks even better at the 1-year review appointment than at appliance removal.

Concluding Remarks

The type of tooth movement and mechanics required for orthognathic surgery, particularly in patients with facial asymmetries, is oftentimes different to standard orthodontics. It is imperative that the treating orthodontist is conversant with the principles and technical mechanical requirements in the management of such patients. Surgeons should also have a working knowledge of modern orthodontics and what is realistically achievable.

References

1. Naini FB. Facial aesthetics: concepts and clinical diagnosis. Oxford: Wiley-Blackwell; 2011.
2. Naini FB, Gill DS (Eds). Orthognathic surgery: principles, planning and practice. Oxford: Wiley-Blackwell, 2017.
3. Andrews LF. The straight-wire appliance, origin, controversy, commentary. J Clin Orthod. 1976;10:99–114.
4. Naini FB, Gill DS (Eds). Preadjusted edgewise fixed orthodontic appliances: principles and practice. Oxford: Wiley-Blackwell, 2021.
5. Lee R, Kirschen R. Space planning for the dentition (space analysis). In: Gill DS, Naini FB, editors. Orthodontics: principles and practice. Oxford: Wiley-Blackwell; 2011.
6. Reitan K. Tissue rearrangement during retention of orthodontically rotated teeth. Angle Orthod. 1959;29:105–13.
7. Reitan K. Principles of retention and avoidance of post-treatment relapse. Am J Orthod. 1969;55:776–90.
8. Collins JM, Witcher TP, Jones VS, Noar JH, Naini FB. An alternative retainer design for cleft patients: the 'aesthetic' retainer. Cleft Palate Craniofac J. 2010;47(6):597–9.

Management of Asymmetric Dentofacial Deformities with Digital Planning

Brian B. Farrell

Abstract

Virtual planning is regarded as the standard of care for the correction of dentofacial deformities. The presence of craniofacial asymmetry frequently increases the complexity of surgical correction placing greater emphasis on treatment planning through surgical simulation. Virtual planning provides tremendous advantage in the management of asymmetric deformities compared to traditional planning methods. The multidimensional nature of the deformity can be readily appreciated, provides preoperative insight into the anatomic repositioning, and aids in improving the efficiency of the intraoperative experience that can lead to the delivery of a sound clinical outcome for patients. This chapter describes the application of virtual planning directed toward the correction of asymmetric dentofacial deformities.

Keywords

Facial asymmetry · Dentofacial deformity · Virtual planning · Orthognathic surgery · Cutting guides and templates

B. B. Farrell (✉)
Private Practice and Director of Fellowship Program, Carolinas Center for Oral and Facial Surgery, Charlotte, NC, USA

Department of Oral and Maxillofacial Surgery, Louisiana State University Health Sciences Center, New Orleans, LA, USA
e-mail: bfarrell@mycenters.com

P. Mehra, L. M. Wolford (eds.), *Management of Facial Asymmetry*,
https://doi.org/10.1007/978-3-030-44971-1_4

Introduction

Virtual planning is regarded as the standard of care for the correction of dentofacial deformities. The presence of craniofacial asymmetry frequently increases the complexity of surgical correction placing greater emphasis on treatment planning through surgical simulation [1, 2]. The broad perspective of skeletal anatomy combined with the occlusion expands the narrow focus offered with model surgery to provide tremendous advantage in the management of asymmetric deformities [3–7]. The multidimensional nature of the deformity can be readily appreciated, provides preoperative insight into the anatomic repositioning, and aids in improving the efficiency of the intraoperative experience that can lead to the delivery of a sound clinical outcome for patients [8–13].

History

Virtual planning has evolved with advances made in imaging modalities of the head and neck region. Three-dimensional imaging and subsequent development of planning modalities has been successfully applied throughout the scope of oral and maxillofacial surgery including implant rehabilitation to total joint replacement as well as tumor ablation and reconstruction via osteocutaneous flaps [14–18]. The application of virtual planning to orthognathic surgery is a revolution similar to the advent of rigid internal fixation applied to stabilize bony osteotomies decades prior [19–21] (Fig. 1).

Clinical records and plain films including panoramic radiographs and lateral cephalometric imaging were the mainstays in the management of dentofacial deformities. The addition of PA cephs and submental vertex films were advantageous in asymmetrical cases to quantify deviation of the occlusal plane, chin, mandibular angles, and pattern of ramus divergence. The pattern of ramus divergence aided in determining the best surgical technique for addressing mandibular ramus osteotomies, vertical ramus osteotomies, or sagittal split osteotomies, respectively. Traditional model surgery conducted in a dental laboratory was often time consuming and tedious even with straightforward treatment plans [22]. Inaccuracy at

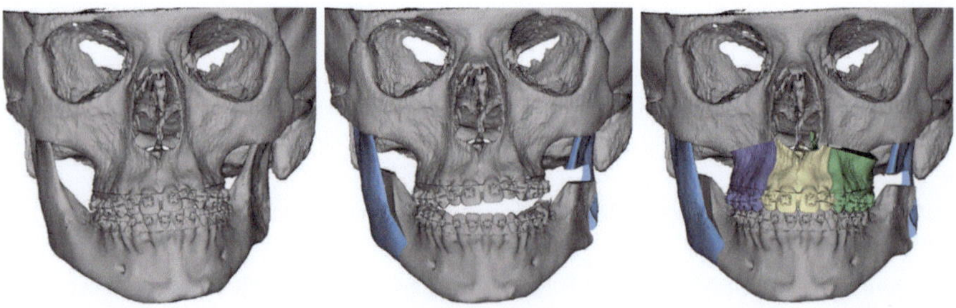

Fig. 1 Appreciation of the malocclusion and multidimensional dentofacial deformity with subsequent reorientation of the maxilla and mandible to establish facial symmetry via virtual planning

any point of data collection whether it be face bow record or transfer, centric relation record, or mounting errors was often unrecognized. The failure to appreciate an inaccuracy allowed the error to be carried unnoticed throughout the steps of the presurgical workup. An inaccurate centric relation record from displacement of the condyle can lead to a departure from the planned repositioning of the maxilla often appreciated as a skewed midline. The first indication of deviation from the intended plan unfortunately might be intraoperatively forcing a modified plan of "best judgment" to reorient the mobile segment. A more troubling outcome is the discovery of a planning error postoperatively that may require revision.

Inherent human nature is also at play when managing the presurgical workup with traditional model surgery even when the casts have been mounted accurately. The occlusion represented with mounted stone models on an articulator lacks perspective and reference when on a lab bench. The absence of anatomic references with conventional model surgery may result in the required movements to establish multidimensional symmetry to be over or under positioned, most frequently the latter. The lack of reference that stems from measurement of cusp tips to fixed points on an articulator is the root of surgeons' second guessing their proposed movements that can lead to under treating the correction of asymmetric dentofacial deformities. The undertreatment of asymmetry might commonly be perceived as a persistent midline disparity, residual chin deviation, failure to fully address yaw deformity, as well as management of occlusal cant (Fig. 2).

The loss of spatial perspective on an articulator can frequently affect the correction of occlusal plane in multiple dimensions. Changes in pitch such as clockwise rotation for Class III individuals or counterclockwise rotation to maximize advancement of the lower facial third in obstructive sleep apnea might not always be moved according to plan from improper mounting (Fig. 3a, b).

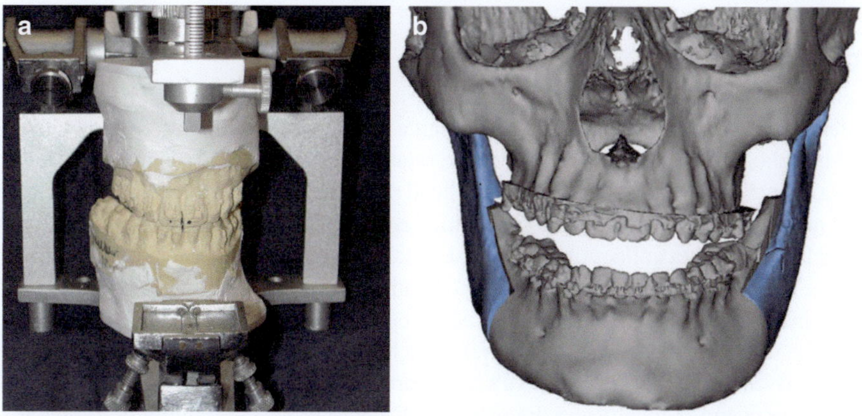

Fig. 2 (**a**) The lack of reference to facial skeletal and soft tissue anatomy in traditional model surgery could lead to errors in achieving anticipated skeletal movements. The narrow focus of the dentition referenced to the articular frequently led to undercorrection of asymmetric deformities. (**b**) The necessary movement required to level the occlusal plane appreciated with virtual planning

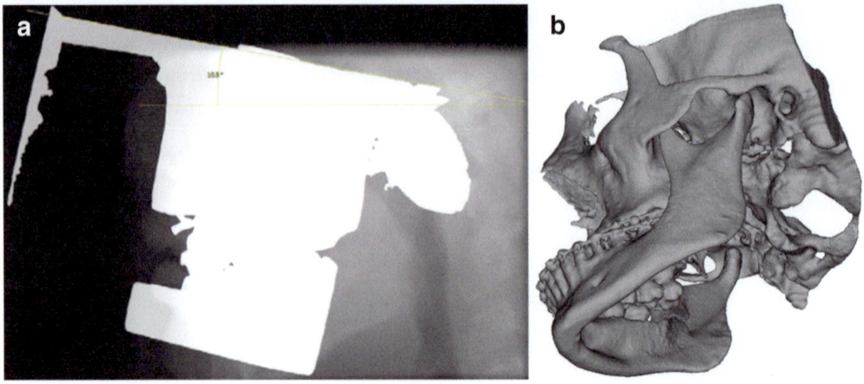

Fig. 3 (**a**) Inaccurate transfer of maxillomandibular position in traditional model surgery can result in insufficient correction when reorienting the occlusal plane. (**b**) Inaccurate centric relation record with displaced condyle identified in the presurgical virtual workup

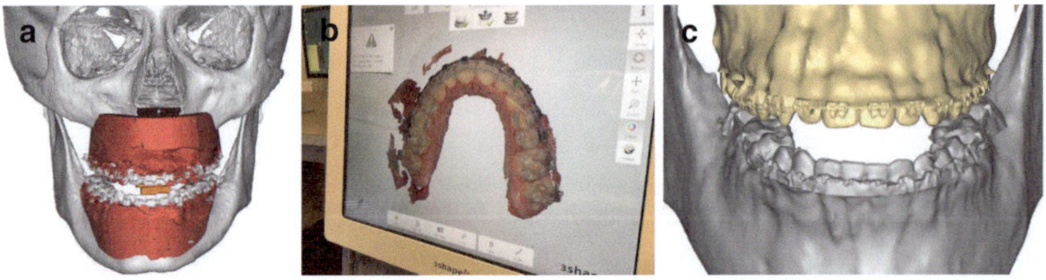

Fig. 4 (**a**) Occlusal anatomy from scanned stone models merged with CBCT skeletal data to allow bite correction and splint fabrication. (**b**) Intraoral optical scan. (**c**) Optical scanned occlusion (STL) merged DICOM data of CBCT to generate the most accurate representation of the skeleton and occlusion

Data Collection

Planning surgical correction through a digital medium has continued to evolve from its initial origin [23]. Bite jigs for centric relation record, fiducials to aid in merging data, as well as a gyroscope for natural head position have been replaced with clinical photos, local scanning of models with CBCT, and optical scanning of the occlusion [24–27]. Data collection requires skeletal information through either a medical grade CT scan or more commonly cone beam CT scans within the oral and maxillofacial surgery office. The accuracy at the occlusal level, however, is not captured via the scans of the maxillomandibular skeleton requiring the addition of dental anatomy. Stone models mailed to a service provider and subsequently laser scanned offsite or scanned locally via the office CBCT and transferred digitally allows for the occlusal topography to be merged with the skeletal data. A complete digital workflow is completed from the use of an optical scanner to record the occlusal topography via an STL file with accuracy to aid in the establishment of postsurgical occlusions as well as form accurate fitting splints (Fig. 4a–c).

The time allotment required for data collection has been drastically reduced with the digital workflow from that of traditional model surgery. A cone beam CT scan to collect skeletal anatomy and occlusal registration via optical scanning can be now collected in minimal time. The current workflow for data collection is efficient and handled entirely by a surgical assistant.

The completion of mandibular surgery first is advantageous as it removes the need for a centric relation record with one less opportunity to induce error into planning. The reorientation of the distal mandible to the existing position of the maxilla via an intermediate splint is independent of the condyle position on the proximal segment. An improperly seated condyle during record collection will result in a deviation in skeletal measurements over the osteotomy gap, but properly seating the condyle intraoperatively should deliver accuracy to the virtual plan (Fig. 5).

Reviewing records carefully is needed to ensure natural head position is verified prior to the initiation of treatment planning. Many surgeons have moved to orienting

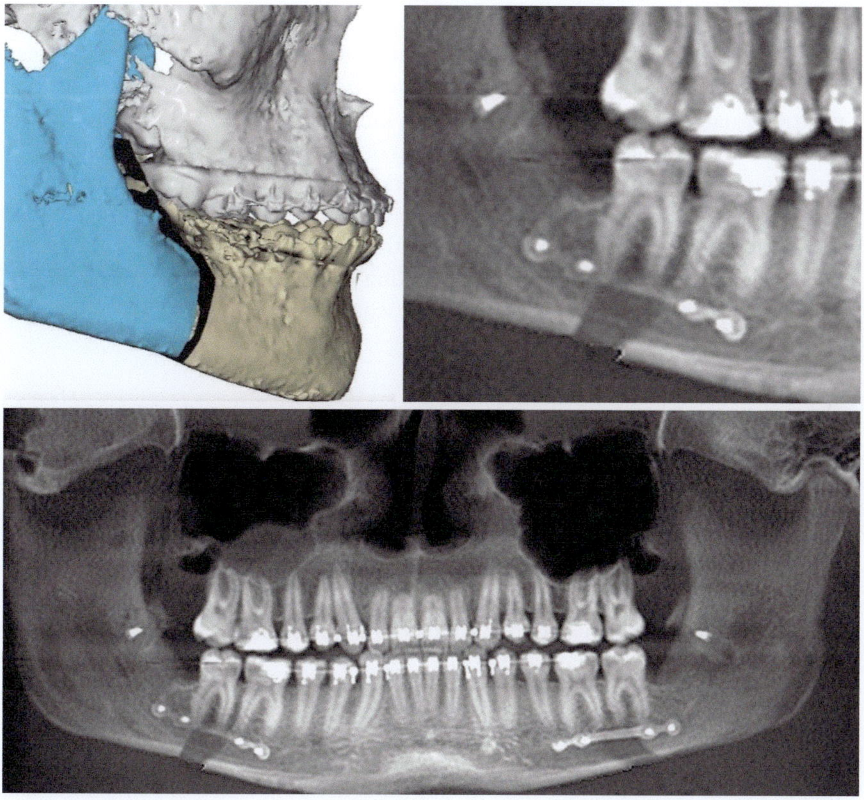

Fig. 5 Virtual planning illustrates advancement between the proximal and distal segment that does not sync with that appreciated on postoperative radiograph after mandibular advancement. The anticipated occlusal correction was achieved with sound seating of the condyle intraoperatively, but the discrepancy can be traced to an inaccurate centric relation record during data collection

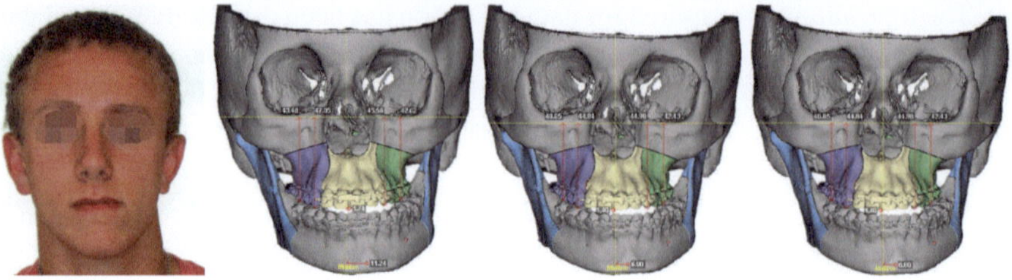

Fig. 6 *Orbital dystopia.* Variation of maxillary midline based on head position. The perceived midline is to the left with the orbital rims "leveled." True head position taking into account the existing orbital dystopia has the midline residing to the right. An inaccurate head position results in the perception the midline needs to be moved to the right to orient it on the midsagittal plane. In true head position with orbital dystopia taken into account, moving the midline further right only deviates it further from the philtrum of the upper lip

head position via clinical photos from past iterations of face bows, laser levels, fiducials, and gyroscopes. Sound reproduction of natural head position is vital to ensure accurate correction as individuals who possess asymmetry may be inclined to posture their head in compensation. Fortunately, most patients hold their head in a neutral or natural position even with an asymmetric dentofacial deformity. These individuals are amenable to the establishment of natural head position prior to initiating planning based on their clinical photographs. Individuals who possess craniofacial deformities such as hemifacial microsomia or orbital dystopia require detailed confirmation to ensure appropriate head position. An error in orienting natural head position can result in an inaccurate perception of the anatomic layout including midline displacement or canting that will subsequently lead to an inappropriate surgical plan as discussed previously (Fig. 6).

Planning

The planning session conducted by experienced engineers allows visualization of the occlusal and skeletal discrepancies with an opportunity to review linear measurements to quantify midline deviation, skeletal asymmetry, cant referenced to the orbital rims, and calculation of yaw based on variation from the midsagittal plane. Treatment planning is focused on establishing a functional occlusion while maximizing smile and facial esthetics (Fig. 7).

Setting of the occlusion is accomplished through conventional haptic efforts with the surgeon articulating stone models or digital through virtual manipulation of the occlusion in software platforms. Digital planning can provide similar insight seen with inspection of traditional dental models as underlying arch form anomalies and residual dental compensation may be noted with asymmetric deformities of the skeleton. A digital workflow is greatly enhanced through engineer experience and repetition with a surgeon to initially grossly establish the bite based on the deformity, specifically setting an open bite deep against the opposing brackets, a class II

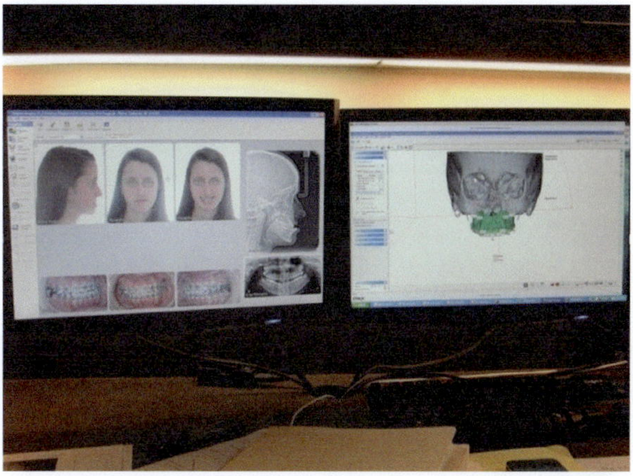

Fig. 7 Inspection of skeletal and occlusal discrepancies through visual and linear measurements via a webinar guided by biomedical engineers manipulating imported data via planning software. Natural head position oriented through comparison of clinical photos

deep bite via a tripod, or providing some relief in overjet with a Class III correction. The desired occlusion is refined and subsequently confirmed by the surgeon at the onset of planning prior to proceeding with skeletal correction (Fig. 8a–d).

The skeletal correction through digital planning is initiated as the occlusion, is set haptically or digitally, and is manipulated from the baseline natural head position. The movement of the entire occlusion is in contrast with repositioning a single arch with reference to the opposing arch experienced with traditional model surgery and surgery itself. The ideal position of the central incisors remains the mainstay of treatment planning. Multidimensional reorientation of maxillary incisor position influences the necessary skeletal correction of the bony foundation as virtual osteotomies of the maxilla and mandible are manipulated.

The correction of the malocclusion through digital osteotomies allows tremendous preoperative insight into situations that will be encountered during the surgical intervention. The digital movement of the occlusion and associated skeleton, contrasted to the narrow focus with traditional model surgery, allows bony interferences and osteotomy gaps to be visualized providing insight into intraoperative mitering or grafting requirements, respecitvely (Fig. 9).

A canted occlusal plane can be leveled to ensure appropriate incisor position for smile esthetics through rotation about either the midline or respective canines based on whether they wish to impact a side that is inferiorly positioned versus moving a canine and posterior maxilla inferiorly when necessary. Virtual planning allows the opportunity to visualize yaw associated with the dentition and maxillomandibular complex. The evaluation of yaw in relationship to both the mobilized Le Fort to the anterior maxillary wall and proximal and distal segments in the mandible can be reviewed (Fig. 10).

In cases without excessive asymmetry, the distal mandible may be oriented clockwise or counterclockwise to control the yaw to provide a more passive relationship of the segment. This passive relationship is advantageous as it allows a smoother intraoperative experience with minimizing or elimination of bony mitering. Subtle asymmetry of a millimeter or several degrees is likely not clinically

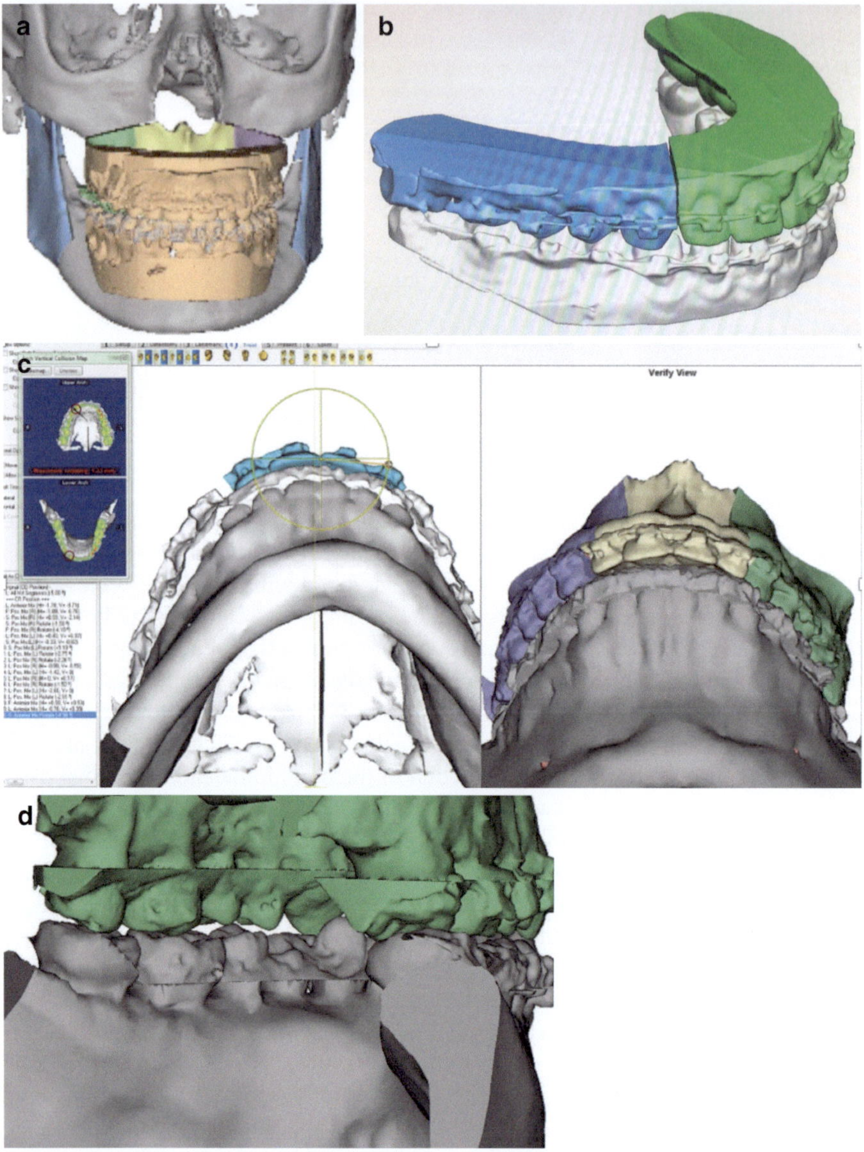

Fig. 8 (**a**) Models of surgeon established occlusion imported into virtual planning for correction of dentofacial deformity. (**b**) Digital establishment of the occlusion. (**c**) Orientation of maxillary incisor for appropriate overbite and overjet with segmental maxillary surgery. (**d**) Inspection of posterior occlusion to review intercuspation and transverse concerns

identifiable or creates an esthetic consequence, but the orientation of the proximal and distal segments to provide a passive relationship preoperatively can aid in moving efficiently through the surgical intervention. The need to recontour and miter bone segments to allow a passive relationship was common with traditional model surgery as focus was limited to the dentition. Failure to address interferences could

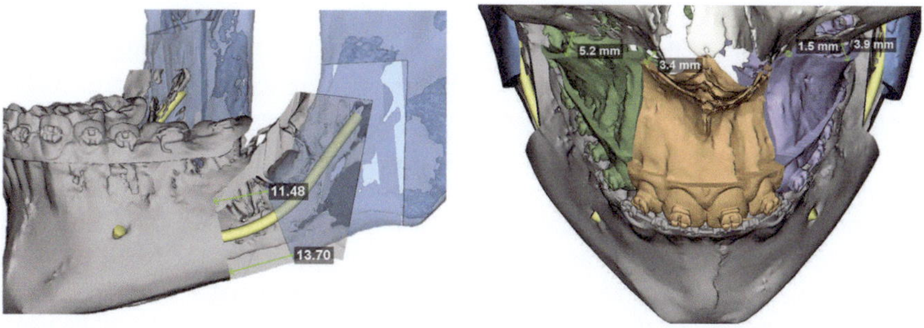

Fig. 9 Preoperative insight into the anticipated osteotomy gaps, rigid internal fixation requirements, and bone grafting needs

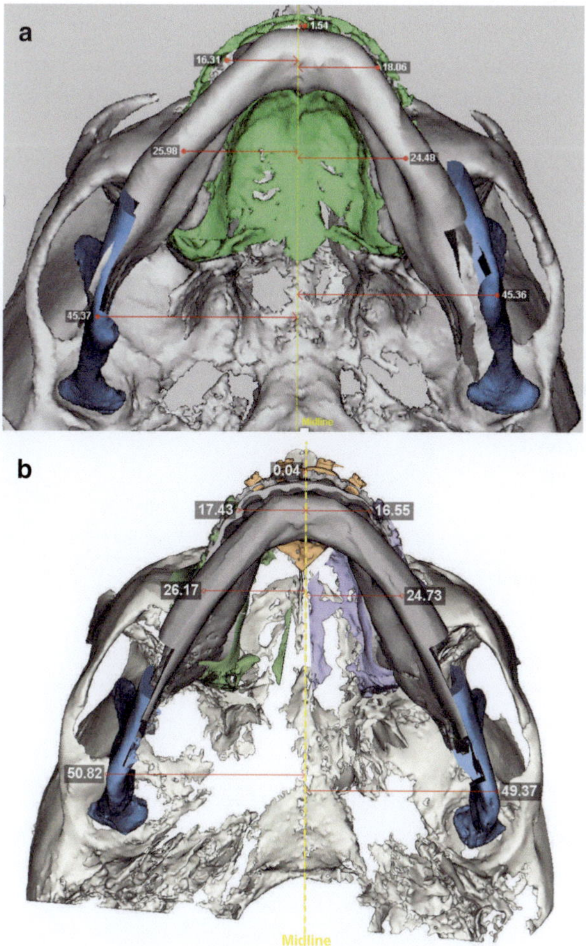

Fig. 10 (**a**) Evaluation of yaw with illustration of the proximal and distal segment relationship. (**b**) Illustration of reorientation of the distal mandible will allow a more passive positioning of the segments reducing the need for substantial bony mitering and allowing a more efficient intraoperative procedure

result in displacement of the condyle that could ultimately lead to dysfunction. Sound positioning of the proximal and distal segment passively on a planning session can reduce the apprehension that often surrounds lag screw fixation to stabilize the segments without fear of displacement of the condyle medial or lateral (Fig. 11).

In cases involving significant asymmetry, there may be an advantage to leaving the segment "proud" or allowing a side to collapse to balance the mandibular angles to a more skeletally symmetrical position. Measurement from each mandibular angle to a midsagittal plane can be readily calculated to ensure the facial width or projection is approximate. Despite the establishment of symmetry with the skeletal scaffold, asymmetry of the face may persist from soft tissue. Patients with long-standing facial asymmetry may have resultant soft tissue changes that include varying thickness of the masseter muscles or overlying superficial tissue. During planning the opportunity to review the soft tissue thickness overlying the midface, zygomatic arches, or mandible may lead to the use of stock or patient-specific custom implant to compensate for some soft tissue decreased bulk. The use of a compensatory implant to increase tissue projection and fullness may be placed over the orbital rim, zygoma, and mandibular angle or body to provide facial symmetry (Fig. 12a–e).

The gross perspective of the facial skeleton through digital planning allows the opportunity to visualize skeletal asymmetry that persists despite the correction of the malocclusion. The presurgical insight provides the opportunity to discuss adjunctive measures with patients and family preoperatively with a visual reference to aid in informed consent. A common example is asymmetry of the mandible and chin that is greater than the midline deviation at the dentition. Persistent asymmetry in the chin despite the correction of the malocclusion through osteotomies in the

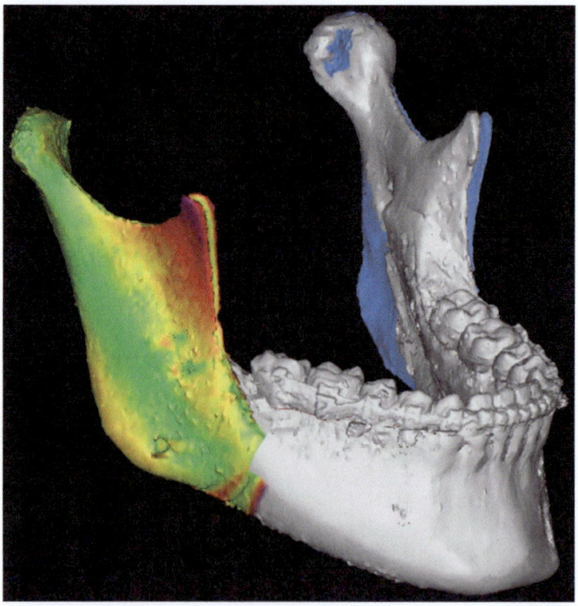

Fig. 11 Postoperative imaging superimposed over digital planning illustrates accuracy of mandibular repositioning and maintenance of condylar position without deviation after the use of lag screw fixation to stabilize the segments

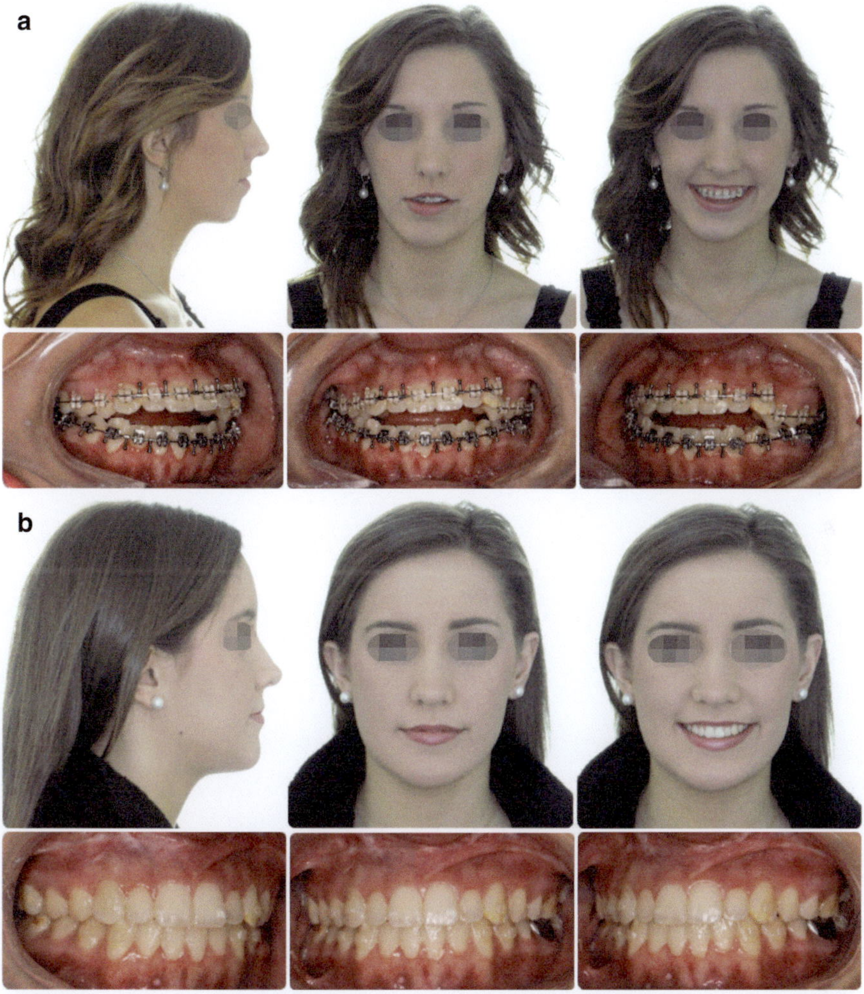

Fig. 12 (**a**) Asymmetric Class II openbite malocclusion. (**b**) Postoperative photo illustrates sound occlusal result with persist facial asymmetry. (**c**) Residual asymmetry related to bony irregularities and varying soft tissue thickness. (**d**) Custom implant over the mandibular angle to provide improved facial symmetry. (**e**) Final esthetic outcome

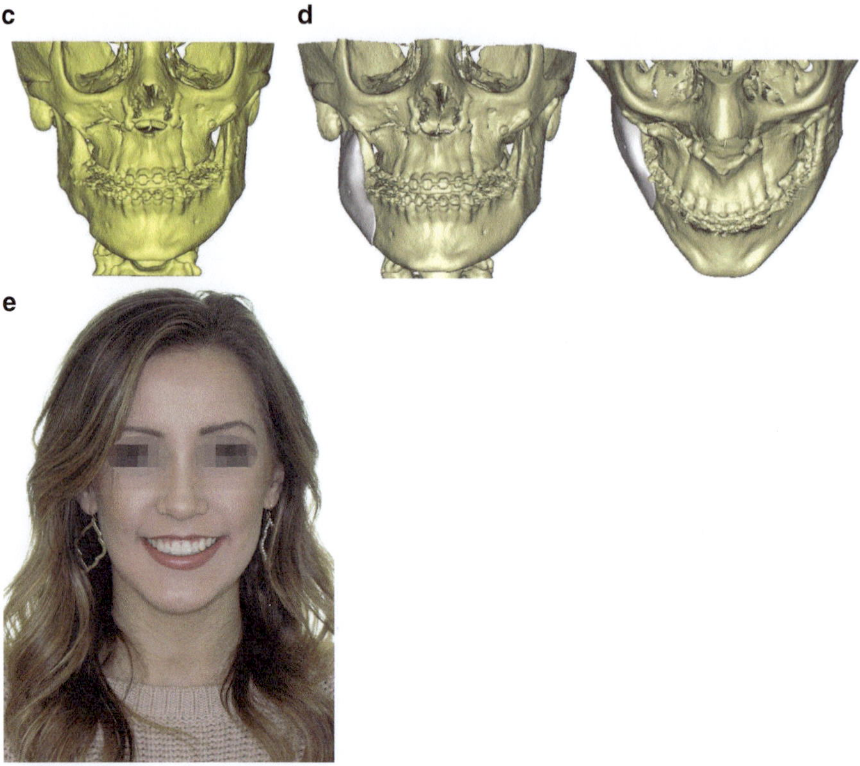

Fig. 12 (continued)

ramus will require an additional procedure to establish skeletal symmetry. An anterior segmental osteotomy allows the opportunity to reorient the chin into a symmetrical position in all three dimensions. Occlusal-borne or bone-borne guides can be used initially to provide predictive hole placement and cutting guidance. A second guide is then positioned to reorient the mobilized anterior mandible clinically to that established in the planning session (Fig. 13a–d).

Occlusal splints generated for cases involving vertical asymmetry and canting of the occlusal plane can be combined with additive manufactured adjuncts to aid in the establishment of skeletal symmetry [13]. Virtual planning can identify persistent asymmetry at the inferior border and assist in the surgical correction and accuracy of skeletal symmetry by reference to the opposing side. Hemimandibular hyperplasia frequently may have a greater discrepancy at the inferior border than that noted at the level of the occlusion. With the occlusal cante corrected, virtual planning allows visualization of the inferior borders to gauge and quantify a persistent skeletal disparity. The visualization of the skeletal disproportion can aid in determining

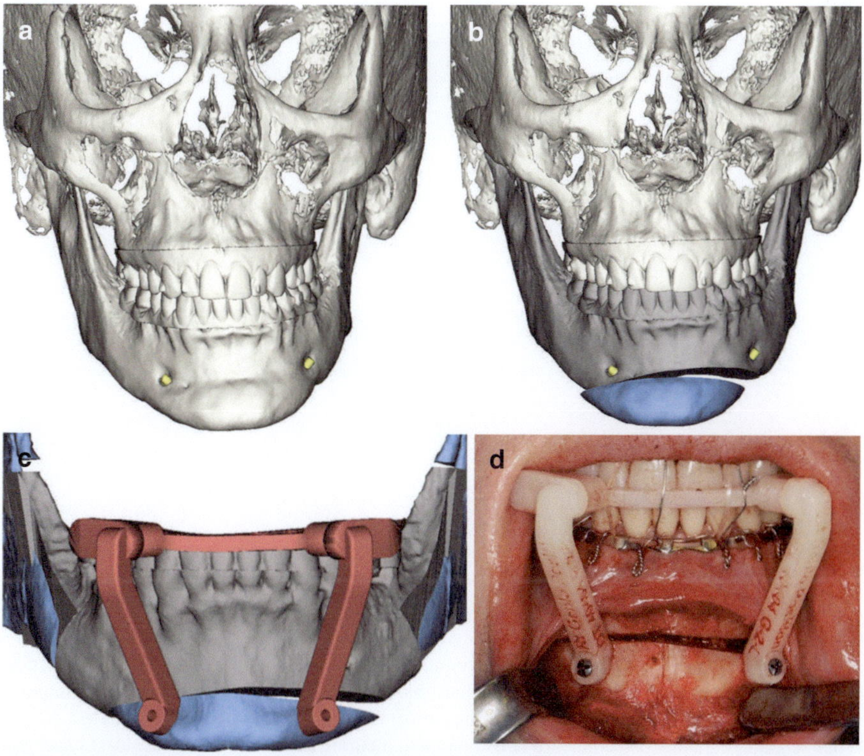

Fig. 13 (**a**) Asymmetric dentofacial deformity. (**b**) Digital planning of anterior segmental osteotomy to establish skeletal symmetry. (**c**) Digital plan to guide chin repositioning to through occlusal-borne splint and predictive holes. (**d**) Clinical reorientation of anterior segmental osteotomy

if planning will require reduction of the inferior border that remains vertically displaced versus additive to the nonaffected side that may be deficient. In cases where the inferior border remains vertically excessive, an occlusal-borne splint connected to a cutting fence guides the bony ostectomy allowing for resection that mirrors the opposing side (Fig. 14). The imaging can illustrate the course of the inferior alveolar nerve and aid in treatment planning whether decortication is necessary prior to completing any bony ostectomy. Both the planning session and subsequent case report can provide immense insight into the approaching surgical intervention. The bony relationships with the maxilla and mandible reoriented provide the ability to appreciate the surgical involvement.

The skeletal reorientation of the Le Fort referenced to the superior maxilla provides an appreciation of bony interferences likely to be encountered and potential grafting requirements within the osteotomy gap. When establishing the occlusion digitally, the position of interdental cuts in cases with transverse or vertical

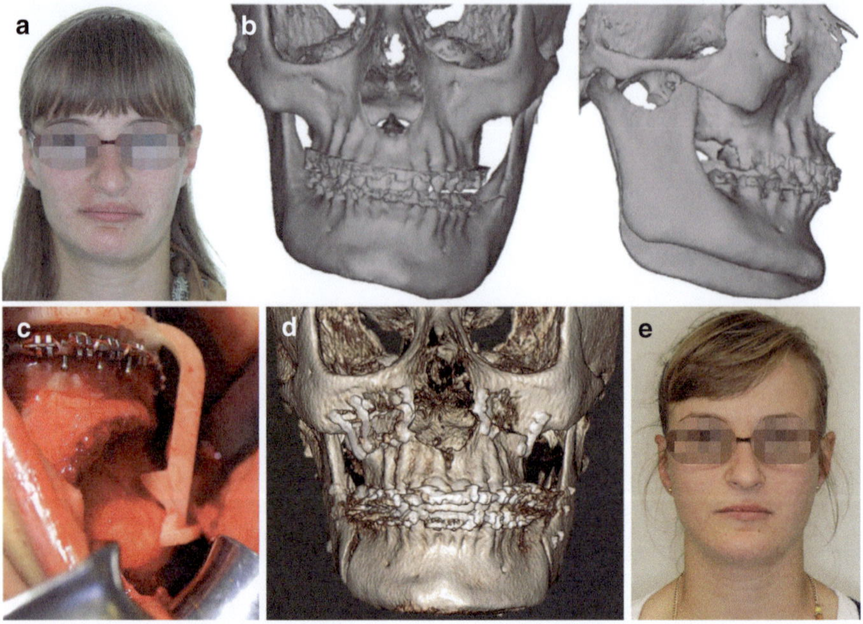

Fig. 14 (**a**) Clinical photo of facial asymmetry related to hemimandibular hyperplasia. (**b**) Vertical asymmetry at the inferior borders greater than that appreciated with the occlusal cant requires adjunctive measures to achieve skeletal symmetry. (**c**) Occlusal-borne splint connected to a cutting fence to guide the bony ostectomy. (**d**) Postoperative imaging illustrates a level occlusal plane and inferior border alignment after guided bony resection. (**e**) Postoperative clinical photo with skeletal and soft tissue symmetry

concerns necessitating segmental surgery can be created (lateral incisor to canine or canine to first premolar) with awareness of arch form and divergence of tooth roots. Oftentimes, segmental surgery may be necessary to address the occlusal arch form that may be distorted from skeletal asymmetry despite orthodontic efforts to decompensate. In cases where the necessary interdental cut is anatomically challenged from close proximity of tooth roots, an occlusal-borne guide with a cutting fence can help orient the sagittal saw through the alveolus and aid in avoiding injury to tooth roots (Fig. 15). The concept of skeletal surgery "first" or "early" can limit the interval our orthodontic colleagues have to adequately diverge tooth roots making the fabrication of the cutting guide advantageous for efficiency and accuracy [28].

Skeletal planning provides insight into the ideal method to correct asymmetry in the mandible. Ramus anatomy can guide whether the osteotomy is best addressed via sagittal split, intraoral vertical ramus osteotomy, or an inverted L osteotomy based on the required movements and subsequent relationship of the segments. The orientation of the proximal and distal segments can be appreciated to ensure passive positioning and quantify the osteotomy gap for anticipated

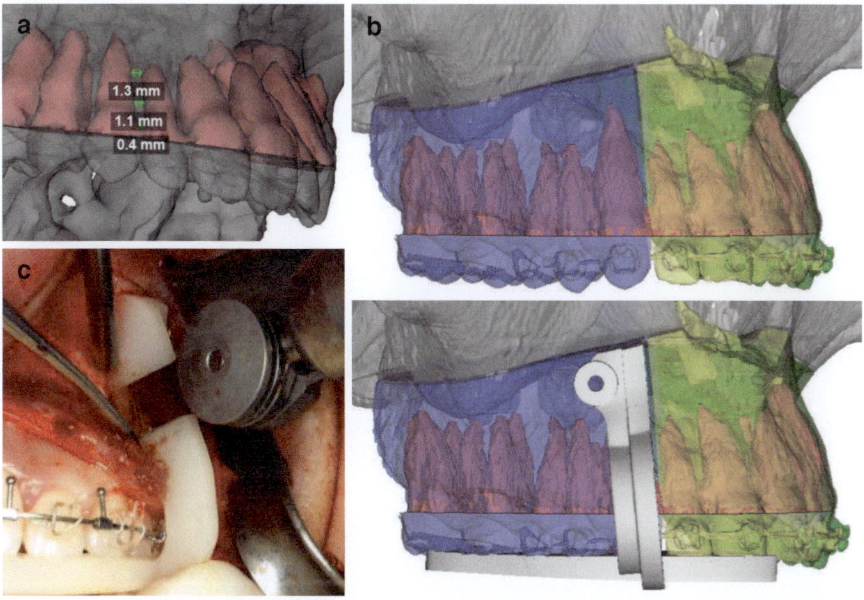

Fig. 15 (**a**) Evaluation of root divergence to position interdental cuts in segmental surgery. (**b**) Virtual cutting fence to aid in guidance of interdental cut between canine and lateral incisor. (**c**) Clinical use of interdental cutting guide to assist in orienting sagittal saw through the alveolus and avoid injury to adjacent tooth roots

fixation needs. The avoidance of unfavorable fractures in mandibular surgery via a sagittal split osteotomy is frequently based on the cut through the inferior border. Maintaining a sound inferior border to ensure structural integrity of the proximal segment aids in the avoidance of unfavorable fractures. The anatomy of the inferior alveolar nerve within the body of the mandible is traditionally included in the case report to allow reference to the inferior border and lateral vertical osteotomy. The appreciation of the course of the neurovascular structure may carry even greater importance when there is warping and a skewed nature of the mandible (Fig. 16).

The insight gained through virtual planning can aid in providing a smoother intraoperative experience. The surgeon should possess confidence with the knowledge that the transfer of the surgical plan to clinical outcome in the correction of dentofacial deformities has been proven accurate although deviation from the expected certainly can occur which can result in the failure to accurately deliver correction of the asymmetric deformity [4, 8–10].

Virtual planning is a mainstay in the management of asymmetric dentofacial deformities and truly, the standard of care. Virtual planning provides tremendous insight into the multidimensional nature of asymmetric dentofacial deformities and the required skeletal repositioning to correct the malocclusion and potential adjunctive procedures to establish facial symmetry. The technologic advances

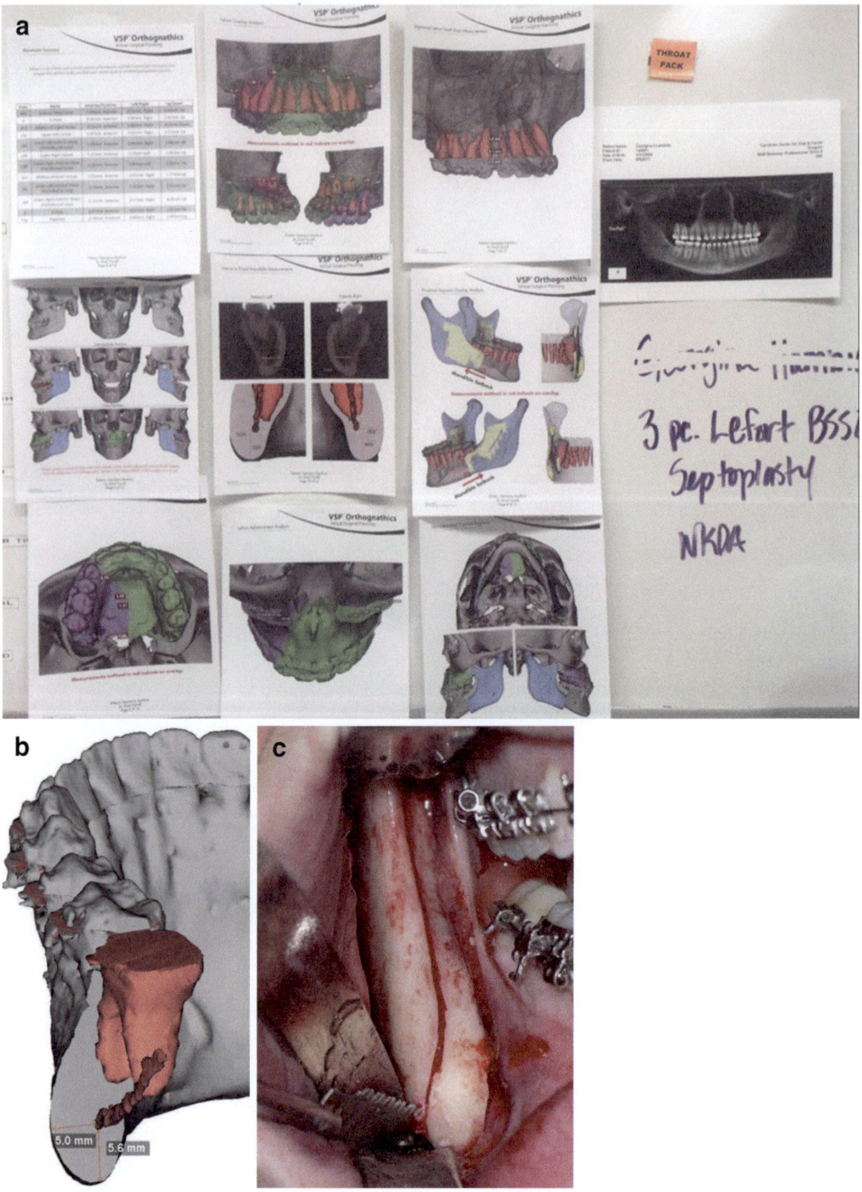

Fig. 16 (**a**) Surgeon preference "card" displayed in the operating room to provide reference to skeletal movements, anatomy and stages of occlusal change with double jaws surgery. (**b**) Course of the inferior alveolar nerve in the body of the mandible identified to provide insight for completion of a sound cut through the inferior border. (**c**) Inferior border osteotomy with reciprocating saw

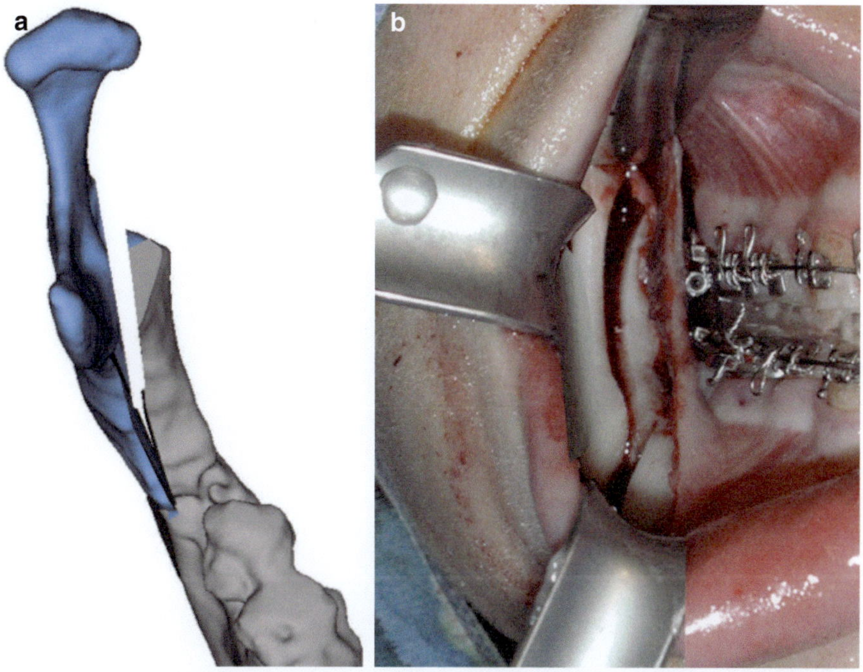

Fig. 17 Improved intraoperative efficiency can be garnered from preoperative insight. (**a**) Virtual understanding of segment alignment after addressing a severe asymmetric deformity. The avoidance of condyle displacement medially during bicortical screw fixation can be illustrated from planning the skeletal correction digitally. (**b**) The clinical representation of the surgery with segment alignment mirroring that visualized through planning. A bone shim collected from bony mitering of the proximal segment was placed to maintain the position of the segment and avoid compression during fixation. Complex asymmetric dentofacial deformities can be managed through virtual planning efficiently and accurately

and innovation have aided in managing cases commonly designated as a more complex routine with less stress as the skeletal repositioning has been reviewed and inspected prior to delivering care. The ability to appreciate the anatomic relationships at the osteotomy sites can aid in moving methodically and efficiently through the surgical procedure that can lead to cost savings and a smoother recovery for patients with less operative time and anesthesia requirements [28, 29]. (Fig. 17).

Virtual planning of surgery will continue to evolve in the management of dentofacial deformities. The digital workflow and planning of occlusal and skeletal correction will continue to be refined, and patient-specific customized plates within the maxilla and mandible that aid in mirroring the surgical outcome to that planned on the computer are available the accuracy of the three-dimensional soft tissue predictions improve, we will be provided with a greater understanding of the tissue response as the skeletal scaffolding is repositioned.

Case Report

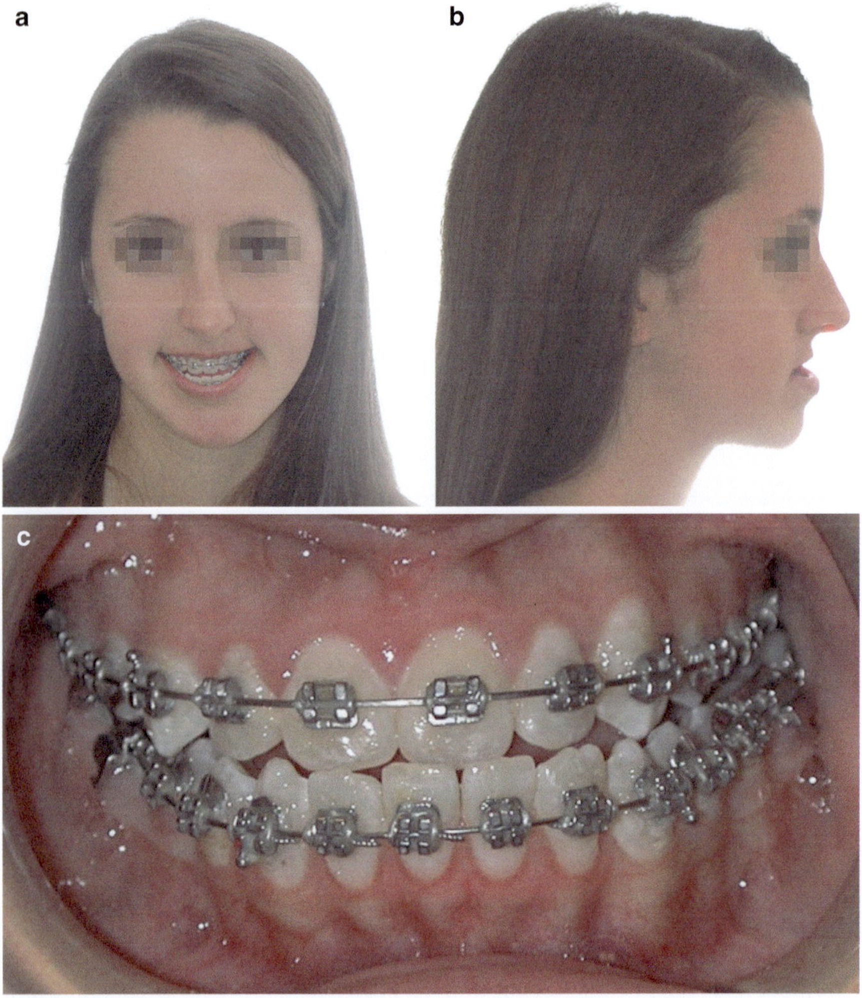

17.1- year-old female with asymmetric dentofacial deformity. A, B. Maxillary hypoplasia and asymmetry resulting in a canted occlusal plane and concomitant mandibular hyperplasia with asymmetry. C. Asymmetric Class III malocclusion. D. Multiple rows of teeth and distinct inferior borders of the mandible illustrate vertical asymmetry. E. Profile view with virtual planning after merging of skeletal and occlusal data. F. Multidimensional skeletal discrepancy. G, H. Facial photographs illustrate good facial symmetry and facial balance and proportion after surgery. I. Esthetic and functional postoperative occlusion

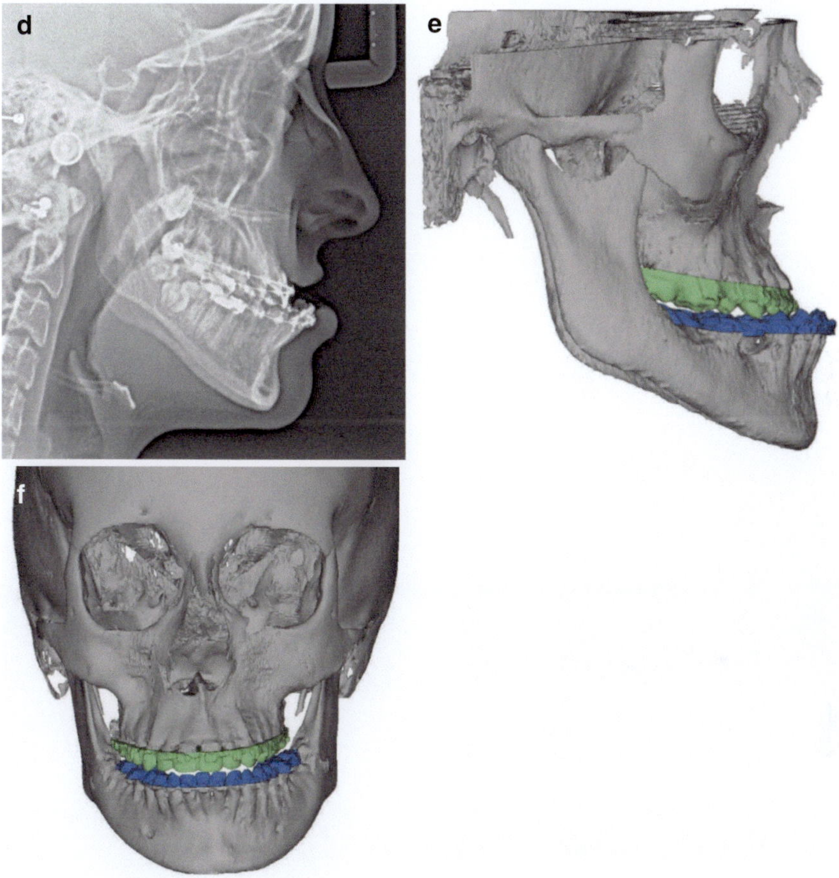

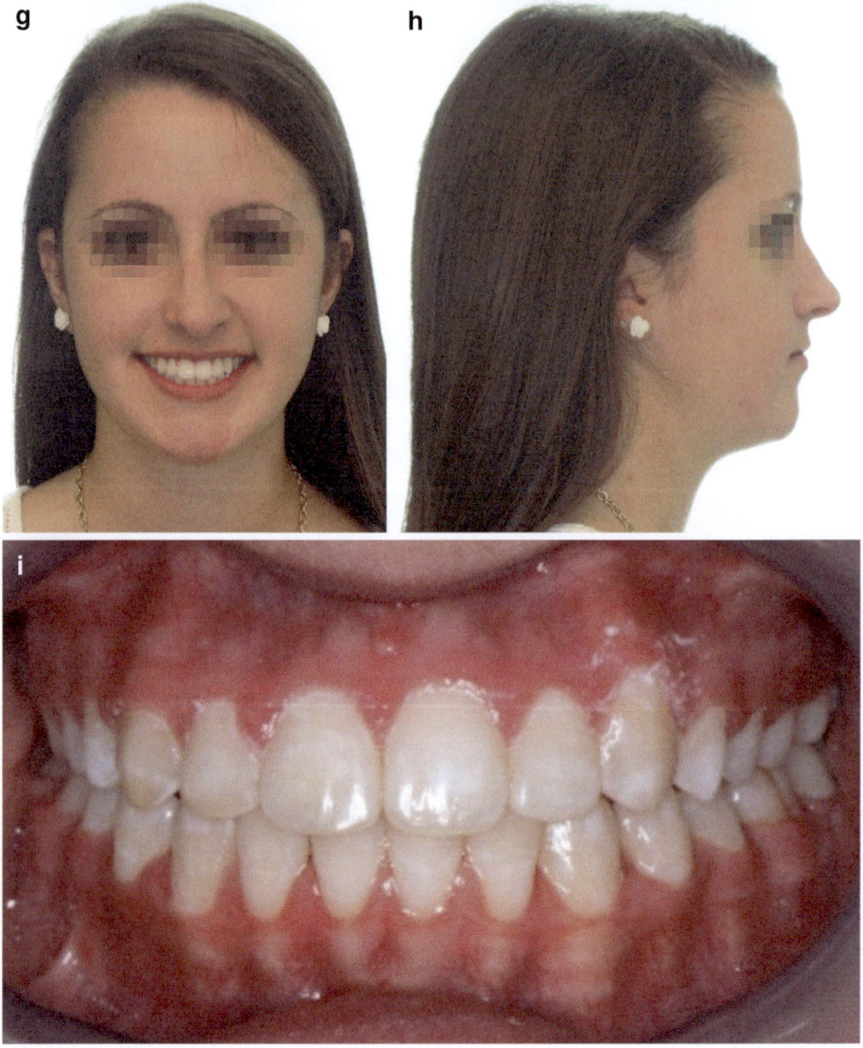

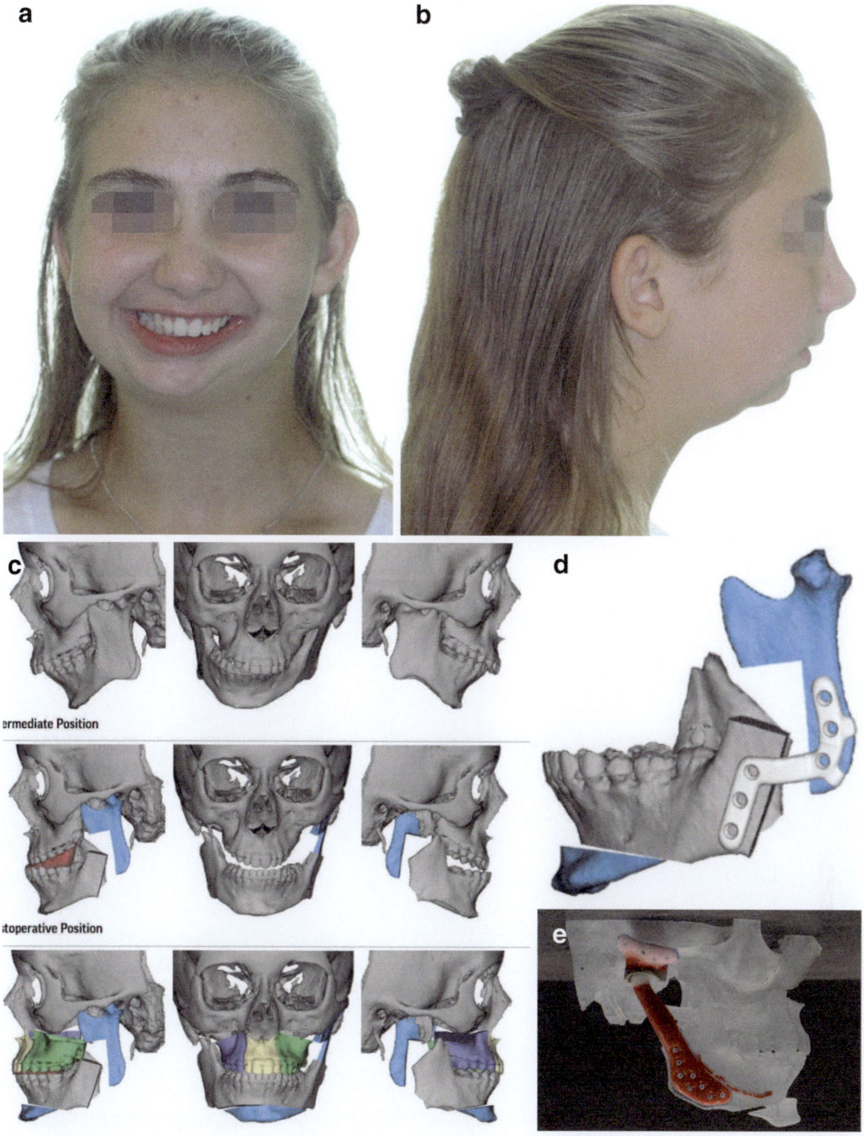

17- year-old female with pathology that led to ankylosis of the right temporomandibular joint. A, B. Asymmetry and deficiency of the lower facial third. C. Digital planning of the asymmetrical dentofacial deformity with orthognathic surgery and joint replacement. D. Planning of patient-specific custom plate with inverted L osteotomy. E. TMJ Concepts total joint replacement. F. Condylar prosthesis stabilized to the mandible through classic transcutaneous approach. G. Cadaveric bone grafting of inverted L osteotomy delivered intraorally. H. Postoperative appearance in the operating room prior to extubation. I. Initial postoperative imaging. J. Superimposition of radiographic imaging over clinical photo at 6 weeks. K. Postoperative facial esthetics and symmetry. I. Range of motion after correction of ankylosis

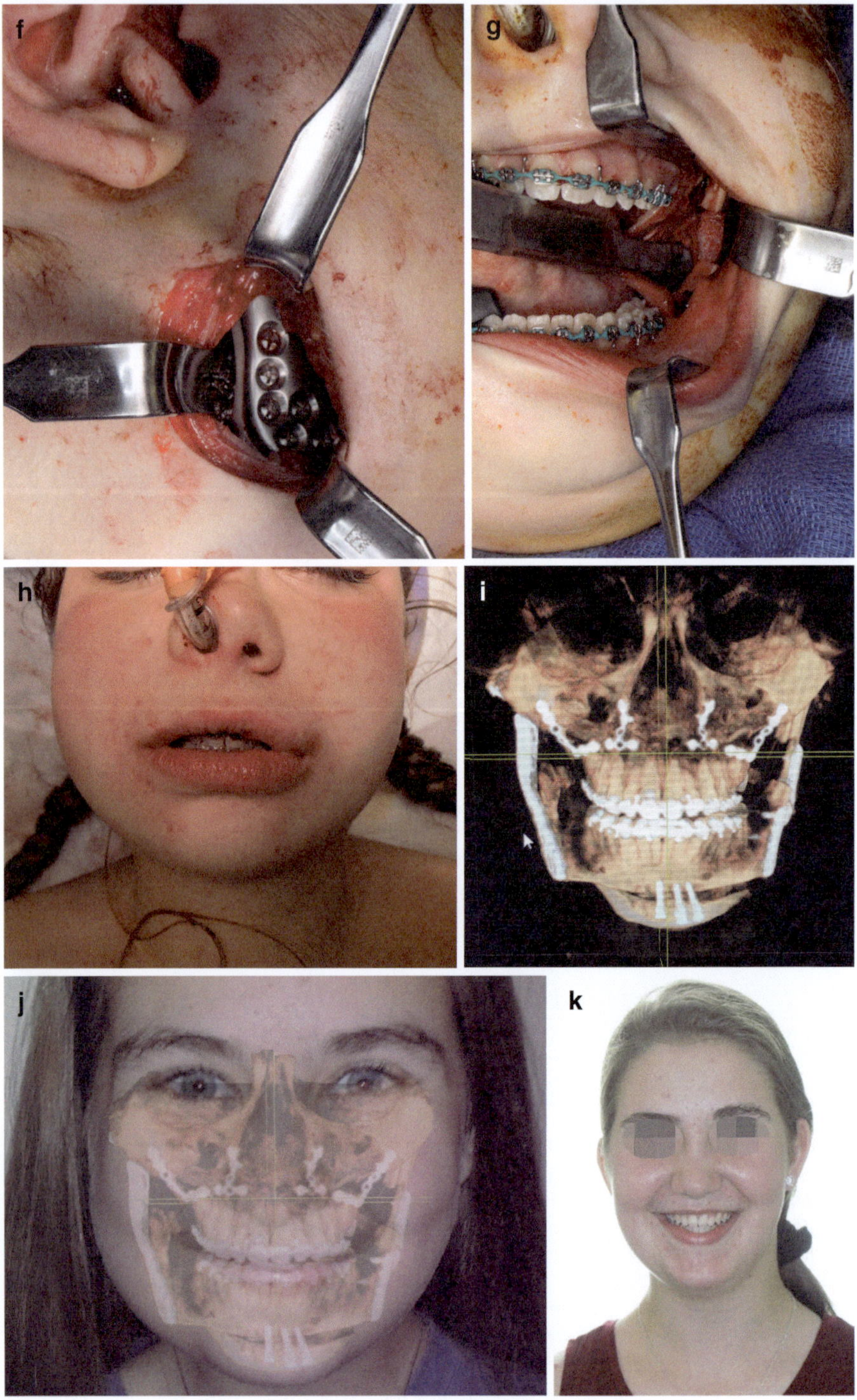
f
g
h
i
j
k

I

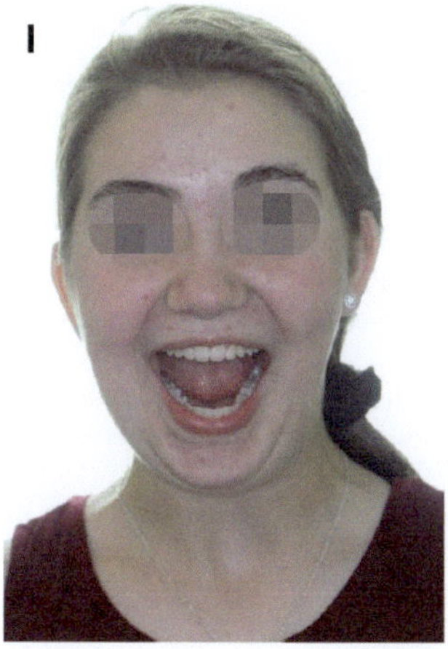

References

1. Bell WH, editor. Surgeon correction of dentofacial deformities. Philadelphia: WB Saunders; 1980.
2. Bell WH, editor. Modern practice in orthognathic and reconstructive surgery. Philadelphia: WB Saudners; 1992.
3. Xia JJ, Gateno J, Teichgraeber JF. New clinical protocol to evaluate craniomaxillofacial deformity and plan surgical correction. J Oral Maxillofac Surg. 2009;67:2094.
4. Bobek S. Farrell Br, Choi C, Farrell Ba, Weimer K, Tucker M: virtual surgical planning for orthognathic surgery using digital data transfer and an intraoral fiducial marker: the Charlotte method. J Oral Maxillofac Surg. 2015;73:1143.
5. Xia JJ, Teichgraeber J, Gateno J. Computer aided surgical simulation in orthognathic surgery. Chapter 74. Bell RB, Bagheri SC, Ali Kahn H, editors. Current therapy in oral and maxillofacial surgery. St. Louis (MO): WB Saunders; 2012.
6. Gelesko S, Markiewicz M, Weimer K, et al. Computer-aided orthognathic surgery. Atlas Oral Maxillofac Surg Clin North Am. 2012;20:107–18.
7. Levine JP, Patel A, Saadeh PB, et al. Computer-aided design and manufacturing in craniomaxillofacial surgery: the new state of the art. J Craniofac Surg. 2012;23(1):288–93.
8. Hsu S, Gateno J, Bell R, Hirsch D, Markiewicz M, Teichgraeber H, Zhou X, Xia J. Accuracy of a computer-aided surgical simulation protocol for orthognathic surgery: a prospective multicenter study. J Oral Maxillofac Surg. 2013;71(1):128–42.
9. Gateno J, Xia J, Teichgraeber J, Christensen A, Lemoine J, Liebschner M, Gliddon M, Briggs M. Clinical feasibility of computer-aided surgical simulation in treatment of complex cranio-maxillofacial deformities. J Oral Maxillofac Surg. 2007;65:728–34.
10. Xia J, Phillips C, Gateno J, Teichgraeber J, Christensen A, Lasky R, Lemoine J, Liebschner M. Accuracy of a computer-aided surgical simulation (CASS) system in the treatment of complex cranio-maxillofacial deformities. J Oral Maxillofac Surg. 2007;65(12):248–54.
11. Xia J, Sheychenko L, Gateno J, Teichgraeber J, Taylor T, Lasky R, English J, Kau C, Mcgrory K. Outcome of computer-aided surgical simulation in the treatment of patient with craniomaxillofacial deformities. J Oral Maxillofac Surg. 2011;69(7):2014–24.
12. Gateno J, Xia J, Teichgraeber J. The precision of computer generated surgical splints. J Oral Maxillofac Surg. 2003;61:814–7.

13. Farrell B, Franco P, Tucker M. Virtual surgical planning in orthognathic surgery. Oral Maxillofacial Surg Clin N Am. 2014;26:459–73.
14. Orentlicher G, Goldsmith D, Abboud M. Computer-guided planning and placement of dental implants. Oral Maxillofacial Surg Clin N Am. 2012;20:53–79.
15. Haq J, Patel N, Weimer K, Matthews NS. Single stage treatment of ankylosis of the temporomandibular joint using patient-specific total joint replacement and virtual surgical planning. Br J Oral Maxillofac Surg. 2014;52(4):350–5.
16. Tepper OM, Sorice S, Hershman GN, Saadeh P, Levine JP, Hirsch D. Use of virtual 3-dimensional surgery in post-traumatic craniomaxillofacial reconstruction. J Oral Maxillofac Surg. 2011;69(3):733–41.
17. Broer PN, Tanna N, Franco PB, Thanik VD, Levine SM, Garfein ES, Saadeh PB, Ceradini DJ, Hirsch DL, Levine JP. Ten-year evolution utilizing computer-assisted reconstruction for giant ameloblastoma. J Reconstr Microsurg. 2013 Mar;29(3):173–80.
18. Hirsch DL, Garfein ES, Christensen AM, Weimer KA, Saddeh PB, Levine JP. Use of computer-aided design and computer-aided manufacturing to produce orthognathically ideal surgical outcomes: a paradigm shift in head and neck reconstruction. J Oral Maxillofac Surg. 2009;67(10):2115–22.
19. Tucker MR. Rigid fixation for maxillofacial surgery. Philadelphia: Lippincott; 1991.
20. Patel A, Karlis V. Chapter 33: Principles of Fixation for Maxillofacial Trauma. In: Fonseca R, editor. Oral and Maxillofacial Trauma. 4th ed. St Louis: WB Saunders; 2013. p. 816–35.
21. Prein J, editor. Manual of internal fixation in the craniofacial skeleton. Springer; 1998.
22. McCormick S, Drew S. Virtual model surgery for efficient planning and surgical performance. J Oral Maxillofac Surg. 2011;69:638–44.
23. Xia J, Gateno J, Teichgraeber J. Three-dimensional computer-aided surgical simulation for maxillofacial surgery. Atlas Oral Maxillofac Surg Clinics. 2005;13:25–39.
24. Damstra J, Fourie Z, Ren Y. Simple technique to achieve a natural position of the head for cone beam computed tomography. Br J Oral Maxillofac Surg. 2010;48:236.
25. Serag M, Nassar T, Avondoglio D, Weiner S. A comparative study of the accuracy of dies made from digital intraoral scanning vs. elastic impressions: an in vitro study. J Prosthodont. 2016;27:88.
26. Aragon M, Pontes L, Bichara L, Flores-Mir C, Normando D. Validity and reliability of intraoral scanners compared to conventional gypsum models measurements: a systematic review. Euro J of Orthodontics. 2016:429–34.
27. Nilsson J, Richards R, Thor A, Kamer L. Virtual bite registration using intraoral digital scanning, CT and CBCT: in vitro evaluation of a new method and its implication for orthognathic surgery. J Cranio-Maxillo-Facial Surg. 2016;44:1194.
28. Farrell B, Tucker M. Safe efficient and cost-effective orthognathic surgery in the outpatient setting. J Oral Maxillofacial Surg. 2009;67:2064–71.
29. Farrell B, Tucker M. Orthognathic surgery in the office setting. Oral Maxillofacial Surg Clin N Am. 2014;26:611–62.

Facial Asymmetry: Management of the Oculoauriculovertebral Spectrum (OAVS)

Bernard J. Costello, Kristopher R. Cooper, and Samuel Liu

Abstract

Oculoauriculovertebral spectrum (OAVS) is a condition characterized by hypoplasia as a result of disrupted development in the first and second branchial arches. Its craniofacial manifestations are often unilateral and the term hemifacial microsomia has been frequently used. Because the phenotypes of OAVS patients are extremely diverse, treatments are individualized and based on the needs of patients on a case-by-case basis. In the absence of significant functional deficits or severe psychosocial esthetic concerns, surgical intervention is the most stable and predictable when performed at or near the completion of growth of the functional unit to be treated. For patients with a severe phenotype, staged reconstruction involving multiple surgeries at various stages of development may be indicated. Others may never require surgical intervention. The skeletal facial asymmetries commonly seen in patients with OAVS are often most successfully managed with traditional orthognathic jaw surgery near the completion of growth of the facial skeleton.

Keywords

Hemifacial microsomia · Goldenhar syndrome · Oculoauriculovertebral spectrum

B. J. Costello (✉) · K. R. Cooper · S. Liu
Department of Oral and Maxillofacial Surgery, University of Pittsburgh, Pittsburgh, PA, USA
e-mail: Bjc1@pitt.edu; cooperkr@upmc.edu

P. Mehra, L. M. Wolford (eds.), *Management of Facial Asymmetry*,
https://doi.org/10.1007/978-3-030-44971-1_5

Introduction

Oculoauriculovertebral spectrum (OAVS) is a congenital three-dimensional hypoplasia that results from disruption of the development of the first and second branchial arches and neural crest migration. Significant phenotypic variability is seen, from patients presenting with isolated ear anomalies to complex lateral facial clefting with significant functional concerns and disrupted development of the lateral facial structures (Figs. 1, 2, and 3). The term "hemifacial microsomia" has been

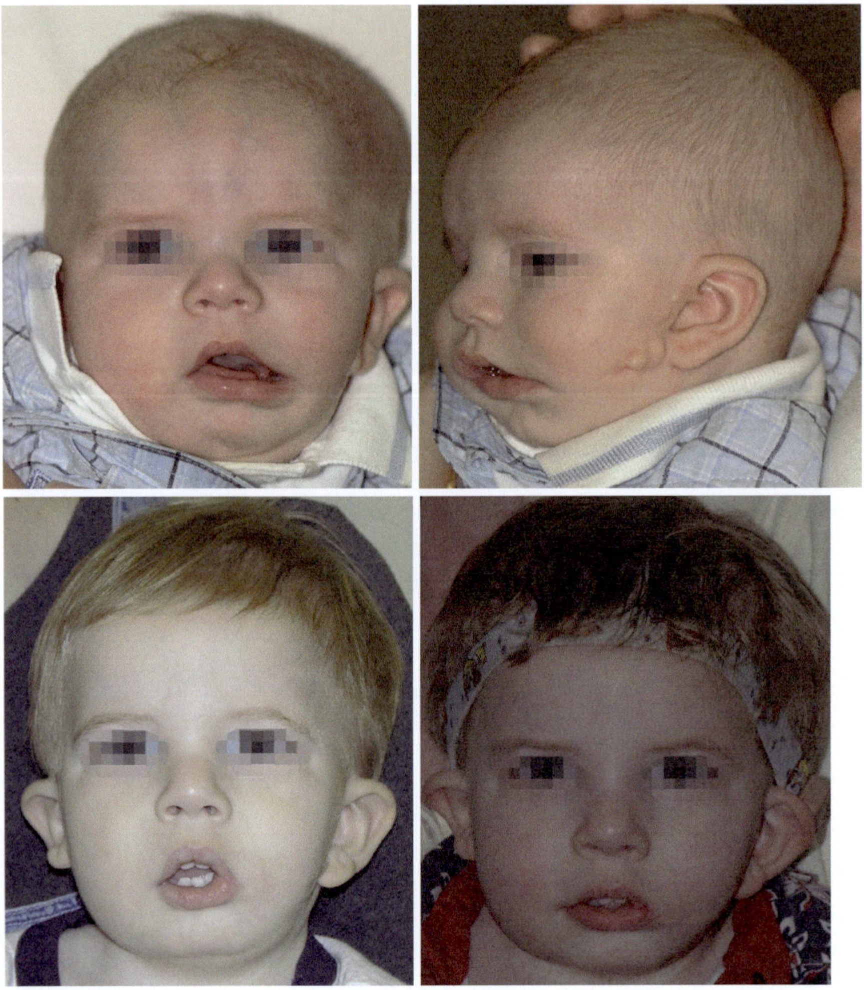

Fig. 1 This male patient demonstrates OAVS primarily affecting the left face. A left-sided Tessier 7 cleft is the most salient soft tissue feature. The cleft was repaired and a functional and esthetic result achieved. Reprinted with Permission: Costello BJ, Ruiz RL, Caccamese JF. "Oculoauriculovertebral Spectrum: Staged Reconstruction." Oral and Maxillofacial Surgery, 3rd Edition. Elsevier, 2018. Ch 39. Pg 687–702

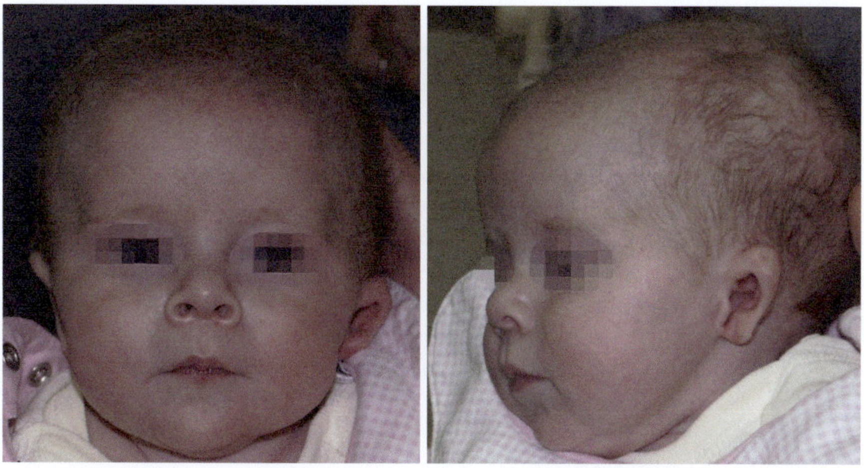

Fig. 2 Infant female patient demonstrating a mild phenotype of OAVS affecting the left face. Ear involvement is the only salient feature of her condition. Reprinted with Permission: Costello BJ, Ruiz RL, Caccamese JF. "Oculoauriculovertebral. Spectrum: Staged Reconstruction." Oral and Maxillofacial Surgery, 3rd Edition. Elsevier, 2018. Ch 39. Pg 687–702

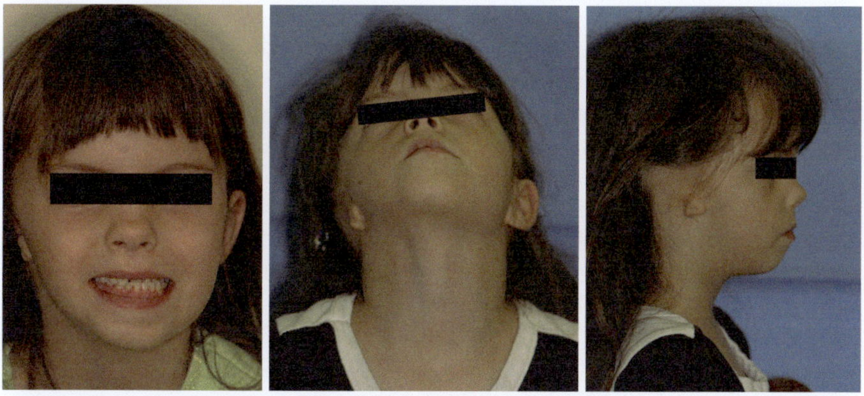

Fig. 3 Female patient with OAVS affecting the right face more significantly than the left. She shows atresia of the right external ear, along with right facial soft tissue hypoplasia. Her skeletal asymmetry includes orbital, zygomatic, and maxillary hypoplasia. Her mandibular hypoplasia is classified as Kaban IIB. At the time of these images, she had previously undergone distraction osteogenesis with another surgeon as a small child but her asymmetry remains significant. Reprinted with Permission: Costello BJ, Ruiz RL, Caccamese JF. "Oculoauriculovertebral Spectrum: Staged Reconstruction." Oral and Maxillofacial Surgery, 3rd Edition. Elsevier, 2018. Ch 39. Pg 687-702

used to describe the hypoplasia seen in these patients, and Goldenhar syndrome has been used denote the most severe phenotypes usually with multisystem involvement. The term "OAVS" has largely replaced other nomenclature as it accurately characterizes the eye, ear, jaw, and spinal involvement. It also correctly indicates that the degree of hypoplasia occurs on a spectrum, and in a heterogenous fashion.

The functional and esthetic challenges faced by patients with OAVS are generally best approached by a team of specialists who are involved in the patient's care at various developmental stages. Surgeons caring for these patients must understand the biologic basis for the malformation as well as the esthetic and functional issues that may arise throughout the child's growth and development. Team care is essential for benchmarking growth and development and guiding parents through a treatment algorithm. As team cleft-craniofacial care is becoming the norm, multispecialty coordination has improved. Successful OAVS treatment planning requires a staged reconstructive approach with a special emphasis on timing of interventions and respecting the growth of normal and abnormal facial structures. In this chapter, we review the pathogenesis and phenotypic variability of clinical presentation and describe approaches to staged reconstruction tailored to the individual patient's needs.

Historical Perspective

OAVS and the related disorders were described in the1950s and redefined by Gorlin in the 1960s [1, 2]. The impressive heterogeneity and phenotypic variability of this condition exist along a spectrum; therefore, the term oculoauriculovertebral spectrum (OAVS) is now commonly used [3]. OAVS has also been known as hemifacial microsomia, craniofacial microsomia, otomandibular dysostosis, and facio-auriculo-vertebral dysplasia. It is likely that only about 10% of OAVS patients have phenotypes consistent with Goldenhar syndrome [4–6]. Goldenhar syndrome has often been considered a phenotypically severe variant of hemifacial microsomia characterized by facial asymmetry with mandibular hypoplasia, ocular dermoids, and vertebral abnormalities. Patients may also present with cardiac and/or renal abnormalities. There has been discussion regarding oculo-auriculo-frontonasal syndrome (OAFNS) as possibly being considered a part of the oculoauriculovertebral spectrum as well, though recent studies by Gabbett in 2008 and Evans in 2013 have supported classifying OAFNS as a distinct entity [5, 7].

Epidemiology, Genetics, and Pathogenesis

Examinations of the incidence of OAVS in the population have been varied, with studies ranging from Morrisen et al. estimating a prevalence of 1 in 45,000 in a Northern Ireland study [8] to Hennekam et al. estimating prevalence of about 1 in 5600 [9]. Given the variable expressivity and diversity of populations affected by OAVS, these figures are only estimates and it is very difficult to pinpoint the actual prevalence. There have been multiple etiologies implicated in the development of OAVS which likely involves both environmental and genetic causes. The majority of OAVS cases seem to result from sporadic mutations and/or chromosomal abnormalities, but there are case reports describing families with OAVS and inheritance patterns that follow autosomal dominant, autosomal recessive, and x-linked patterns [3, 4]. Twin studies in OAVS-affected individuals seem to reveal discordance in

OAVS most often, although occasional concordance with variable expressivity has been noted [10–12]. Multiple chromosomal abnormalities including 5q deletion, trisomy 18, and 7q duplication have been associated with OAVS, as have other genetic abnormalities such as cri-du-chat and trisomy 22 [13–15].

Environmental factors also have been shown to have an association with the incidence of OAVS including exposure to thalidomide, primidone, and retinoic acid [4]. Isotretinoin has also been shown to be associated with OAVS in addition to its other well-known teratogenic effects [16]. Vasoactive drugs such as nonsteroidal anti-inflammatory drugs were examined by Werler et al., and maternal exposure was shown to pose a potential 1.5–2x increased risk of having children with OAVS [17]. Additionally, Wang et al. demonstrated that infants born to mothers with poorly controlled diabetes were more likely to be affected by OAVS [18]. Furthermore, it has been shown that infants conceived with the aid of reproductive technologies (IVF) are more likely to exhibit signs of OAVS [19].

In examining the pathogenesis of the development of OAVS, it has been widely agreed upon that the event(s) likely occurs early in pregnancy at about 30–45 days of gestation [20]. Poswillo has suggested that at this time stapedial artery anastomosis is interrupted in affected individuals and resultant hematoma formation disrupts development [21, 22]. Poswillo also famously used an animal model to reproduce the aforementioned pathosis by introducing maternal thalidomide. This environmental exposure model does not, however, explain familial inheritance or the other associated malformations associated with OAVS.

Johnston and Bronsky suggest that OAVS pathogenesis is more likely associated with a malformation sequence of neural crest cells. They describe that while mandibular changes may be associated with the hemorrhages described by Poswillo, the cerebral hemispheres and mandibular arches were already severely underdeveloped before the hemorrhage occurred. The authors also compare OAVS with syndromes known to involve neural crest cell death or disrupted neural crest migration such as retinoic acid syndrome, DiGeorge syndrome, Down syndrome, and Treacher Collins syndrome [23, 24].

Physical Findings

Patients presenting with OAVS can manifest a number of different findings and abnormalities of the facial bones and soft tissues. At their most subtle, signs can involve only microtia or periauricular abnormalities such as skin tags [3]. Patients can also exhibit underdevelopment (or absence) of structures such as the mandibular ramus, condyle, or the glenoid fossa. Orbital structures including bony orbits and periorbital soft tissues can be involved, along with the external and/or internal ear. Other facial bones such as the zygoma and maxilla can be affected [3, 12, 25]. The hypoplasia seen in these patients is generally unilateral, but asymmetric bilateral involvement can be appreciated in up to 15% of cases [3]. Regarding the relationship between soft tissue deformities and bony deformities, it has been shown that the extent of muscle hypoplasia is predictive of the level of bony abnormality at the site of the muscle insertion [26]. Abnormalities are also common outside the craniofacial region with renal, genitourinary, cardiac, and skeletal abnormalities also being reported [12, 25].

Prenatal imaging and evaluation of these patients has been described, with detection of abnormalities on the OAV spectrum via ultrasound or magnetic resonance imaging possible as early as 14 weeks of gestational age. Early on, oligo- or polyhydramnios can indicate swallowing difficulties that may be suggestive of facial abnormalities. More severe phenotypic variants tend to be detectable earlier in gestation, whereas less severe variants often cannot be detected by prenatal ultrasound; these abnormalities are only discovered on clinical exam after birth [27].

Systems of Classification

There are several systems of classification to describe various aspects of OAVS-associated malformations. Classifications have largely been based on mandibular and temporomandibular joint morphology, and classification systems have been developed and improved over time [28–34]. Classification systems such as those developed by Pruzansky [29], Kaban [35], and others allow for characterization of the temporomandibular joint dysmorphology. These systems are used to classify abnormalities seen in patients for the purpose of developing a well-timed and successful reconstruction.

The Kaban classification was developed and first published in 1981 as a modification to the Pruzansky classification system [29, 35]. It describes the degree of deformity associated with the TMJ and ramus unit. Kaban type I skeletal defects involve mild hypoplasia of the structures within the TMJ complex in which all structures are still present. Patients with type II OAVS have more significant hypoplasia than type I and are separated into type IIA and type IIB deformities. In type IIa, mandibular structures are present but hypoplastic and *abnormal in shape*, but normal function is largely maintained. In addition to the IIa criteria described, type IIb shows marked abnormality in the TMJ morphology, though the condyle (or pseudocondyle in many cases) articulates with the temporomandibular fossa. Patients with IIb abnormalities generally have functional limitations as a result of the deformity. Type III deformities are characterized by the complete absence of the condyle or mandibular ramus. These patients may also demonstrate abnormalities of the temporal bone at the glenoid fossa such as flattening or absence of the fossa altogether. Type I and IIa defects may not lead to significant malfunction and, if surgery is indicated, can usually be managed with standard orthognathic surgical techniques. Type IIb and III malformations typically require more involved reconstructive techniques such as rib grafting or prosthetic joint replacement [36]. In 2010, Madrid and colleagues described a type IV deformity which involves a type III malformation plus ipsilateral mandibular body hypoplasia associated with the absence of the ramus and/or condyle [37].

Vetno et al. described and published an updated classification in 1989 known as the OMENS classification. The acronym OMENS is used to organize deformities in

OAVS by anatomic site: (O for orbital hypoplasia and malposition; M for mandibular hypoplasia; E for ear anomaly; N for facial nerve involvement; and S for soft tissue hypoplasia). Each of the regions described is assigned a number to quantify and describe the deformity (Box 1) [32]. The OMENS-Plus classification system was first described and published in 1995 by Horgan and colleagues, and it includes additional consideration for abnormalities outside of the craniofacial area [33, 34]. The OMENS and OMENS-Plus systems are helpful because they are more comprehensive, quantifying abnormalities in multiple systems in addition to the mandible and TMJ.

Box 1

Orbit	0	Normal morphology
	1	Abnormal size
	2	Abnormal position
	3	Abnormal size + position
Mandible/ TMJ	0	Normal
	1	Hypoplastic mandible, shortened ramus
	2A	Hypoplastic mandible/condyle with acceptable glenoid fossa position
	2B	Severely hypoplastic mandible/condyle with glenoid fossa displaced from functional position
	3	Absence of ramus and/or glenoid fossa
Ear	0	Normal
	1	Hypoplasia of structures, all of which are present
	2	Absent EAC, hypoplasia of auricle
	3	Absent cartilaginous auricle, lobe may remain and be displaced anteriorly and inferiorly
Nerve (CN VII)	0	Normal
	1	Upper branch involvement (temporal/zygomatic)
	2	Lower branch involvement (buccal/marginal mandibular/cervical)
	3	Upper and lower branch involvement
Soft tissue	0	Normal (no deficiency)
	1	Mild
	2	Moderate
	3	Severe deficiency

Growth

An area of ongoing study has been the growth of patients with OAVS and its relationship to timing and strategies of operative intervention. Several authors [38–41] have examined facial growth over time and found evidence suggesting that the natural history of OAVS generally does not involve progressive worsening of the asymmetry over time. This means that the degree of hypoplasia seen at a young age is expected to be similar to the hypoplasia seen in the patient when they reach their teen years. Thus, the tendency is to recommend against operative intervention in young children with ongoing growth with the hope of allowing as much potential growth as possible before interfering surgically. At the time of surgery, traditional orthognathic techniques may be used to achieve a predictable result that is unlikely to relapse because the patient has completed the majority of growth.

Conversely, some providers have advocated surgical intervention early in childhood to correct asymmetry in an effort to prevent the potential for progressive worsening of the malformation and its effect on the rest of the facial skeleton. The treatment employed is usually distraction osteogenesis in an effort to reduce secondary asymmetries that may be attributable to the original defect [35, 36, 42]. There have been studies presenting data suggesting that OAVS deformities are progressive, and studies suggesting the opposite. The studies that suggest OAVS worsens over time were not longitudinal and thus carry the potential for flaws that seriously weaken the case for progressive deformity [35, 36, 38, 43]. In fact, patients who have early operations and do not have a progressive deformity often are converted to patients who have a progressive growth disturbance that is iatrogenic in nature—due to the surgical intervention during the growth phase.

Both early intervention and intervention in the teen years have been used with success. In the opinion of the authors, definitive intervention in the teen years offers the patient the opportunity to undergo fewer procedures and offers more stable and predictable outcome. These procedures are generally orthognathic surgeries very similar to those commonly used to treat non-syndromic patients. It is crucial, however, to consider the unique needs of all patients on the OAV spectrum; surgical intervention in the young child should be considered for management of significant functional and psychosocial concerns. Early intervention is always weighed against the biological consequence of intervening early.

Treatment Overview

The management approaches to OAVS vary among patients, each of whom has unique functional and esthetic needs. The remaining sections describe craniofacial anomalies commonly seen in OAVS and options for approaching their surgical treatment. If significant functional concerns are present, these often are addressed without delay to facilitate the development of normal function. Of *early* concern are the airway, feeding/swallowing, hearing, speech, and vision [44]. Intervention to correct or restore function in these areas often cannot be delayed even if growth is ongoing. As an example regarding speech: a cleft palate should be repaired at a time that allows for the development of functional speech but also respects growth concerns in the maxilla. Additionally, significant esthetic concerns that could lead to psychosocial problems (such as severe facial clefting) may be addressed early. Other concerns, including the treatment of skeletal and dental malocclusions, may be treated during the teen years, when a stable and predictable result is achievable with less of a risk for needing subsequent surgical revision.

Early Intervention + Airway Management

In newborns who fall on the OAVS spectrum, ensuring a patent airway is of paramount importance to avoid life-threatening complications. Mandibular hypoplasia, maxillary hypoplasia, and choanal atresia can all be associated with OAVS and lead to airway concerns including sleep apnea [45]. If OAVS has been diagnosed on ultrasound during fetal evaluation, it is important to consider the importance of immediate postpartum airway management. Urgent surgical intervention (such as an ex utero intrapartum treatment aka EXIT procedure or immediate tracheostomy) is rarely required, but other interventions may be necessary to assist the newborn with his/her airway management. Interventions as simple as repositioning to lateral or prone can be used, and it may also be necessary to introduce a nasal airway/stent temporarily. However, the delivery room should be equipped for a difficult intubation in case other interventions are unsuccessful. Practitioners may consider eventual tracheostomy or a temporary nasopharyngeal airway if polysomnography or clinical exam suggests significant obstruction [46, 47]. In children who require tracheostomy for airway management, decannulation should be planned as motor coordination improves so that the development of normal speech is not impaired. Other surgical interventions to improve the airway can include surgical lengthening of the mandible through distraction osteogenesis, which is usually employed in an effort to expedite decannulation. Poor outcomes are often seen with neonatal distraction though some authors have used it successfully when other techniques have failed [48]. In addition to causing problems with skeletal growth, and presenting a risk of infection, recent studies have suggested that there is an association between distraction osteogenesis and adverse outcomes on the child's future dentition [49]. Other surgical interventions have been described to avoid tracheostomy in children with airway compromise such as tongue reduction, hyoid suspension, tongue-lip adhesion, and adenoidectomy, but these are poorly studied in the setting of OAVS [50].

Cleft Lip and Palate

Facial clefting is a common feature seen in patients with OAVS, at least 35% of whom present with Tessier 7 clefts [3, 20, 51] (Fig. 1). In the setting of a Tessier No. 7 cleft, failure of fusion of the lateral commissure of the lip may include feeding difficulties and esthetic challenges with a significant psychosocial component necessitating early repair. Surgical management requires excision of tissues at both sides of the cleft and repair and approximation of orbicularis oris and associated commissure musculature. After muscular repair, the oral mucosa can be closed and the vermillion of the lip appropriately approximated and closed. Various other protocols for soft tissue management have been described and used successfully including z-plasty, straight-line closure, and transpositional flaps [52]. An excellent esthetic and functional outcome is achievable in most cases though revision may be necessary as the patient continues to grow. The modiolus should be reconstructed as completely as possible to gain function in this area, if the muscular structures are present.

Many providers are familiar with management strategies for unilateral or bilateral clefts of the lip and palate, similar to those seen in non-syndromic patients, though these overt clefts are seen in only about 7–15% of OAVS cases. More often, OAVS patients present with submucous cleft palate (SMCP) which is seen in up to 30% of cases [3]. SMCP repair in these patients is usually deferred until the age of 3–5 years old, when a speech evaluation is usually possible. Because speech is often not significantly affected in the setting of many patients with SMCP, patients may not require surgical intervention to correct it. Others however may present with velopharyngeal dysfunction and speech abnormalities, usually characterized by hypernasal speech. For these patients, repair of the cleft palate should be considered. This may be done in conjunction with pharyngeal flap or pharyngoplasty if indicated to address persistent velopharyngeal insufficiency [6]. It is worth noting that the velopharyngeal insufficiency (VPI) in OAVS patients is seen about 35% of the time, but is usually not associated with clefting but rather with hemipalatal neuromuscular abnormalities leading to poor palatal motion [53]. These abnormalities of palatal innervation and resultant VPI are usually best managed with a pharyngeal flap procedure, rather than with traditional cleft palate repair techniques [20, 54]. A careful speech evaluation along with any indicated imaging or advanced examination techniques (nasendoscopy and/or videofluoroscopy) is helpful in determining the presence or absence of clefting or innervation abnormalities which lead to VPI. The flap may be customized to address unilateral innervation issues as needed.

Mandibular Ramus and Temporomandibular Joint Reconstruction

Patients with OAVS can exhibit abnormalities of the temporomandibular joint that vary greatly between patients from subtle changes to complete absence of joint structures [29, 35]. Patients with mild hypoplasia and no functional concerns (Kaban type I or IIa) may not require treatment as they rarely develop complications such as internal derangements or degenerative joint disease as they grow [35, 36]. Patients missing major functional units of the TMJ (Kaban type III) usually require reconstruction at some point. Even with a missing condyle/fossa or mandibular ramus, some patients exhibit surprisingly functional speech and mastication. As with other procedures for skeletal treatment, the patient's age and remaining growth potential must be carefully considered. Many surgeons prefer to delay surgical treatment until growth has been completed when possible. Other patients, unfortunately, may experience significant functional obstacles or psychosocial challenges associated with their deformity, warranting surgical treatment prior to the completion of growth [20, 44].

One method of reconstruction for the condyle/fossa unit has been the use of a costochondral rib graft. If a patient has a compelling reason to intervene early, such as severe obstructive sleep apnea or inability to masticate, this type of graft can be considered after age 5. The growth of the costochondral graft has been studied and examined extensively in animal models by Peltomaki and has been used with variable success in OAVS patients [55, 56]. This autogenous rib graft is often selected due to its appropriate size, acceptable donor site morbidity, and cartilage cap. The graft is typically harvested from the contralateral side of the patient as it has a closer anatomic shape to the condyle being replaced [57]. Prior to 5 years of age, the rib tends to be too small for adequate fixation and carries a significant potential for resorption. The grafts may also, on the other hand, continue to grow disproportionately leading to a mandibular hyperplasia-like picture with ipsilateral open bite and deviation to the unaffected side [57]. In these cases, patients often require orthognathic surgery for treatment of the asymmetry—an asymmetry that often may be worse than the defect would have been if it was left uncorrected. Thus, it is important to carefully consider whether early intervention and costochondral grafting in the growth period is the most beneficial to the patient.

Another option for autogenous grafting is the fibular free flap, although this graft comes without any growth potential. Thus, it may be utilized after the growth period is completed and if the costochondral graft is not a possibility (cartilage has been used to reconstruct the ear, concern for donor site morbidity, chest wall deformity otherwise preventing harvest). Because this flap is vascularized and can be harvested along with fascia and other soft tissue, it has the added benefit of offering tissue for reconstruction of associated soft tissue defects in the face. Restoration of TMJ function and intelligible speech has been described in the literature; thus, when indicated, the fibular flap is a viable option for reconstruction [58]. Ongoing research in the area of regenerative medicine may provide opportunities for the use of multi-tissue graft without the need for a donor site. Engineering a construct of the TMJ ex vivo may be achievable with these regenerative medicine techniques. It is unclear when such approaches will be possible to enter clinical trials, but could conceivably serve as the future standard for tissue grafting in patients who have significant deficiencies or asymmetries [59].

For some patients, a prosthetic total temporomandibular joint replacement can be used as a method of primary reconstruction or for revision for prior TMJ graft. If the patient presents with a large area of mandibular deficiency, then grafting with autogenous bone from the rib, iliac crest, or fibula may also be considered. This option has mostly been reserved for patients at or near growth completion because, as with the free fibula, the TMJ prosthesis does not grow with the patient. Given the unpredictable growth of the costochondral graft, prosthetic joints may provide an attractive alternative for patients at or near skeletal maturity.

Transport distraction osteogenesis is a technique in which an osteotomy is performed and a transport "disc" of bone is gradually moved toward the glenoid fossa with the hope of bone fill behind it and eventual articulation of the disc with the fossa. This technique has been employed by some surgeons to reconstruct the ramus/TMJ unit in patients with Kaban type III OAVS, but limited success has been reported [60–70]. One of the primary challenges facing surgeons who use this technique surrounds vector control and the difficulty of guiding the distracted disc of bone to grow and articulate with the skull base at an anatomically appropriate point. As with all distraction techniques, infections, trismus, traumatic odontomas, and non-unions have also been described. Additionally, these techniques require lengthy treatment and patient compliance [68–70]. A major drawback is that these techniques can lead to scarring and significant growth restriction, both of which make the necessary future operative intervention much more difficult (Fig. 4). The growth restriction caused by transport distraction can be significant, particularly if the surgery is performed in very young patients. This technique has been used for several decades, but no substantial functional outcomes of this technique have been described in a clinical trial or case series. Given this lack of successful reported outcomes, and the known myriad of complications and challenges associated with this technique, the use of transport distraction osteogenesis is not recommended by the authors. Aforementioned techniques such as costochondral rib grafting offer more predictable results and thus, transport distraction has largely fallen out of favor.

Distraction Osteogenesis

For some patients with OAVS, mandibular distraction osteogenesis in the early years has been utilized in an attempt to improve symmetry during active growth. For very young patients whose OAVS involves a significant component of hypoplasia, these procedures have been utilized to successfully avoid tracheostomy or to eliminate trach dependence [48]. For others, the rationale for intervening at an early age was to improve symmetry, form, occlusion, and overall function, but many of these approaches were hampered by unpredictable growth and challenges controlling vectors. Operating on young children also carries the potential to impair future bone growth of the affected mandible, likely exacerbating the initial hypoplasia. Unfortunately, there is no evidence that early intervention via distraction can improve bone growth [64, 71, 72]. Furthermore, there is no evidence that this approach provides better outcomes than waiting until the teen years and performing traditional orthognathic surgery. For patients who likely have a nonprogressive deformity, distraction techniques could create a deformity that *is* progressive (Fig. 3). These asymmetries can best be surgically addressed at or near the completion of growth with the use of standard orthognathic surgical techniques. Completing surgery at this time allows for more definitive and predictable reconstruction. Additionally, it is important to mention that distraction techniques are not without significant risk of other complications [49, 50, 68, 71, 73]. Unwanted effects on the permanent dentition, infection, and malunion have been noted along with the need for repeat distraction as a result of relapse. Distraction approaches require careful patient compliance and can also lead to scarring and limit the effectiveness of definitive orthognathic surgery later on (Fig. 4).

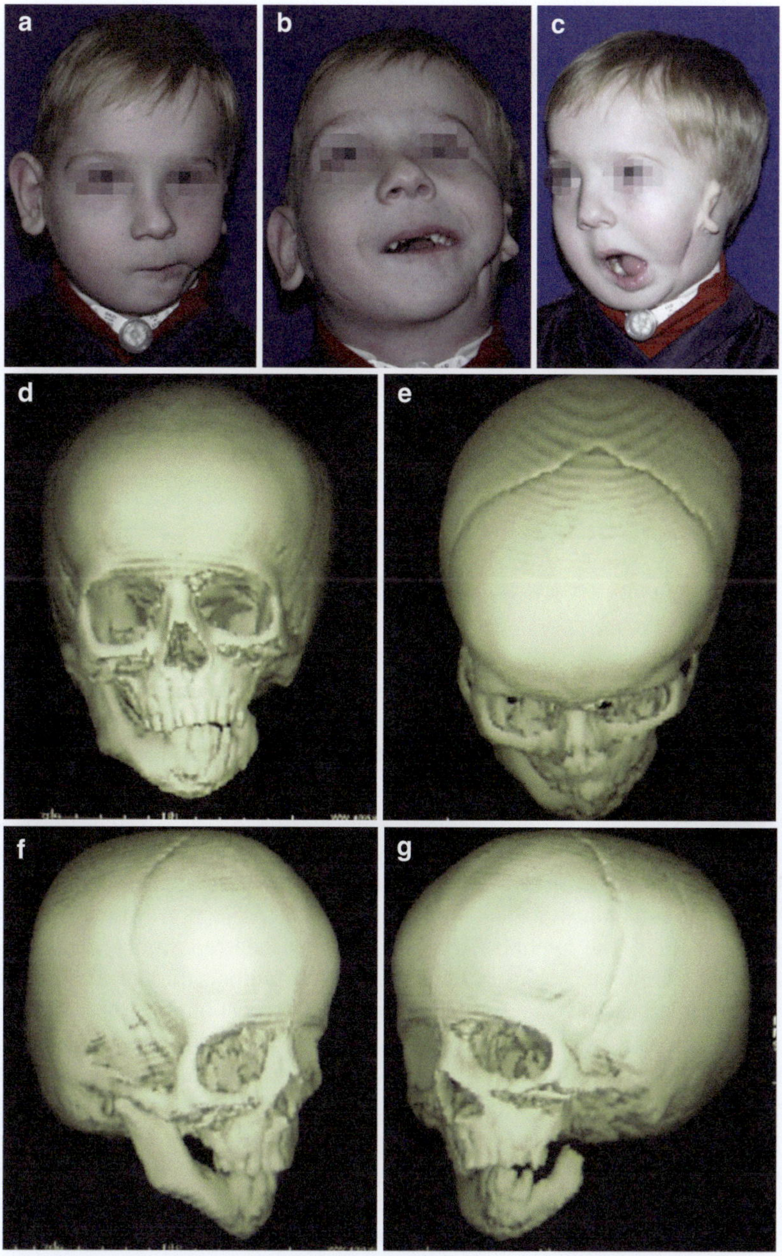

Fig. 4 (**a–c**), A young boy with OAVS with bilateral involvement. The right mandible is classified as type IIA and the left as type III (note the lack of functional condyle/fossa unit in (**g**). He has already undergone several surgeries including distraction and attempts to use transport distraction to create a condyle on the right. The 3D reconstructions of his post-op CT scans (**d–i**) help illustrate the severity of the remaining defect. Reprinted with Permission: Costello BJ, Ruiz RL, Caccamese JF. "Oculoauriculovertebral Spectrum: Staged Reconstruction." Oral and Maxillofacial Surgery, 3rd Edition. Elsevier, 2018. Ch 39. Pg 687–702

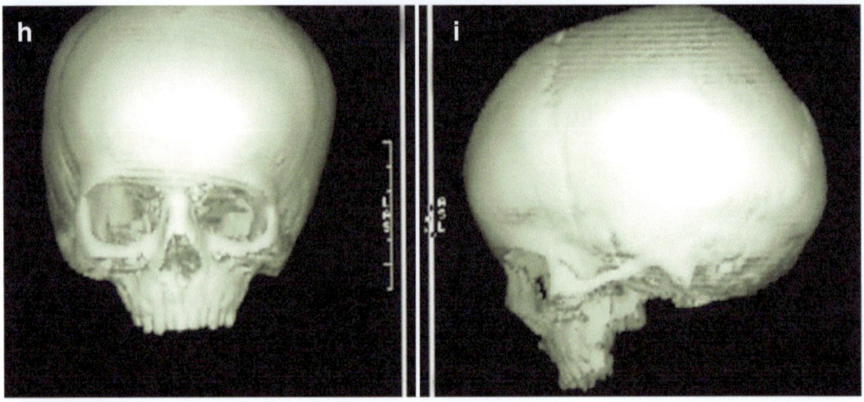

Fig. 4 (continued)

Zygomatic and Orbital Reconstruction

Many patients with OAVS exhibit hypoplasia of the mid- and upper face involving the zygoma and other bones of the orbit. Hypoplasia of the zygoma may be severe enough to pose a significant esthetic and/or functional concern, thus warranting osteotomy and bone grafting. These procedures may be completed after age 5 to 7 when most upper facial bone growth is complete, but reconstruction may be completed later in the absence of compelling functional deficits such as visual impairment as a result of globe malposition.

Various techniques for augmentation and grafting of the zygoma have been described. The surgical approach to the zygoma is usually through a coronal incision. If a significant deformity is present, the zygoma itself can be repositioned by way of formal osteotomy in an attempt to attain facial projection symmetric with the contralateral side. The hypoplastic zygoma, even when repositioned, is often too small or malformed to achieve an adequate result without further augmentation. Onlay bone graft can be used for this purpose and is most often harvested from the cranial vault which is exposed with a coronal incision. Another advantage of performing the procedures after the age of 7 is that the cranial vault should be bicortical by this time, allowing for the option of a split thickness harvest. It is important to plan for the fact that autografts do not grow with the patient and tend to resorb somewhat unpredictably over time. If autogenous grafting is not desired or not possible, porous polyethylene or poly-ether-ether-ketone materials can be custom made and implanted to achieve a similar result. In less severe cases, custom implant materials or bone grafts can be used to achieve projection without the need for osteotomies of the zygoma or orbit/zygoma complex. [71]

One of the crucial functional considerations of the hypoplastic orbital/zygomatic area is the patient's vision. Hypoplasia of the orbital bones, including the zygoma, can lead to enophthalmos. This malposition of the globe may lead to ophthalmologic complications that indicate repair at an earlier age than previously discussed for typical zygomatic reconstruction. Polyethylene implants and autogenous bone have been described for use in orbital floor repair to improve globe position. Other ophthalmologic conditions associated with OAVS include epibulbar dermoids, colobomata, blepharophimosis, and strabismus. Ophthalmologic evaluation should be completed in the OAVS patient, and a pediatric ophthalmologist and/or oculoplastic surgeon should play a role in the ongoing care of patients with relevant eye and periorbital manifestations [3, 71].

Orthognathic Surgery

Patients with OAVS disorders often present with dental malocclusions, missing or malpositioned posterior teeth, enamel or dentin malformations, and abnormal tooth eruption patterns [3, 74]. The role of orthognathic surgery as part of staged reconstruction for treatment of skeletal dental malocclusions has been well described [20, 35, 44, 51, 71]. Because OAVS and similar deformities involve complex three-dimensional deformities, the surgical management is most commonly approached with the use of multiple osteotomies commonly including LeFort I osteotomy and bilateral sagittal split osteotomies, with or without genioplasty (Figs. 5, 6, and 7). It is recommended that patients undergoing orthognathic surgery for treatment of OAVS deformities wait until they are near or at skeletal maturity to avoid ongoing changes and potential relapse associated with growth. In order to best control the occlusion, these surgeries should be done in conjunction with orthodontic treatment [20, 44].

For patients with severe deformities including Kaban class IIb or III deformities, it is often necessary to consider other surgical procedures and other osteotomy approaches. For the mandible, inverted L osteotomy, vertical ramus osteotomy, or other straight osteotomies may be used, often in conjunction with interpositional bone grafting techniques to achieve the desired reconstructive result. Some patients may have had procedures as children such as condylar reconstruction with costochondral rib graft which is often considered the best first-stage option for type III deformities [20, 36, 44]. Others may have undergone distraction osteogenesis of the mandible. Prior surgical interventions like these will often affect the eventual reconstructive plan, and additional maxillomandibular reconstructive procedures will usually be indicated after skeletal maturity (Figs. 5, 6, and 7).

In certain cases, maxillomandibular surgery and temporomandibular reconstruction can be performed simultaneously at skeletal maturity if no significant functional concerns are present at a younger age that indicated earlier intervention. Vascularized free fibula microvascular transfer may be used for interpositional grafting and is often used for vertical ramus reconstruction. The soft tissues that can be transferred with the fibula such as skin, muscle, and fascia can be used to provide

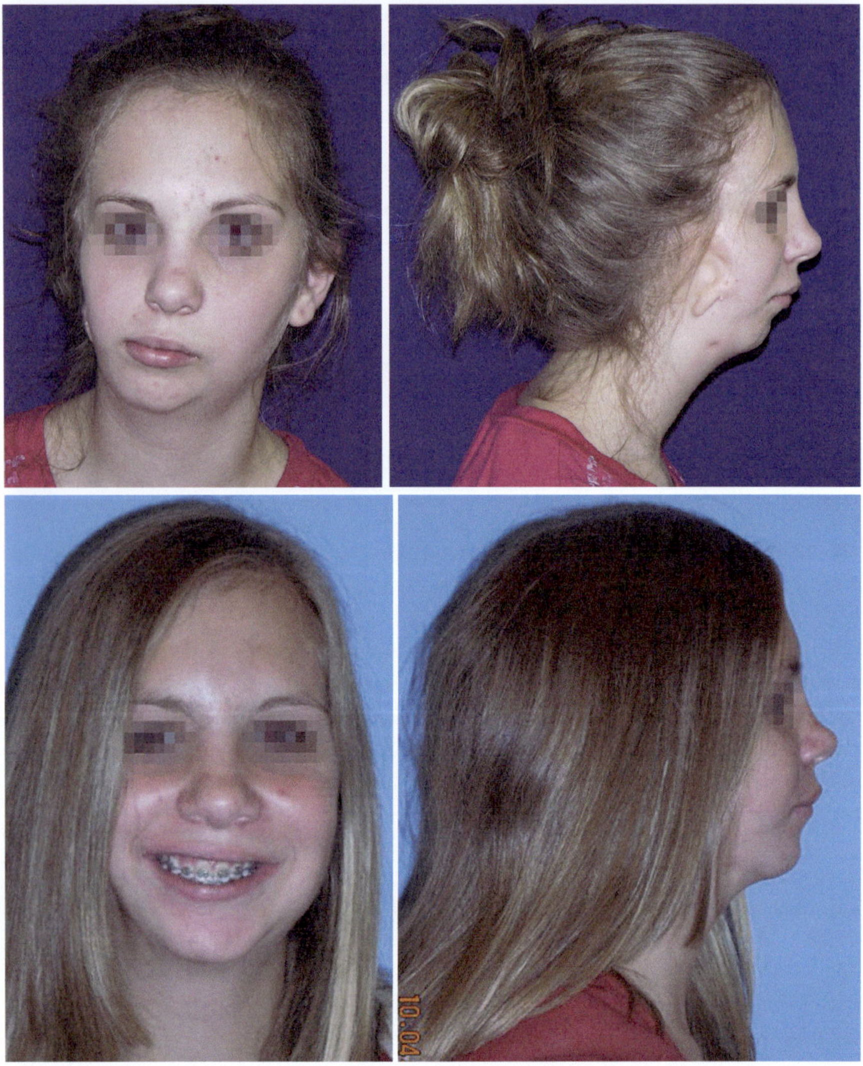

Fig. 5 A teenage female who was initially treated for type III OAVS with a rib graft to the right TMJ as a child. She later underwent several distraction procedures of the rib graft site with another surgeon. After growth completion, she underwent Le Fort I osteotomy, left-sided sagittal split osteotomy, and right-sided modified sagittal osteotomy through the previous distraction site with removal of an impacted tooth, as well as asymmetric genioplasty with bone grafting. Pre- and post-op photographs from the latter procedure are shown. Reprinted with Permission: Costello BJ, Ruiz RL, Caccamese JF. "Oculoauriculovertebral Spectrum: Staged Reconstruction." Oral and Maxillofacial Surgery, 3rd Edition. Elsevier, 2018. Ch 39. Pg 687–702

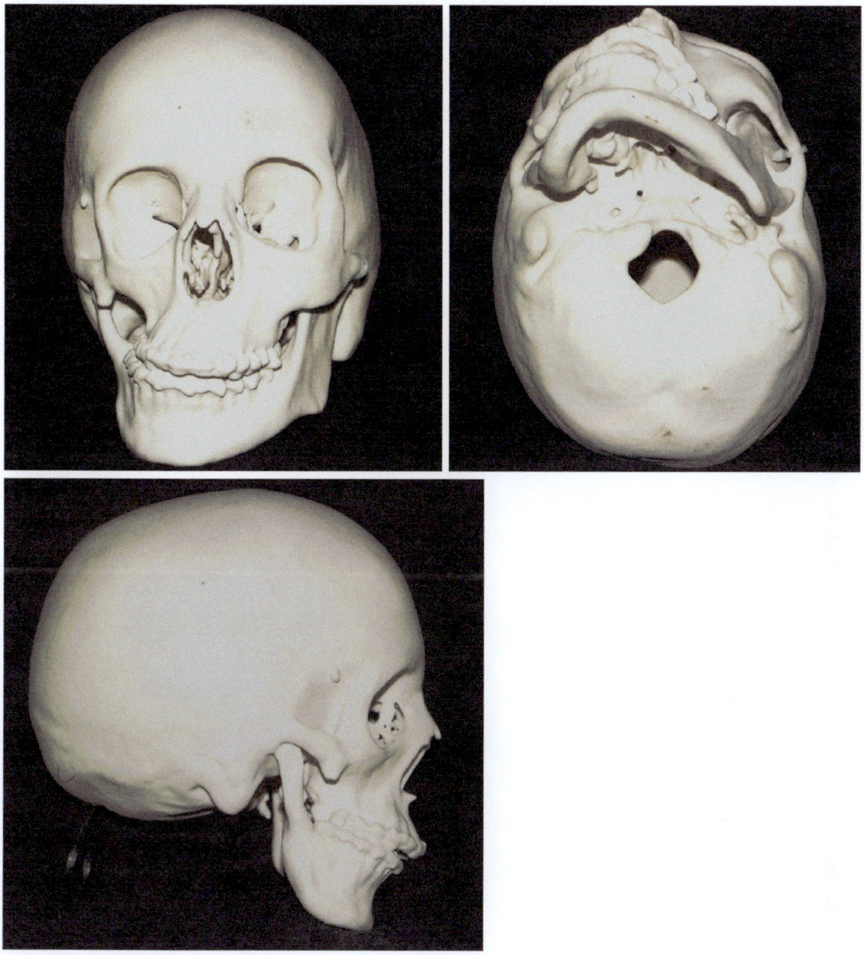

Fig. 5 (continued)

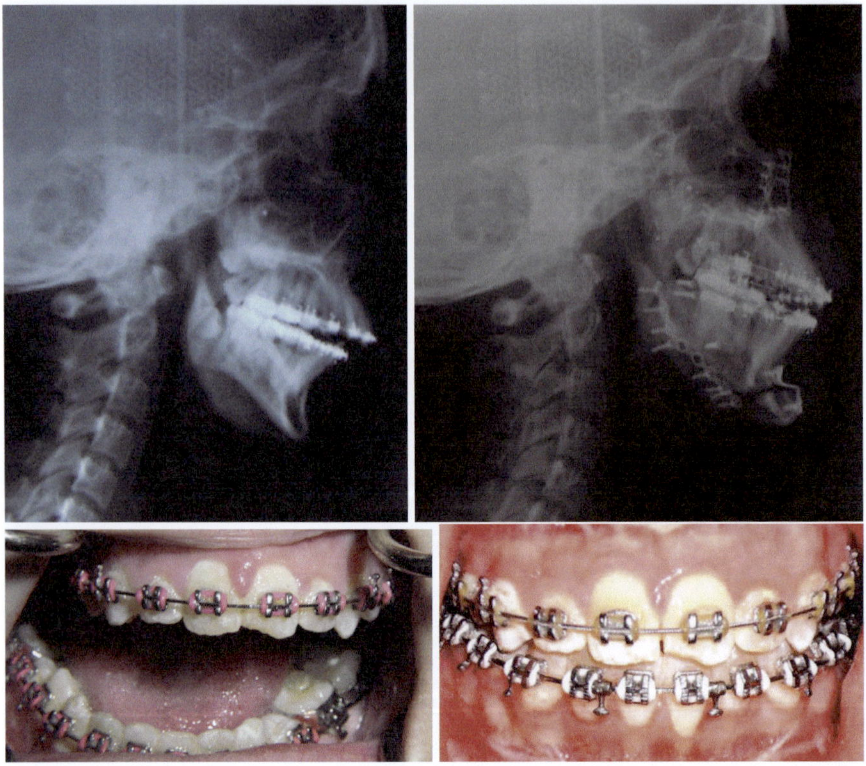

Fig. 5 (continued)

bulk to the lateral facial soft tissues if necessary. A custom-fabricated total joint TMJ prosthesis can be used to replace a missing or severely deficient joint and can be introduced in conjunction with orthognathic surgery. Virtual surgical planning allows for the simultaneous planning of custom joint prosthesis and the maxillary and mandibular osteotomies with a high degree of precision (Figs. 8, 9, 10, 11, 12, and 13).

Orthognathic surgical techniques are almost always preferable when compared with techniques based on distraction osteogenesis because of the predictability, precision, and stability offered by orthognathic surgery completed at skeletal maturity. This is especially true considering advances in three-dimensional virtual planning. Additionally, complications of distraction techniques have been described and include infection, malocclusion, trismus, and device failure, with complication rates that are still being underreported [73, 75].

In terms of imaging and surgical planning, it is often helpful to use virtual surgical planning from three-dimensional computed tomography images and stereolithographic models to precisely plan surgical movements for patients with complex

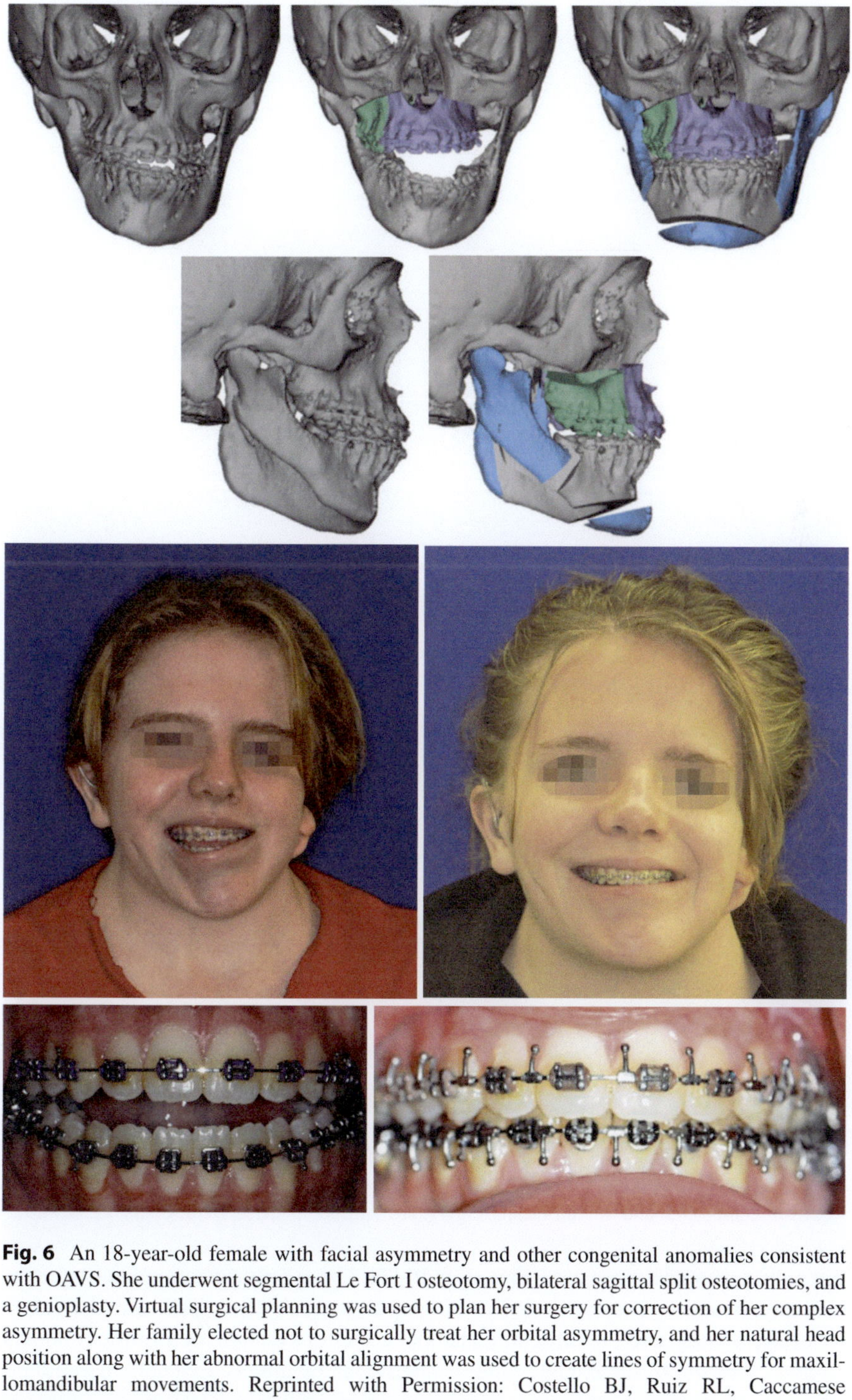

Fig. 6 An 18-year-old female with facial asymmetry and other congenital anomalies consistent with OAVS. She underwent segmental Le Fort I osteotomy, bilateral sagittal split osteotomies, and a genioplasty. Virtual surgical planning was used to plan her surgery for correction of her complex asymmetry. Her family elected not to surgically treat her orbital asymmetry, and her natural head position along with her abnormal orbital alignment was used to create lines of symmetry for maxillomandibular movements. Reprinted with Permission: Costello BJ, Ruiz RL, Caccamese JF. "Oculoauriculovertebral Spectrum: Staged Reconstruction." Oral and Maxillofacial Surgery, 3rd Edition. Elsevier, 2018. Ch 39. Pg 687–702

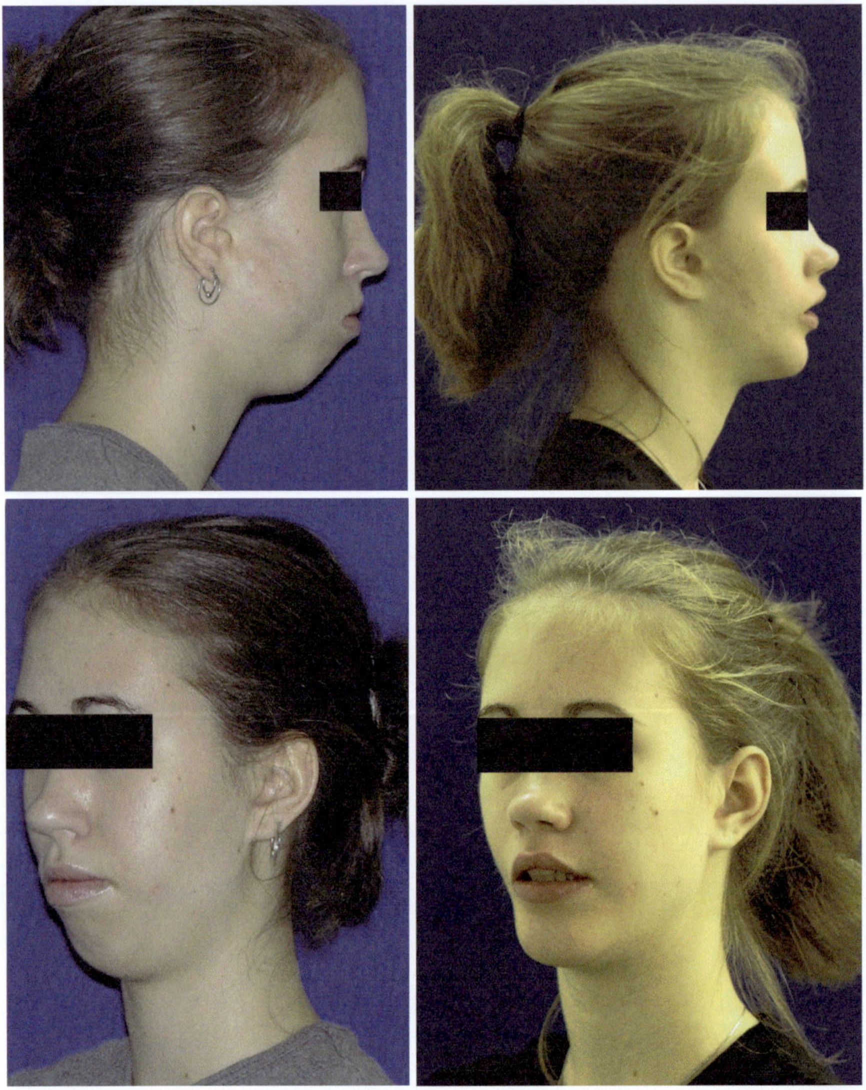

Fig. 7 A teenage female with type IIA oculoauriculovertebral spectrum (OAVS) and a Tessier No. 7 cleft (repaired by another surgeon) is seen preoperatively and postoperatively. She underwent Le Fort I osteotomy, bilateral sagittal split osteotomies, and a double-stack genioplasty. Reprinted with Permission: Costello BJ, Ruiz RL, Caccamese JF. "Oculoauriculovertebral Spectrum: Staged Reconstruction." Oral and Maxillofacial Surgery, 3rd Edition. Elsevier, 2018. Ch 39. Pg 687–702

three-dimensional asymmetry (Figs. 5, 6, 9, 11). Using only posterior anterior cephalometric and lateral cephalometric radiographs generally underestimates the severity of asymmetry and the three-dimensional complexity of the deformities and has largely fallen out of favor. Obtaining detailed imaging data is especially paramount

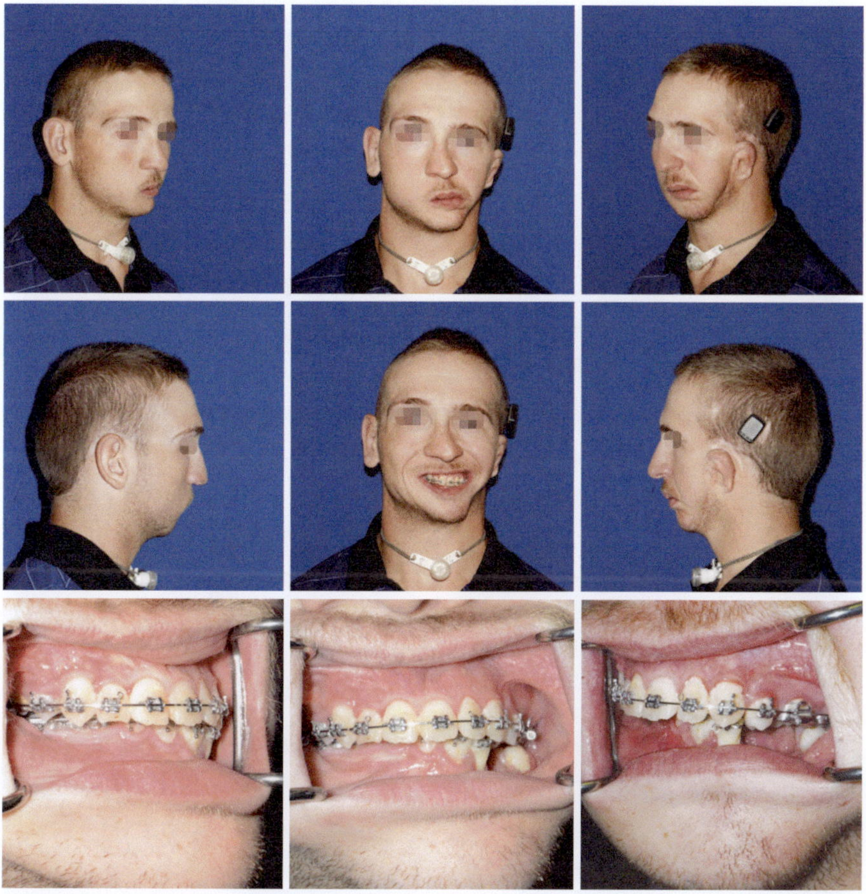

Fig. 8 A 17-year-old male patient with Goldenhar syndrome and associated symptoms of hypoplasia of multiple structures on the left face including ear, midface, and mandibular deformities. The patient previously underwent three rounds of mandibular distraction during early childhood as well as a costochondral graft to treat the left TMJ and mandible deformities. Note that the mandibular tooth under the left maxillary canine is actually the right lateral incisor, which has been shifted leftward due to disproportionate growth. At this point, the patient's maximal opening was no greater than 15 mm

for patients in whom previous reconstruction or distraction techniques have been attempted, but their asymmetry is still significant. These patients may be excessively long in the vertical dimension but still hypoplastic in the transverse and sagittal dimensions, making the postoperative deformity more difficult to reconstruct than the original presentation [6].

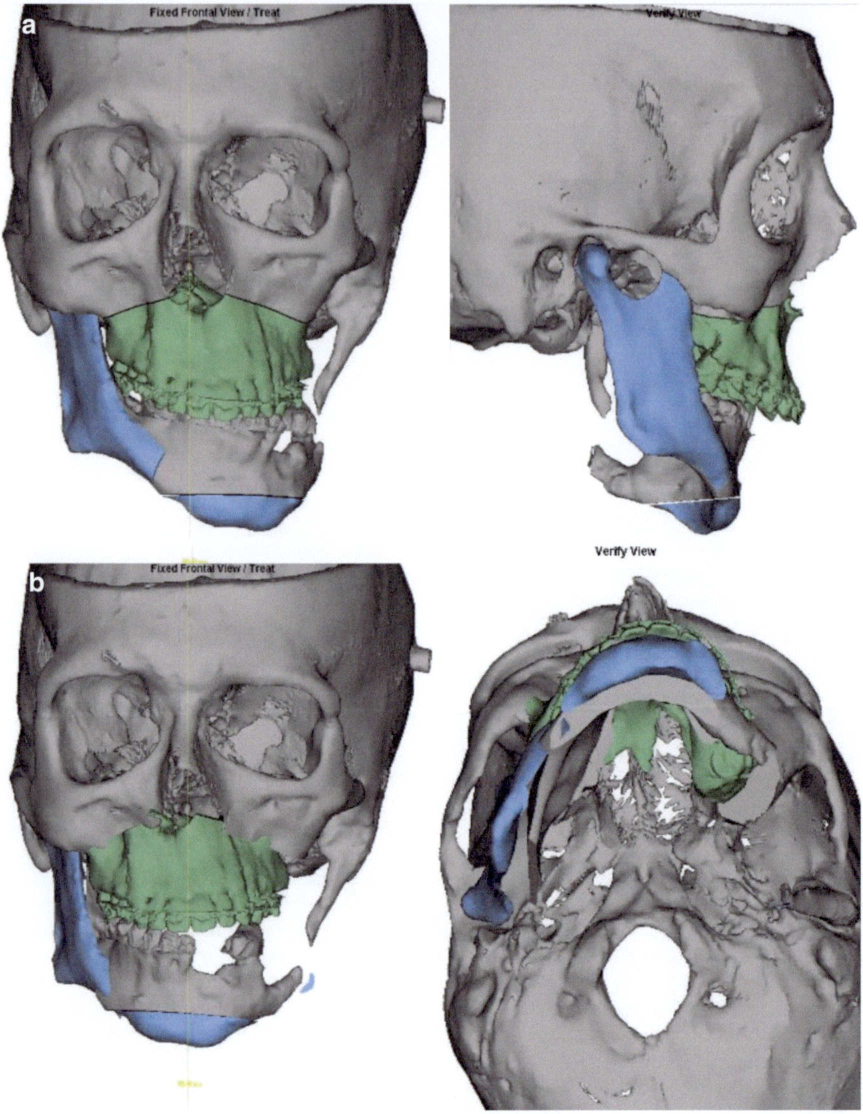

Fig. 9 (**a**, **b**) Three-dimensional renditions of the patient during virtual surgical planning. Virtual surgical planning was used in treatment planning and involved moving the lower incisor 28 mm to the right and 23 mm anteriorly. This surgery was intended to be the first stage of a two-stage surgery involving also a total joint replacement using TMJ Concepts to replace the nonfunctioning costochondral graft

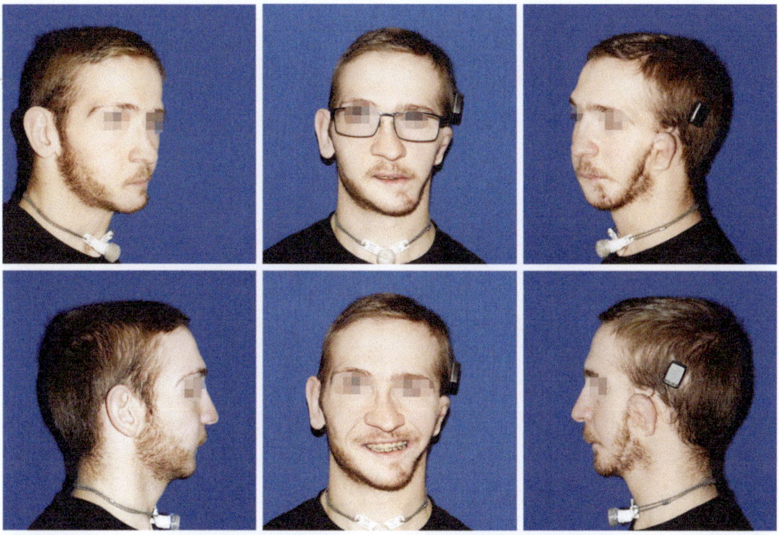

Fig. 10 The same patient after orthognathic surgery involving LeFort 1, bilateral sagittal split and genioplasty osteotomies. Note that the patient's mandible deviates to the left at rest

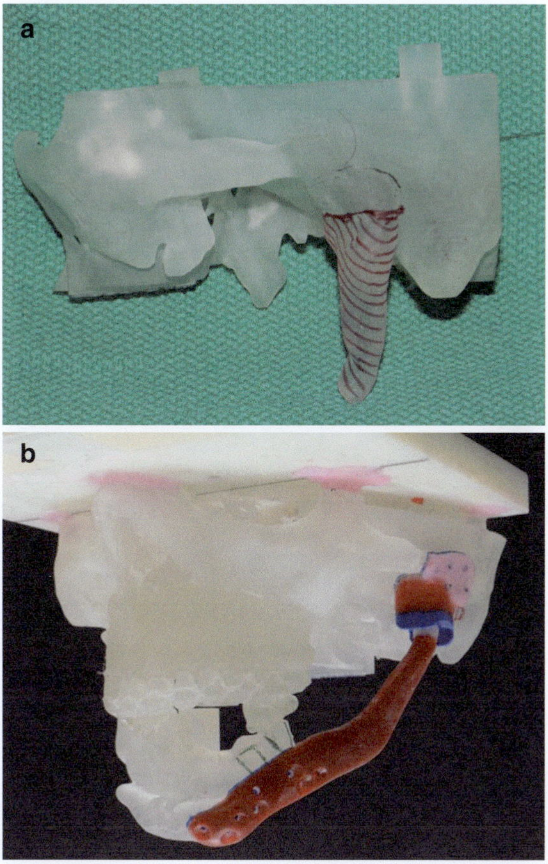

Fig. 11 (**a**, **b**) Stereolithographic models showing the fused costochondral graft with the highlighted portion denoting bone to remove prior to inserting total joint prosthesis. Wax-up model of TMJ total joint prosthesis shows more favorable mandibular positioning and symmetry

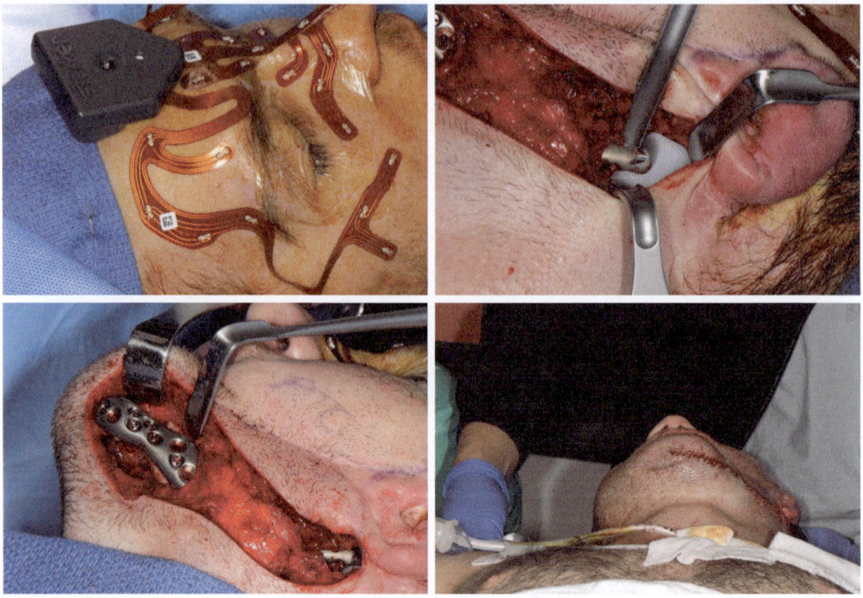

Fig. 12 Intraoperative images of the second surgery, undertaken 1 year after the initial orthognathic surgery. Dynamic navigation was used to assist in the condylectomy of the costochondral graft, which had fused to the skull base. It was found on planning CT scans that the external carotid artery was in extreme proximity to the medial surface of the pseudo-condyle. Adequate seating of the TMJ prosthesis was verified intraoperatively, and the worm's eye view of the immediate postoperative patient shows good midline positioning of the mandible

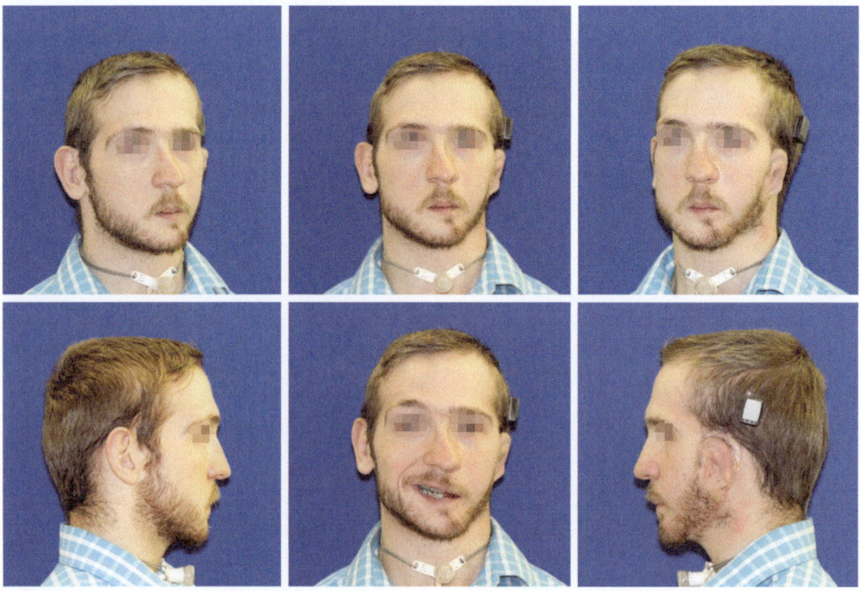

Fig. 13 Patient approximately 1 month after left TMJ total joint replacement showing increased opening well as improved facial symmetry

Management of Soft Tissues

Developmental abnormalities involving the external ear commonly found in OAVS patients, and in some patients, may be the only significant finding (Fig. 2). At their mildest, these ear abnormalities present as small skin tags or preauricular pits which are amenable to simple excision or revision. More commonly, patients present with significant asymmetry, malposition, or malformation of the ear that include deformities of the external helix, microtia, or even complete anotia. Many of these patients will benefit from reconstructive efforts which are often technically challenging, and esthetically acceptable results are difficult to achieve [20, 71].

Several options are currently available for reconstruction of a missing or severely malformed external ear: staged reconstruction with an autogenous cartilage rib graft, temporoparietal fascial flaps or local skin flaps, placement of craniofacial implants to support a maxillofacial prosthesis, and placement of a carefully designed porous polyethylene implant under a skin flap. There are advantages and shortcomings to each option. Chondral grafts require multiple procedures to reconstruct the ear, and considerable experience of an expert is required to achieve an ear with an esthetically acceptable appearance. Cartilage is typically harvested from the contralateral sixth–eighth ribs to reconstruct the external ear. This technique-sensitive procedure is usually completed between the ages of 6 and 10, or later [71, 76–81].

An implant-supported prosthesis can provide excellent esthetics, but it is removable. Additionally, implants placed to support an ear prosthesis require diligent cleaning to avoid irritation and inflammation of the skin. Three-dimensional planning, computer-aided design, and surgical navigation have been used to aid in successful placement of implant-supported prostheses [8].

Implantable prostheses made from porous polyethylene (such as MEDPOR®) can also be used to achieve excellent esthetic results. These products, however, pose a lifetime infection risk and might need to be removed. Removal of an infected prosthesis and the resultant scar renders other reconstructive options more difficult in these cases. Adequate blood flow to the auricular area is crucial for their success, so it may be prudent to complete angiography prior to planning to ensure success. When comparing polyethylene implants to chondral grafts, some surgeons have suggested that polyethylene may provide better esthetic outcomes with fewer surgeries, but at the cost of the aforementioned risk of infection [80].

Some patients with OAVS may exhibit conductive or sensorineural hearing loss. Banded conductive hearing devices can be used to overcome hearing loss in certain cases (Fig. 1). Some patients will present with conductive hearing loss only; in these cases, a bone-anchored hearing device can be considered after the age of 5–7 years. These titanium devices are implanted into the temporal bone posterior to the ear. In some patients, hearing loss is attributed to auditory canal stenosis or atresia. They can also present with ankylosis or absence of the ossicles. A few select patients may be candidates for cochlear implants or other surgical procedures to correct abnormalities of the middle ear. If these interventions are attempted, it is prudent to complete them prior to external ear reconstruction to ensure that the auricle is in the optimal position for functional surgical reconstruction. These middle ear surgeries are usually not undertaken, because most patients with hearing loss as a result of deformities of this type will not regain significant hearing ability on the affected side. They will have to rely on the unaffected side [20, 71]. A pediatric otolaryngologist and audiologist should be involved in the care of these patients from birth as part of the interdisciplinary team to help determine which interventions are possible, and which are necessary.

Other facial soft tissue structures may require augmentation. For example, the soft tissue bulk of the lateral face may be deficient even after treatment of skeletal deformity by orthognathic surgery. When a microvascular fibular flap is used to reconstruct the ramus, a de-epithelializing skin paddle can be brought up with it to contribute to facial bulk. Onlay grafts or alloplastic implants can also be used over the mandibular ramus or body to add to facial bulk in an attempt to provide symmetry. As with alloplastic ear reconstruction, these implants can unfortunately present a lifetime risk of infection. Another technique has been the use of fat transfer to add to facial bulk. Abdominal fat can be used for this application, but these grafts tend to resorb over time and thus may not provide a lasting result, even with specialized techniques [82–84].

Finally, it is important to note that functional and esthetic outcomes will depend heavily on the degree of severity that the patient exhibits. Patients with a severe phenotype often have a reduced potential when compared to their counterparts with only mild hypoplasia. While this may be intuitive to the experience provider, it is crucial to communicate with patients and parents that perfect symmetry may not be possible and is often not present in unaffected individuals in the population either.

Conclusions

OAVS is a complex three-dimensional congenital hypoplasia affecting neural crest migration and the tissues associated with the first and second branchial arches. Often, OAVS does not follow a clear pattern of genetic inheritance and thus is not usually possible to detect early or to plan for. Deformities are unilateral in the majority of cases and can involve the maxilla, mandible, zygoma, eyes, ears, and vertebrae. Treatment of facial abnormalities is best approached in a staged manner, first addressing severe functional concerns and esthetic components that pose psychosocial distress. While there is some ongoing controversy in the area of growth, evidence suggesting that OAVS deformities remain stable over time is more compelling. The most predictable outcomes can be achieved using orthognathic surgery at the completion of growth. With the advent of virtual surgical planning, the precision of these techniques has improved.

References

1. Goldenhar M. Associations malformatives de l'oel et de l'oreille, en particular le syndrome dermoide epimoide epibulbaire-appendices auriculaires-fistula auris congenital et ses relations avec la dysostose mandibulofaciale. J Genet Hum. 1952;1:243–82.
2. Gorlin RJ, Jue KL, Jacobsen NP, Goldschmidt E. Oculoauriculovertebral dysplasia. J Pediatr. 1963;63:991–9.
3. Gorlin RJ, Cohen MM, Hennekam RCM. Syndromes of the head and neck. New York: Oxford Press; 2001. p. 790–8.
4. Cohen MM, Rollnick BR, Kaye CI. Oculoauriculovertebral spectrum: an updated critique. Cleft Palate J. 1989;26:276–86.
5. Gabbett MT, Robertson SP, Broadbent R, Aftimos S, Sachdev R, Nezarati MM. Characterizing the oculoauriculofrontonasal syndrome. Clin Dysmorphol. 2008;17(2):79–85.
6. Costello BJ, Ruiz RL, Caccamese JF. Ch 39: Oculoauriculovertebral spectrum: staged reconstruction. In: Oral and maxillofacial surgery. 3rd ed. Elsevier; 2018. p. 687–702.
7. Evans KN, Gruss JS, Khanna PC, Cunningham ML, Cox TC, Hing AV. Oculoauriculofrontonasal syndrome: case series revealing new bony nasal anomalies in an old syndrome. Am J Med Genet A. 2013;161A(6):1345–53.
8. Morrison PJ, Mulholland HC, Craig BG, Nevin NC. Cardiovascular abnormalities in the oculo-auriculo-vertebral spectrum (Goldenhar syndrome). Am. J. Med. Genet. 1992;44:425–8.
9. Hennekam RCM, Krantz ID, Allanson JE. Branchial arch and oral-acral disorders. Gorlin's Syndromes of the Head and Neck. 5th ed. New York: Oxford Univ Press (pub.); 2010. p. 879–87.
10. Connor JM, Fernandez C. Genetic aspects of hemifacial microsomia. (Letter). Hum Genet. 1984;68:349 only.
11. Boles DJ, Bodurtha J, Nance WE. Goldenhar complex in discordant monozygotic twins: a case report and review of the literature. Am. J. Med. Genet. 1987;28:103–9.
12. Rollnick BR, Kaye CI, Nagatoshi K, et al. Oculoauriculovertebral dysplasia and variants: phenotypic characteristics of 294 patients. Am J Med Genet. 1987;26:361–75.
13. Burck U. Genetic aspects of hemifacial microsomia. Hum Genet. 1983;64:291–6.
14. Choong YF, Watts P, Little E, Beck L. Goldenhar and cri-du-chat syndromes: a contiguous gene deletion syndrome? J. AAPOS. 2003;7:226–7.
15. Kobrynski L, Chitayat D, Zahed L, McGregor D, Rochon L, Brownstein S, Vekemans M, Albert DL. Trisomy 22 and facioauriculovertebral (Goldenhar) sequence. Am J Med Genet. 1993;46:68–71.
16. Lammer E. Preliminary observations on isotretinoin-induced ear malformations and pattern formation of the external ear. J Craniofac Genet Dev Biol. 1991;11:292–5.
17. Werler MM, Sheehan JE, Hayes C, Mitchell AA, Mulliken JB. Vasoactive exposures, vascular events, and hemifacial microsomia. Birth Defects Res A Clin Mol Teratol. 2004a;70:389–95.
18. Wang R, Martinez-Frias ML, Graham JM Jr. Infants of diabetic mothers are at increased risk for the oculo-auriculo-vertebral sequence: a case-based and case-control approach. J Pediat. 2002;141:611–7.
19. Wieczorek D, Ludwig M, Boehringer S, Jongbloet PH, Gillessen-Kaesbach G, Horsthemke B. Reproduction abnormalities and twin pregnancies in parents of sporadic patients with oculo-auriculo-vertebral spectrum/Goldenhar syndrome. Hum Genet. 2007;121:369–76.
20. Posnick JC. Craniofacial and maxillofacial surgery in children and young adults. Philadelphia: WB Saunders; 2000. p. 419–45.
21. Poswillo DE. The pathogenesis of the first and second branchial arch syndrome. Oral Surg. 1973;35:302–29.
22. Poswillo DE. Otomandibular deformity: pathogenesis as a guide to reconstruction. J Maxillofac Surg. 1974;2:64–72.
23. Johnston MC, Bronsky PT. Prenatal craniofacial development: new insights on normal and abnormal mechanisms. Crit Rev Oral Biol Med. 1995;6:368–422.

24. Johnston MC, Bronsky PT. Craniofacial embryogenesis: abnormal developmental mechanisms. In: Mooney MP, Siegel MI, editors. Understanding craniofacial anomalies: the etiopathogenesis of craniosynostosis and facial clefting. New York: Wiley and Sons; 2002. p. 61–124.
25. Avon SW, Shively MD. Orthopedic manifestations of Goldenhar syndrome. J Pediatr Orthop. 1988;6:683–6.
26. Kane AA, Lo LJ, Christensen GE, Vannier MW, Marsh JL. Relationship between bone and muscles of mastication in hemifacial microsomia. Plast Reconstr Surg. 1997;99(4):990–7.
27. Castori M, Brancati F, Rinaldi R, Adami L, Mingarelli R, Grammatico P, Dallapiccola B. Antenatal presentation of the oculo-auriculo-vertebral spectrum (OAVS). Am J Med Genet Part A. 2006;140A:1573–9.
28. Rahbar R, Robson C, Mulliken JB, et al. Craniofacial, temporal bone, and audiologic abnormalities in the spectrum of hemifacial microsomia. Archiv Otolaryngol Head Neck Surg. 2001;127:265–71.
29. Pruzansky S. Not all dwarfed mandibles are alike. Birth Defects. 1969;4:120.
30. Murray JE, Kaban LB, Mulliken JB. Analysis and treatment of hemifacial microsomia. Plast Reconstr Surg. 1984;74:186–99.
31. Meurman Y. Congenital microtia and meatal atresia. Arch Otolaryngol. 1957;66:443.
32. Vento AR, LaBrie RA, Mulliken JB. OMENS classification of hemifacial microsomia. 1989;28:312–7.
33. Horgan JE, Padwa BL, LaBrie RA, Mulliken JB. OMENS-plus: analysis of craniofacial and extracraniofacial anomalies in hemifacial microsomia. Cleft Palate Craniofac J. 1995;32:405–12.
34. Poon C, Meara JG, Heggie A. Hemifacial microsomia: use of the OMENS-Plus classification at the Royal Children's Hospital of Melbourne. Plast Reconstr Surg. 2003;111:1011–8.
35. Kaban LB, Mulliken JB, Murray JE. Three-Dimensional approach to analysis and treatment of hemifacial microsomia. Cleft Palate Craniofac J. 1981;18:90–9.
36. Kaban LB, Padwa BL, Mulliken JB. Surgical correction of mandibular hypoplasia in hemifacial microsomia: the case for treatment in early childhood. J Oral Maxillofac Surg. 1998;56:628–38.
37. Madrid JRP, Montealegre G, Gomez V. A New Classification Based on the Kaban's Modification for Surgical Management of Craniofacial Microsomia. Craniomaxillofacial Trauma & Reconstruction. 2010;3(1):1–7.
38. Polley JW, Figueroa AA, Liou EJ, Cohen M. Longitudinal analysis of mandibular asymmetry in hemifacial microsomia. Plast Reconstr Surg. 1997;99(2):328–39.
39. Meazzini MC, Mazzoleni F, Bozzetti A, Brusati R. Comparison of mandibular vertical growth in hemifacial microsomia patients treated with early distraction or not treated: follow up till the completion of growth. J Craniomaxillofac Surg. 2012;40(2):105–11.
40. Ongkosuwito EM, Van Vooren J, Van Neck JW, et al. Changes of mandibular ramal height, during growth in unilateral hemifacial microsomia patients and unaffected controls. J Craniomaxillofac Surg. 2013;41(2):92–7.
41. Ongkosuwito EM, Van Neck JW, Wattel E, Van Adrichem LN, Kuijpers-Jagtman AM. Craniofacial morphology in unilateral hemifacial microsomia. Br J Oral Maxillofac Surg. 2013;51(8):902–7.
42. Kaban LB, Moses MH, Mulliken JB. Surgical correction of hemifacial microsomia in the growing child. Plast Reconstr Surg. 1988;82(1):9–19.
43. Kearns GJ, Padwa BL, Mulliken JB, Kaban LB. Progression of facial asymmetry in hemifacial microsomia. Plast Reconstr Surg. 2000;105(2):492–8.
44. Posnick JC. Surgical correction of mandibular hypoplasia in hemifacial microsomia: A personal perspective. P J Oral Maxillofac Surg. 1998;56(5):639–50.
45. Cohen SR, Levitt CA, Simms C, Burstein FD. Airway disorders in hemifacial microsomia. Plastic Reconstruct Surg. 1999;103(I):27–33.
46. Chang AB, Masters IB, Williams GR, Harris M, O'neil MC. A modified nasopharyngeal tube to relieve high upper airway obstruction. Pediatr Pulmonol. 2000;29(4):299–306.

47. Wagener S, Rayatt SS, Tatman AJ, Gornall P, Slator P, Slator R. Management of infants with Pierre Robin sequence. Cleft Palate Craniofac J. 2003;40:180–5.
48. Sesenna E, Magri AS, Magnani C, Brevi BC, Anghinoni ML. Mandibular distraction in neonates: indications, technique, results. Italian Journal of Pediatrics. 2012;38:7. https://doi.org/10.1186/1824-7288-38-7.
49. Peacock ZS, et al. Long-term effects of distraction osteogenesis of the mandible. J Oral Maxillofac Surg. 1998;76(7):1512–23.
50. Burstein FD, Cohen SR, Scott PH, Teague GR, Montgomery GL, Kattos AV. Surgical therapy for severe refractory sleep apnea in infants and children: application of the airway zone concept. Plast Reconstr Surg. 1995;96(1):34–41.
51. Caccamese JF, Costello BJ, Mooney MP. A novel deformity of the mandible in oculo-auriculovertebral spectrum: a case report and literature review. J Oral Maxillofac Surg. 2006;64:1278–82.
52. Woods RH, Varma S, David DJ, Tessier no. 7 cleft: a new subclassification and management protocol. Plast Reconstr Surg. 2008;122(3):898–905.
53. Dentino KM, Valstar A, Padwa BL. Cleft characteristics and treatment outcomes in hemifacial microsomia compared to non-syndromic cleft lip/palate. Int J Oral Maxillofac Surg. 2016;45(6):679–82.
54. Shprintzen RJ, Lewin ML, Croft BC, et al. A comprehensive study of the pharyngeal flap surgery: tailor made flaps. Cleft Palate Craniofac J. 1979;16:46–55.
55. Peltomaki T, Vahatalo K, Ronning O. The effect of a unilateral costochondral graft on the growth of the marmoset mandible. J Oral Maxillofac Surg. 2002;60(11):1307–14.; discussion 1314–1315.
56. Peltomaki T. Growth of a costochondral graft in the rat temporomandibular joint. J Oral Maxillofac Surg. 1992;50(8):851–7.
57. Padwa BL, Mulliken JB, Maghen A, Kaban LB. Midfacial growth after costochondral graft construction of the mandibular ramus in hemifacial microsomia. J Oral Maxillofac Surg. 1998;56:122–7.
58. Wax MK, Winslow CP, Hansen J, et al. A retrospective analysis of temporomandibular joint reconstruction with free fibula microvascular flap. Laryngoscope. 2000;110(6):977–81.
59. Chu TM, Hollister SJ, Halloran JW, et al. Manufacturing and characterization of 3-D hydroxyapatite bone tissue engineering scaffolds. Ann NY Acad Sci. 2000;961:114–7.
60. Zhu S, Hu J, Li J, Ying B. Reconstruction of mandibular condyle by transport distraction osteogenesis: experimental study in rhesus monkey. J Oral Maxillofac Surg. 2006;64:1487–92.
61. Polley JW, Figueroa AA. Distraction osteogenesis: its application in severe mandibular deformities in hemifacial microsomia. J Craniofac Surg. 1997;8:422–31.
62. Stucki-McCormick S. Reconstruction of the mandibular condyle using transport distraction osteogenesis. J Craniofac Surg. 1997;8:48–52.
63. Hijiki H, Takato T, Matsumato S, Mori Y. Experimental study of reconstruction of the temporomandibular joint using a bone transport technique. J Oral Maxillofac Surg. 2000;58:1270–6.
64. Mommaerts MY, Nagy K. Is early osteodistraction a solution for the ascending ramus compartment in hemifacial microsomia?. A literature study. J Craniomaxillofac Surg. 2002;30:201–7.
65. McCarthy JG, Hopper RA, Hollier LH, et al. Molding of the regenerate in mandibular distraction: clinical experience. Plast Reconstr Surg. 2003;115:1239–46.
66. Huisinga-Fischer CE, Vaandrager JM, Prahl-Andersen B. Longitudinal results of mandibular distraction osteogenesis in hemifacial microsomia. J Craniofac Surg. 2003;14:933–4.
67. Kunz C, Brauchli L, Moehle T, et al. Theoretical considerations for the surgical correction of mandibular deformity in hemifacial microsomia patients using multifocal distraction osteogenesis. J Oral Maxillofac Surg. 2003;61:364–8.
68. Troulis MJ, Kaban LB. Complications of mandibular distraction osteogenesis. Oral Maxillofacial Surg Clin N Am. 2003;15:251–64.
69. Heffez LB, Kirton M. Vector control in transportation osteogenesis. J Oral Maxillofac Surg. 2005;63:737–46.

70. Neelakandan RS, Bhargava D. Transport Distraction Osteogenesis for Maxillomandibular Reconstruction: Current Concepts and Applications. J Maxillofac Oral Surg. 2012;11(3):291–9.
71. Posnick JC. Ch 28: "Hemifacial Microsomia: Evaluation and Treatment". In: Orthognathic Surgery, Principles & Practice. Saunders; 2013.
72. Nagy K, Kujpers-Jagtman AM, Mommaerts MY. No evidence for long-term effectiveness of early osteodistraction in hemifacial microsomia. Plast Reconstruct Surg. 2009;124:2061–71.
73. Verlinden CRA, et al. Complications of mandibular distraction osteogenesis for congenital deformities: a systematic review of the literature and proposal of a new classification for complications. Int J Oral Maxillofac Surg. 2015;44(1):37–43.
74. Farias M, Vargervik K. Dental development in hemifacial microsomia, eruption and agenesis. Pediatr Dentistry. 1998;10(2):140–3.
75. Swennen G, Schliephake H, Dempf R, Schierle H, Malevez C. Craniofacial distraction osteogenesis: a review of the literature. Part 1: Clinical studies. Int J Oral Maxillofac Surg. 2001;30:89–103.
76. Kelley PE, Scholes MA. Microtia and congenital aural atresia. Otolaryngol Clin N Am. 2007;40:61–80. vi.
77. Tanzer RC. The total reconstruction of the auricle: the evolution of a plan of treatment. Plast Reconstr Surg. 1971;47:523.
78. Brent B. The correction of microtia with autogenous cartilage grafts: the classic deformity I+II. Plast Reconstr Surg. 1980;66:1–21.
79. Brent B. Microtia repair with rib cartilage grafts: a review of personal experience with 1000 cases. Clin Plast Surg. 2002;29:251–25.
80. Constantine KK, Gilmore J, Lee K, Leach J Jr. Comparison of microtia reconstruction outcomes using rib cartilage vs porous polyethylene implant. JAMA Facial Plast Surg. 2014;16:240.
81. Weissler JM, Sosin M, Dorafshar AH, Garcia JR. Combining Virtual Surgical Planning, Intraoperative Navigation, and 3-Dimensional Printing in Prosthetic-Based Bilateral Microtia Reconstruction. J Oral Maxillofac Surg. 2017;75(7):1491–7.
82. Reiche-Fischel O, Wolford LM, Pitta M. Facial contour reconstruction using an autologous free fat graft: a case report with 18-year follow-up. J Oral Maxillofac Surg. 2000;58:103–6.
83. Tanna N, Broer PN, Roostaeian J, Bradley JP, Levine JP, Saadeh PB. Soft tissue correction of craniofacial microsomia and progressive hemifacial atrophy. J Craniofac Surg. 2012;23:2024–7.
84. Mazzola RF, Cantarella G, Torretta S, Sbarbati A, Lazzari L, Pignataro L. Autologous fat injection to face and neck: from soft tissue augmentation to regenerative medicine. Acta Otorhinolaryngologica Italica. 2011;31:59–69.

Facial Asymmetry Caused by Condylar Hyperplasia

Larry M. Wolford

Abstract

Hyperplasia indicates the increased production and growth of normal cells in a tissue or organ without an increase in the size of the cells but the affected part becomes larger yet retains its basic form. Condylar hyperplasia (CH) is a generic term describing conditions that cause excessive growth and enlargement of the mandibular condyle. There are a number of suggested etiologies of CH including neoplasia, trauma, infection, abnormal condylar loading, and aberrant growth factors. These condylar pathologies can adversely affect the size and morphology of the mandible, alter the occlusion, indirectly affect the maxilla, with resultant development or worsening of dentofacial deformities such as; mandibular prognathism, unilateral enlargement of the condyle, neck, ramus, and body; facial asymmetry; malocclusion; and pain. Some CH pathologies occur more commonly within particular age ranges and gender. Identifying the specific CH pathology will provide insight to: Its progression if untreated; the clinical, imaging, and histologic characteristics; as well as treatment protocols proven to eliminate the pathological processes and provide optimal functional and esthetic outcomes.

Keywords

Condylar hyperplasia · Condylar hypoplasia · Osteochondroma · Condylectomy Facial asymmetry

L. M. Wolford (✉)
Departments of Oral and Maxillofacial Surgery and Orthodontics, Texas A&M, University College of Dentistry, Baylor University Medical Center, Dallas, TX, USA
e-mail: lwolford@drlarrywolford.com

P. Mehra, L. M. Wolford (eds.), *Management of Facial Asymmetry*,
https://doi.org/10.1007/978-3-030-44971-1_6

Hyperplasia indicates the increased production and growth of normal cells in a tissue or organ without an increase in the size of the cells, but the affected part becomes larger yet retains its basic form. Condylar hyperplasia (CH) is a generic term describing conditions that cause excessive growth and enlargement of the mandibular condyle. There are a number of suggested etiologies of CH including neoplasia, trauma, infection, abnormal condylar loading [1], and aberrant growth factors. These condylar pathologies can adversely affect the size and morphology of the mandible, alter the occlusion, and indirectly affect the maxilla, with resultant development or worsening of dentofacial deformities such as mandibular prognathism; unilateral enlargement of the condyle, neck, ramus, and body; facial asymmetry; malocclusion; and pain. Some CH pathologies occur more commonly within particular age ranges and gender. Identifying the specific CH pathology will provide insight to its progression if untreated; the clinical, imaging, and histologic characteristics; as well as treatment protocols proven to eliminate the pathological processes and provide optimal functional and esthetic outcomes.

Wolford et al. [2] developed a classification system to place patients with mandibular CH into categories based on histology, clinical and imaging characteristics, effects on the jaws and facial structures, and rate of occurrence. Four major categories are defined that reflect the occurrence rate, with CH Type 1A being the most common pathology and CH Type 4 the rarest. CH Type 1 is an accelerated and prolonged growth aberration of the "normal" mandibular condylar growth mechanism, causing a predominantly horizontal growth vector, resulting in prognathism that can occur bilaterally (CH Type 1A) or unilaterally (CH Type 1B). CH Type 2 refers to enlargement of the mandibular condyle caused by an osteochondroma, resulting in predominantly unilateral vertical overgrowth and elongation of the mandible and face. One of the forms has predominantly a vertical growth vector and condylar enlargement, but without exophytic tumor extensions (Type 2A), whereas the other primary form grows vertically but develops horizontal exophytic tumor growth off of the condyle (CH Type 2B). CH Type 3 includes other rare, benign tumors and CH Type 4 includes malignant conditions that originate in the mandibular condyle causing enlargement. This classification system for CH pathology should help the clinician understand the nature of the pathology, progression if untreated, recommended ages for surgical intervention to minimize adverse effects on subsequent facial growth and development in younger patients, and the surgical protocols to comprehensively and predictably treat these conditions. This chapter will focus on the most common forms of CH: Types 1 and 2.

Brief Description of the Condylar Hyperplasia (CH) Classification

CH Type 1: Onset usually occurs during puberty; an accelerated and prolonged growth aberration of the "normal" condylar growth mechanism causing condylar and mandibular elongation (prognathism); 60% female; growth is self-limiting, usually ending by the early to mid-20s, and can occur bilaterally (CH Type 1A) or unilaterally (CH Type 1B).

CH Type 2: A unilateral condylar enlarging pathology caused by an osteochondroma; can develop at any age (although 68% are initiated during the second decade); predominately in females (76%); and with a vertical overgrowth of the mandible. One growth vector causes predominately vertical elongation and enlargement of the condylar head and neck (Type 2A) and the other form additionally has an exophytic tumor growth off of the condyle (CH Type 2 B).

CH Type 3: Other benign tumors causing CH.

CH Type 4: Malignant tumors that originate in the condyle causing enlargement.

There have been other classifications applied to CH. Obwegeser et al. [3] described two different types of CH anomalies that correlate with the Wolford classification. Hemimandibular elongation (HE) describes a deformity creating horizontal displacement of the mandible and chin toward the contralateral side without significant vertical elongation (same as CH Type 1). Obwegeser stated this entity can be bilateral (same as CH Type 1A) or unilateral (same as CH Type 1B). The other anomaly is hemimandibular hyperplasia (HH) (same as CH Type 2) that includes enlargement on one side of the mandible as a tridimensional anomaly, involving the condyle, ramus, and body creating a unilateral vertical elongation deformity with the maxilla usually following the mandible creating a transverse cant in the occlusion and jaws. Obwegeser made a distinction between "exclusive hyperplasia of the condyle" (same as CH Type 2A) and "osseous tumor and exostosis of the condyle" (same as CH Type 2B). Nitzan et al. [4] described CH as a unilateral disorder in which the pathology occurs at the head of the condyle creating facial asymmetry in either the vertical or horizontal direction or a combination of both.

Normal Facial Growth

Two main types of bone play an integral role in the development of the facial skeleton: intramembranous and endochondral ossification. The facial structures are a hybrid of osteogenic mechanisms; the cranial vault, upper face, midface, and majority of the mandible arise from intramembranous ossification, while the cranial base and mandibular condyle are from endochondral sources. Developing bone receives genetic, chemical, hormonal, and/or mechanical signals that induce proliferation and differentiation, as well as impact the contour, shape, and volume of bone in any given area. The mandible is the last element to skeletally mature and is a keystone in the development of the facial skeleton, providing normal occlusion and the maintenance of anteroposterior and vertical facial balance [5]. Alteration or abnormal inflection of any of these stimuli could induce abnormal condylar growth.

Growth of cartilage is interstitial in nature; chondrocytes' multiplication and extracellular matrix synthesis are mainly controlled by interstitial genetics and epigenetic factors. During growth of primary cartilage, the matrix effectively isolates the dividing chondrocytes from the environmental influences. Chondral growth of TMJ cartilage is distinctly different. Because secondary cartilage grows primarily by apposition, with proliferation occurring in progenitor cells that are surrounded by substantial fewer matrixes, mechanical stimulation alters both the growth and differentiation of condylar secondary cartilage cells [6]. Hormonal stimulation from growth hormones and/or sex-based hormones may be a major factor in the development of CH Types 1 and 2. In our studies of CH Type 1 [2, 7], the onset is during the pubertal growth phase (usually between the ages of 11 and 15) and is more common in females (60%), which could indicate a possible female and/or growth hormonal stimulating factors. Our studies of CH Type 2 show that 68% of these cases develop during the second decade (ages 10 to 20) and predominately in females (76%) indicating a more probable relation to female hormonal stimulus [7, 8] perhaps in conjunction with growth hormones.

Although the specific cause of CH Types 1 and 2 has not been clearly identified, the strong predilection for initiation during the teenage years and the dominant occurrence of CH Types 1 and 2 in females support a theory of female and growth hormonal mediation. Estrogen receptors have been identified in the TMJs of female primates [9, 10], human TMJ tissues that appear to correlate to TMJ symptoms [11], and in arthritic knee joints [12]. Estrogen is known to mediate cartilage and bone metabolism in the female TMJ. An increase in receptors may predispose to the initiation of CH conditions. Further studies in this area are indicated to determine cause and effect.

Condylar Hyperplasia Type 1

CH Type 1 occurs in adolescence and the pathological process is usually initiated during the pubertal growth phase suggesting a hormonal etiology. Approximately 1/3 of the cases may be genetically related, but the other 2/3 occur spontaneous [13]. The gender distribution in our study was 60% female [2]. Normal jaw growth is usually 98% complete in females at age 15 years and in males at age 17–18 years [14]. CH Type 1 is an accelerated and excessive growth of the "normal" condylar growth mechanism creating overgrowth of the mandible predominately in a horizontal vector (mandibular prognathism) with the growth often continuing into the patient's early to mid-20s, but CH Type 1 is a self-limiting growth aberration. Patients may begin with a Class I occlusal and skeletal relationship as they enter their pubertal growth phase and grow into a Class III skeletal and occlusal

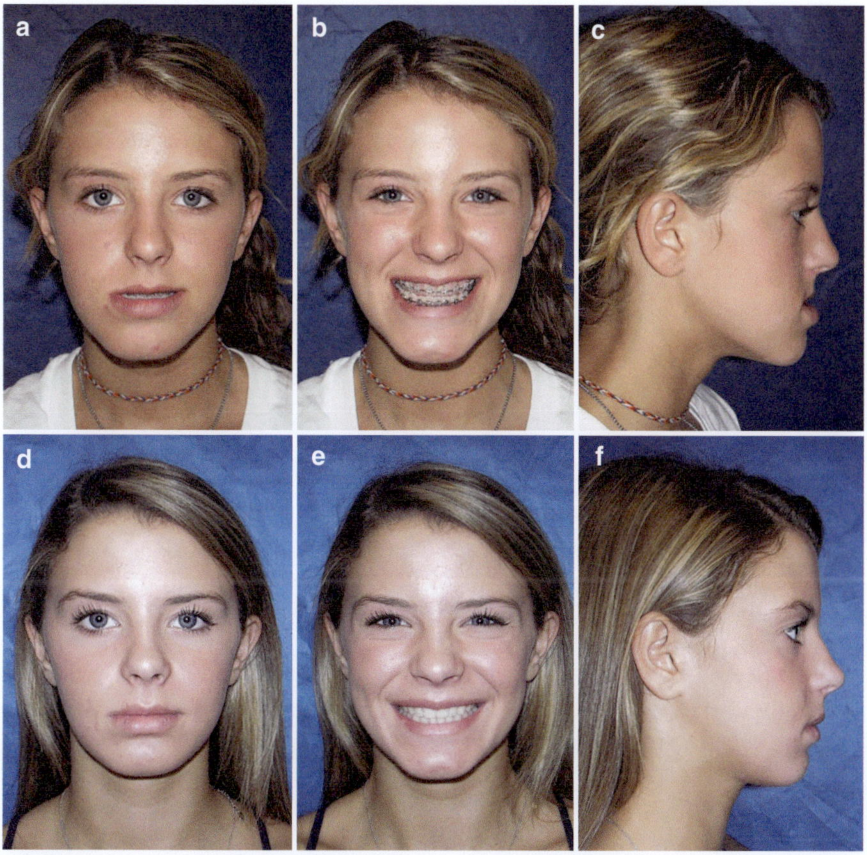

Fig. 1 Case 1, (**a**–**c**) This 14-year and 10-month-old patient reported that over the past 3–4 years, she developed a protruding lower jaw and a worsening bite relationship. The mandible was growing at an accelerated rate, confirmed with serial lateral cephalograms, secondary to CH Type 1A. This patient was treated in a single surgical stage with (1) bilateral high condylectomies and articular disc repositioning with Mitek anchors, (2) bilateral mandibular ramus osteotomies, (3) multiple maxillary osteotomies, (4) removal of impacted third molars, and (5) bilateral partial inferior turbinectomies. (**d**–**f**) At 2 years post-surgery, the patient maintains good facial symmetry and balance as well as a stable Class I skeletal and occlusal relationship

relationship (Figs. 1a–c, 2a–c, 3a) or begin as a Class III and develop into a worse Class III relationship. Condylar and mandibular growth can be accelerated bilaterally (CH Type 1A) or unilaterally (CH Type 1B) in a horizontal or uncommonly a vertical vector. The increase in the mandibular growth rate occurs in the condyle but causes elongation of the condylar head, neck, and mandibular body, which leads to development of a Class III skeletal and occlusal relation as well as dental compensations where the mandibular incisors can become lingually inclined and the maxillary incisors over-angulated [2, 7].

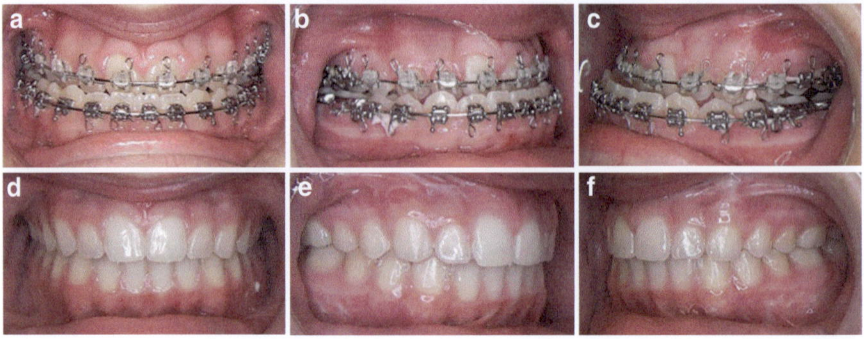

Fig. 2 Case 1, (**a–c**): Presurgery, a Class III occlusion was present, getting progressively worse. (**d–f**): The occlusion remained stable at 2 years post-surgery

Not all prognathic mandibles are caused by CH, but only those demonstrating accelerated, excessive mandibular growth that continues beyond the normal growth years. Differential diagnosis includes (1) Class III skeletal relationship with normal mandibular and maxillary growth, (2) deficient maxillary growth with a normal growing mandible, or (3) CH Type 1 with or without deficient maxillary growth. Differentiation must be clarified between CH Type 1 and maxillary growth deficiency (maxillary hypoplasia). Maxillary hypoplasia can also result in a Class III occlusal and skeletal relationship in the presence of a normal growing mandible with a resultant progressive worsening occlusion through the normal facial growth process (usually completed at age 15 for females and at age 17 to 18 for males) with stability of the jaw and occlusal relationship after that time. Maxillary hypoplasia creating the Class III relationship is usually evident years before the pubertal growth phase. Maxillary hypoplasia can also be present with accelerated mandibular growth (CH Type 1) creating a more extreme dentofacial deformity. However, the accelerated mandibular growth is usually not evident until initiated during pubertal growth. Deviated mandibular prognathism is usually related to bilateral CH Type 1A where one side is growing faster than the opposite side or CH Type 1B where only a unilateral condyle is involved in the accelerated growth process.

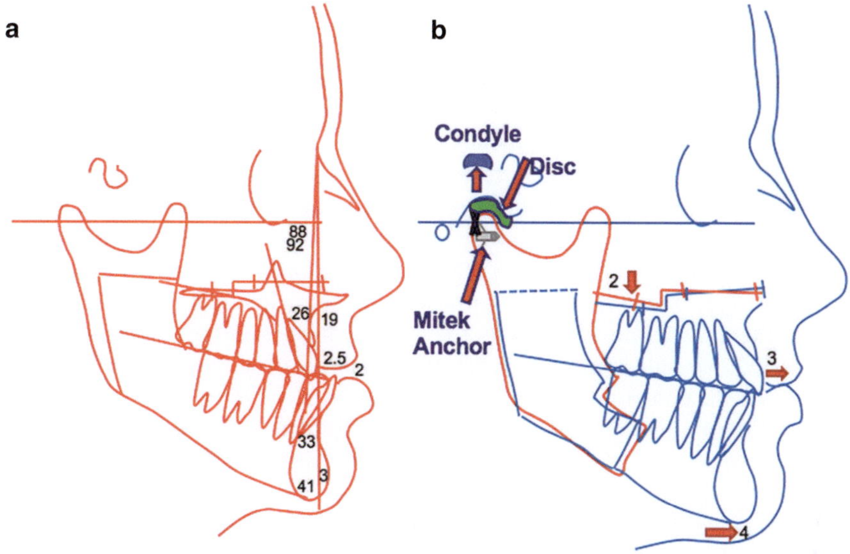

Fig. 3 Case 1, (**a**) Lateral cephalometric radiograph demonstrates the skeletal Class III relationship. (**b**) The surgical treatment objective included (1) bilateral high condylectomies, (2) bilateral disc repositioning with Mitek anchors, (3) bilateral mandibular ramus osteotomies, (4) multiple maxillary osteotomies, (5) removal of impacted third molars, and (6) partial reduction of the hyperplastic nasal inferior turbinates

Analysis of serial lateral cephalometric and lateral tomograms that include the TMJ, ramus, and mandibular body should allow determination of the growth rates of the maxilla and mandible to differentiate the source of the Class III occlusal and skeletal relationship. In CH Type 1, growth can usually be determined by worsening functional, esthetic, skeletal, and occlusal changes with serial assessments (preferably at 6- to 12-month intervals) consisting of clinical, dental model, and radiographic evaluations [2, 7].

During pubertal growth, the normal yearly growth rate of the mandible measuring on the lateral cephalogram from condylion to point B is 1.6 mm for females and 2.2 mm for males [14]. Growth significantly greater than the normal rate indicates accelerated growth likely related to CH Type 1. With asymmetric condylar growth, the amount of growth may be more difficult to determine from the lateral cephalogram because of the mandible shifting toward the side with less growth, essentially hiding some of the forward growth and elongation on the faster growing side. Thus, using lateral TMJ tomograms that include the mandibular body, posterior teeth, ramus, and condyle will allow superimposition of the body, ramus, and posterior teeth to analyze the amount of condylar growth over time for each side. A horizontal mandibular growth vector extending beyond the normal growth years will likely be CH Type 1, and the growth can continue into the mid-20s until cessation.

Bone scintigraphy of the TMJs will usually be nondiagnostic in determining active CH Type 1 growth. Healthy growing TMJs normally light up some in scintigraphy. The growth rate of CH Type 1 is not growing at a tumorous rate, as seen in CH Type 2, but only somewhat faster than the normal condylar growth rate and is confined to the thin proliferative layer; thus, it is usually difficult to differentiate CH Type 1 from normal growth, particularly if both joints are involved. In unilateral cases, it may also be difficult to determine an increased uptake on the involved side, particularly if the contralateral TMJ develops a displaced disc and associated arthritic changes (a common contralateral development) since this contralateral TMJ may also have a slight increased uptake. Wrist/hand radiographs provide no insight to CH Type 1 since there is no correlation between normal physiological development and the CH pathological process affecting the mandibular condyles.

Histology

A normal condyle is approximately 15–20 mm long mediolaterally and 8 to 10 mm wide anteroposteriorly [15]. Histologically, the normal condyle is composed of the following tissue layers beginning from the outside and progressing inward: fibrous connective tissue layer forming the articulating surface, undifferentiated mesenchyme proliferation layer, intermediate layer, cartilage layer, compact bone, and spongy bone. In CH Type 1, histology of the affected condyle commonly looks like a normal growing condyle without any notable pathological abnormalities (Fig. 4a, b). In some cases, the proliferative layer may demonstrate greater thickness in some areas. The activity of the proliferative layer may regulate the rate at which the condyle will grow. In normal condyles, the formation of cartilage from the proliferative layer and the replacement of cartilage by bone ceases by approximately 20 years of age. The marrow cavity is entirely occluded from the remaining cartilage by the closure of the bone plate [16]. The inability of this plate to close in the presence of an active proliferative cartilage layer may be a major etiological factor in CH Type 1 and may correlate to our observation that cessation of growth related to CH Type 1 may not occur until the early to mid-20s [2, 7]. Clinically, we have observed an increased vertical height of condyle covered by the cartilaginous cap compared to the normal condyle. Conditions that initiate excessive accelerated mandibular growth after the pubertal growth phase (age 15 years for females and 17 to 18 years for males) are most often related to an osteochondroma (CH Type 2) or other types of proliferative condylar pathology (CH Type 3 and Type 4).

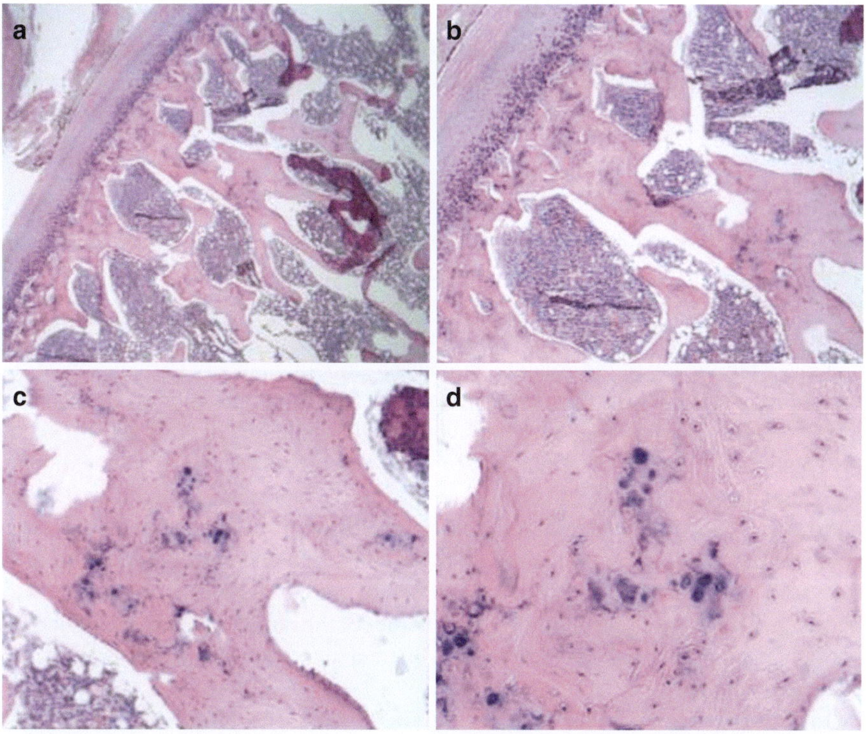

Fig. 4 Histology: Hematoxylin and eosin staining. (**a**, **b**) CH Type 1 (40X and 80X) may appear very similar to a normal growing condyle without any significant pathological abnormalities. In some cases, the proliferative layer may demonstrate an increased thickness along with some subarticular bone hyperplasia. (**c**, **d**) CH Type 2 (40X and 80 X) shows a cartilaginous cap that may not be too dissimilar from the normal growth cartilage, although there can be areas of increased thickness. There are endochondral ossification and cartilaginous islands in the subcortical bone. These deeper regions have isolated aggregates of chondrocytes which resemble a growth plate with endochondral ossification and transition to cancellous bone

CH Type 1A

Clinical Characteristics

Patients with bilateral active CH Type 1A (Figs. 1a, b and 2a–c) may have some or all of the following characteristics: (1) development or progressive worsening of mandibular prognathism, (2) worsening Class III malocclusion, (3) anterior and posterior cross bites, (4) dental compensations including decreased angulation of lower incisors and over-angulation of maxillary incisors, (5) facial shape more triangular and tapered often with weakly defined mandibular angles, (6) masseter muscles having less bulk than normal, and (7) relatively asymptomatic for TMJ symptoms in patients with symmetric growth of the mandible. In asymmetric cases where one side grows faster than the other side, patients may develop (1) facial asymmetry with the mandible shifting toward the slower growing side, (2) anterior and unilateral posterior cross bite on the slower growing side, (3) greater Class III occlusion on the faster growing side, (4) displaced articular disc in the TMJ on the slower growing side and sometimes on the faster growing side, and (5) TMJ symptoms such as clicking, TMJ pain, headaches, masticatory dysfunction, ear symptoms, etc.

Imaging

Lateral cephalometric (Fig. 3a) and tomographic (Fig. 5d–f) analyses will demonstrate the following: (1) Class III skeletal and occlusal relationship, except in patients with high occlusal plane angulation where the occlusion will be Class III but the skeletal relation could be closer to Class I; (2) condylar head and neck are elongated but the top of the condyle will have a smooth relatively normal-appearing morphology (Fig. 5d–f); (3) in the coronal view, the top of the condyle will appear more rounded (domed) than a normal condyle; (4) mandibular body is elongated; (5) gonial angle may be more obtuse; (6) vertical height of the posterior mandibular body may be decreased; (7) A-P thickness of the symphysis and alveolus may be narrower; (8) mediolateral width and A-P dimension of the rami may be narrower compared to normal; (9) cranial base length tends to be decreased and the cranial base angulation (Sella-Nasion to Nasion-Basion) tends to be increased compared to normal; and (10) the slope of the posterior border of the ramus compared to Frankfort horizontal plane may be angled forward greater than normal, particularly in the faster growing cases.

In the MRI (Fig. 6a), the articular discs are commonly thin and may be difficult to identify. Occasionally, the articular discs can be posteriorly displaced (Fig. 6b). Posterior disc displacement occurs in these conditions where there is an increased rate of vertical condylar growth that is faster than the rate of upward migration of the posterior ligament attachment of the disc, thus pulling the disc posterior to the condyle as the condyle continues to grow at an accelerated rate. In asymmetric CH Type 1A, anterior disc dislocation can occur unilaterally (greater risk on the slower growing side) (Fig. 6c) or bilaterally.

Treatment Protocol

Treatment of CH Type 1 depends on whether the growth is still active or arrested. Since CH Type 1 is self-limiting relative to growth, patients in their mid-20s or older will rarely have further jaw growth related to CH Type 1 so that routine orthognathic surgical procedures can usually be performed to correct the dentofacial deformity and malocclusion. However, if the TMJ discs are displaced and salvageable, the discs may require repositioning. If the patient is a teenager or even in their early 20s, the growth process can be active and progressive. If there is active growth and only the orthognathic surgery is performed, then there will be predictable relapse with the mandible growing into a Class III skeletal and occlusal relationship [2, 7]. If growth is active, then there are two predictable treatment options:

Option 1 Wolford's surgical protocol for active CH Type 1A includes (1) high condylectomy removing 4 to 5 mm of the top of the condylar head on the involved

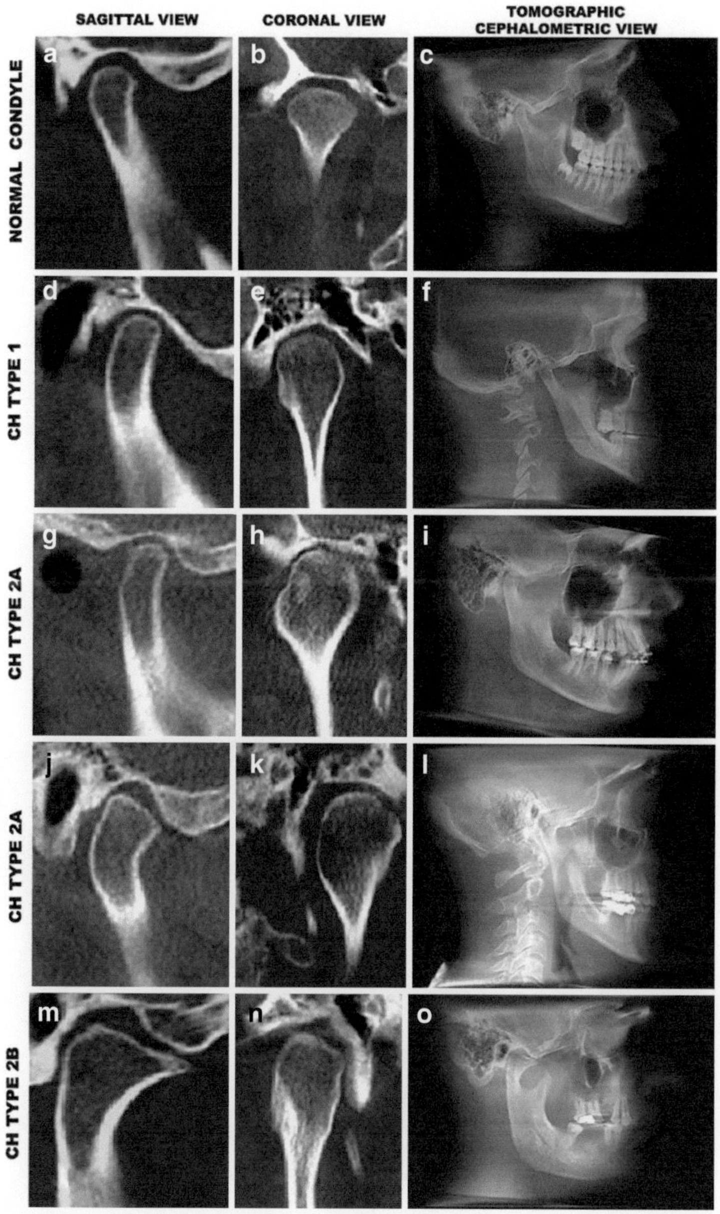

Fig. 5 (**a–c**) CT scan of a normal condyle and TMJ anatomy. (**d–f**) CH Type 1 shows an increased vertical length of the condylar head and neck. In coronal view, the crown of the condyle may be more rounded (domed) than a normal condyle. The mandible is in a Class III position. (**g–i**) CH Type 2A demonstrates increased vertical height of the condylar head and neck with greater deformity in the condyle observed in the coronal view (**h**). (**j–l**) CH Type 2A with larger condyle but still predominantly with a vertical growth vector. (**m–o**) CH Type 2B demonstrates the exophytic growth from the head of the condyle. In the coronal view, the abnormal growth may not be as evident. (**o**) There is significant vertical growth and enlargement of the right mandibular condyle, neck, ramus, and body of the mandible

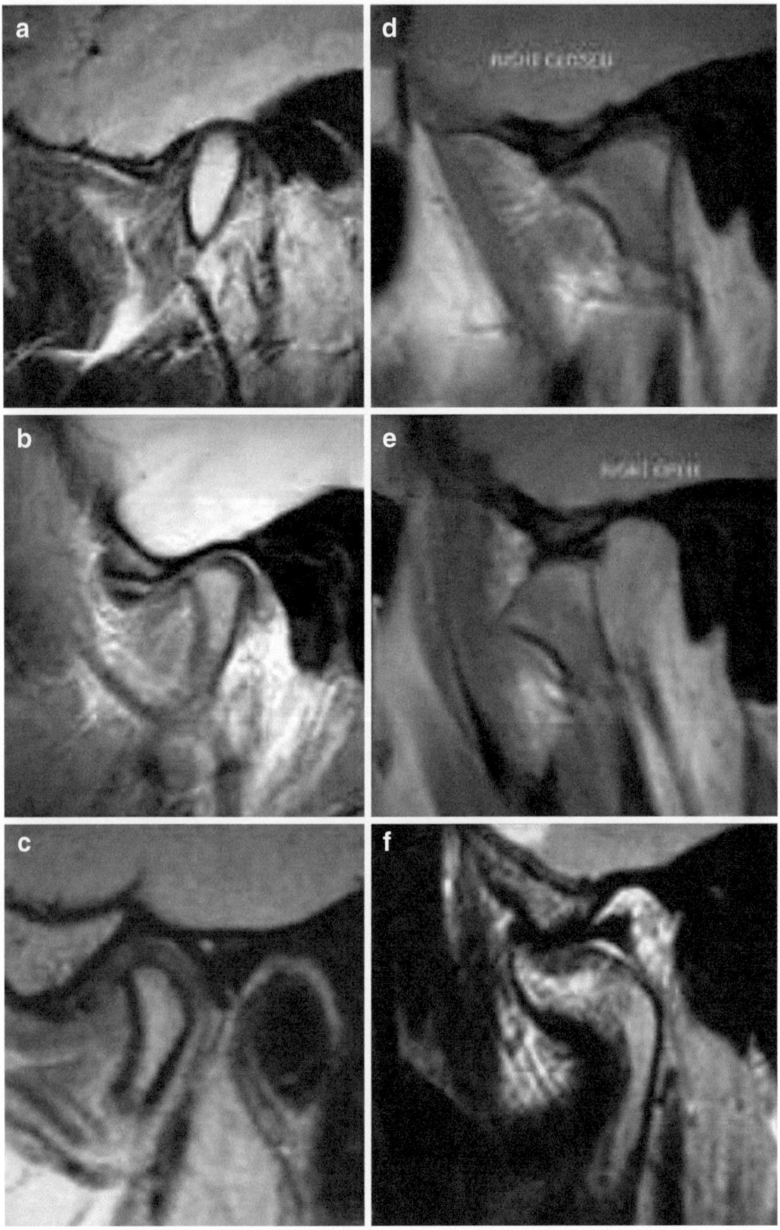

Fig. 6 MRI Evaluation. (**a**) CH Type 1 TMJ with a thin disc that is difficult to identify. (**b**) Posteriorly displaced discs can occur in CH Type 1 and Type 2 A on the ipsilateral side. (**c**) In CH Type 1 B with deviated prognathism and in CH Type 2, the contralateral joint may demonstrate a displaced articular disc and arthritic changes. (**d**, **e**) CH Type 2, the articular disc on the ipsilateral side is seen in two different cases in position in the closed and open views. (**f**) CH Type 2 B, even with large exophytic growth development, the articular disc will commonly be in place. In this particular case, notice the significant downward displacement of the condyle out of the fossa created by the large exophytic tumor growth

side (both sides for CH Type 1A) including the medial and lateral pole areas (Fig. 7a) which will arrest any further A-P growth of the mandible, (2) repositioning the articular discs using the Mitek anchor (Mitek Products Inc., Westwood, MA) technique (Fig. 7b), and (3) performing the appropriate orthognathic surgical procedures including bilateral mandibular ramus osteotomies and maxillary osteotomies if indicated (Figs. 3b and 4). Additional ancillary procedures are completed as indicated (third molar removal, genioplasty, turbinectomies, rhinoplasty, etc.). This protocol will provide predictable and stable results (Figs. 1d–f and 2d–f). These procedures can be done in one operation or divided into two or more operations depending on the surgeon's skills and experience, but the TMJ surgery should be performed first.

Option 2 Delay surgery until growth is complete; then perform orthognathic surgery only. However, since these cases often continue to grow into the mid-20s, the surgery would be delayed until it is confirmed that the growth has stopped. The longer the abnormal growth is allowed to proceed, the worse the facial deformity, asymmetry, and dental compensations will become, affecting both the dento-skeleton and excessive soft tissue development. This may increase the difficulties in obtaining an optimal functional and esthetic result, besides the adverse effects on the occlusion, dental compensations, mastication, speech, and psychosocial development. If the TMJ articular discs are displaced, then TMJ surgery may still be indicated to reposition the discs.

Age of Surgery

Wolford's surgical protocol for treating active CH Type 1A is a highly predictable treatment that will stop the abnormal growth and allow completion of the orthognathic surgery at the same operation with long-term stable functional and

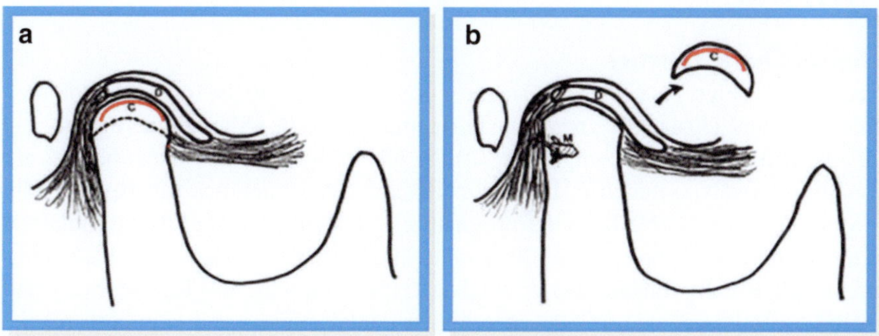

Fig. 7 (**a**) Schematic illustration demonstrates the level of high condylectomy removing the top 4–5 for treatment of CH Type 1. The red line in the condylar head represents the growth center in the proliferative layer of the condyle. (**b**) For CH Type 1 in active growth, a high condylectomy will arrest any further AP mandibular growth. The articular disc is repositioned and stabilized on the condyle with a Mitek anchor

esthetic outcomes [2, 7]. Except in select cases, surgical correction of CH Type 1A requiring double jaw surgery and high condylectomies should be deferred until at least age 14 years in females and age 16 years in males, when normal maxillary and mandibular growth are closer to completion. Since no further A-P growth of the mandible and maxilla can be expected after high condylectomies and Le Fort I osteotomies, residual maxillary and mandibular dento-alveolar vertical growth results in a downward and backward rotation of the maxillo-mandibular complex until normal cessation of alveolar growth, but the occlusion should remain stable [17–20]. If only the high condylectomies and mandibular osteotomies are performed (no maxillary osteotomies), then surgery should be delayed until age 15 years for females and 17 to18 years for males, since the maxilla can continue to grow in the A-P and vertical direction potentially developing a Class II occlusion if surgery is performed earlier because of cessation of mandibular growth from the high condylectomies but continued maxillary growth.

Case 1

This 14-year, 10-month-old patient reported that over the past 3–4 years, she developed a protruding lower jaw and a worsening bite relationship (Figs. 1a–c, 2a–c, and 3a). Serial lateral cephalograms demonstrated the mandible was growing at an accelerated rate secondary to CH Type 1A. This patient was treated in a single surgical stage with (1) bilateral high condylectomies and articular disc repositioning with Mitek anchors, (2) bilateral mandibular ramus osteotomies, (3) multiple maxillary osteotomies (Fig. 3b), (4) removal of impacted third molars, and (5) bilateral partial inferior turbinectomies. At 2 years post-surgery, the patient maintained good facial symmetry and balance as well as a stable Class I skeletal and occlusal relationship (Figs. 1d–f and 2d–f).

CH Type 1B

Clinical Characteristics

CH Type 1B (Figs. 8a–c and 9a–c) is the unilateral form with the following common characteristics: (1) usually grows in a horizontal direction, although there rarely can be a vertical directional component; (2) the left to right vertical facial heights are usually relatively symmetric, but the ipsilateral side sometimes can be vertically longer; (3) the mandible becomes prognathic and deviated toward the contralateral side; (4) increased worsening of the ipsilateral Class III occlusion while the contralateral side usually remains closer to Class I; (5) cross bites develop anteriorly and on the contralateral side; (6) the mandibular dental midline and chin shift off the facial and maxillary dental midlines toward the contralateral side; (7) the mandible continues to grow more asymmetrically beyond the normal growth years but usually will complete its growth in the early to mid-20s; and (8) unilateral CH may cause articular disc displacement, particularly on the contralateral side, creating typical TMJ symptoms. Histology for the ipsilateral CH Type 1B is the same as for CH Type 1A (Fig. 4a, b).

Imaging

Radiographic imaging for CH Type 1 B patients (Figs. 5d–f and 10a) commonly show the following features: (1) mandibular deviated prognathism; (2) mandibular asymmetry primarily in a transverse direction (however, there can occasionally be a vertical component) with the mandible and chin shifted toward the contralateral

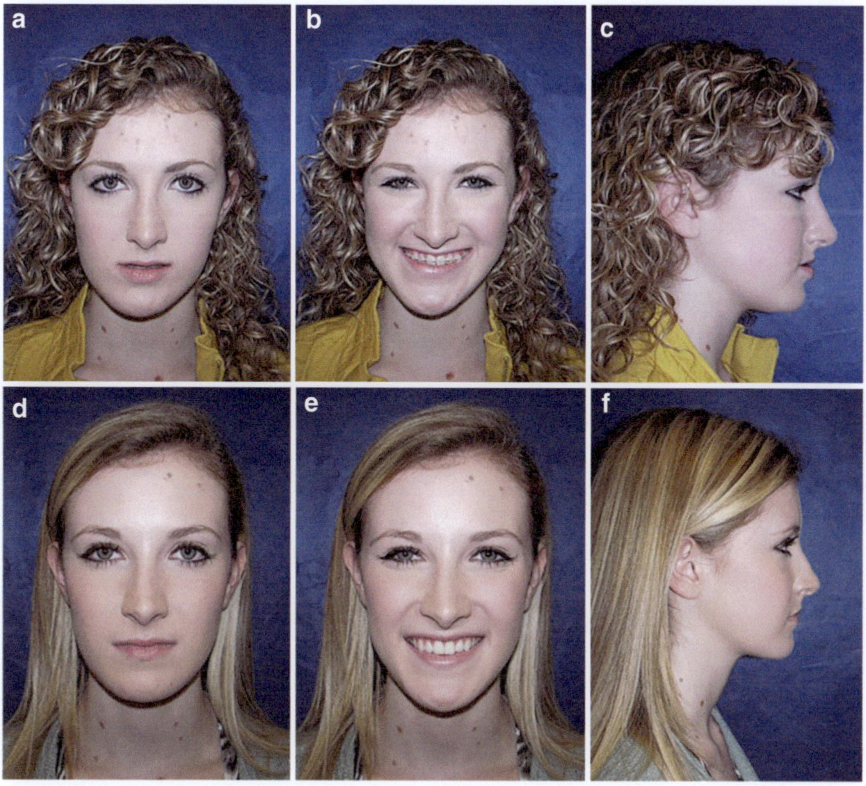

Fig. 8 Case 2, (**a–c**) A 15-year-old female with left-sided CH Type 1B, bilateral displaced articular discs, and significant TMJ pain and headaches. She was treated in a single surgical stage with (1) unilateral left high condylectomy, (2) bilateral disc repositioning, (3) bilateral ramus osteotomies, (4) multiple maxillary osteotomies, (5) nasal partial turbinectomies, and (6) third molar removal x4. (**d–f**) At 3 years post-surgery, the patient has good facial balance and a stable skeletal and occlusal relationships and is pain-free

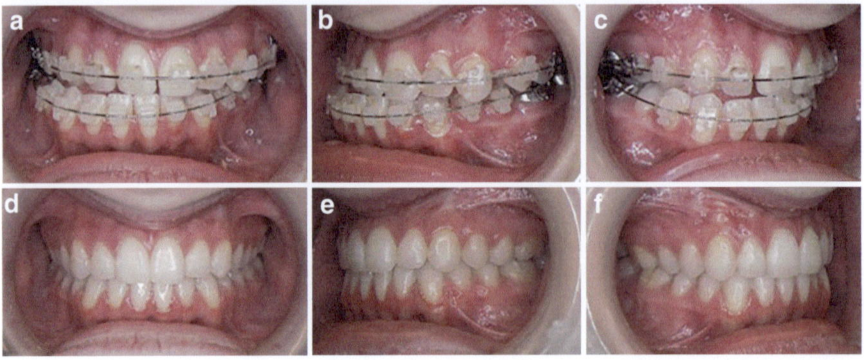

Fig. 9 Case 2, (**a–c**) Presurgery, a unilateral left Class III occlusion is present with a right-sided cross bite and mandibular dental midline shift off to the right side, getting progressively worse, related to the active left mandibular CH. (**d–f**) The occlusion remained stable at 3 years post-surgery

side; (3) condylar head and neck on the involved side are longer in length as compared to the contralateral side; (4) the ipsilateral body of the mandible may be more bowed and the contralateral side may be more flat creating significant asymmetry in the axial plane of the mandible; and (5) bone scans generally are not diagnostic for CH Type 1B because the growth rate, although accelerated, is still relatively slow but continuous on the involved side, and the proliferative layer in the condylar growth center is extremely narrow. In addition, if there is a displaced disc and mild arthritis on the contralateral side, there may not be much differentiation in the amount of isotope uptake comparing one side to the other. Serial radiographs (lateral cephalograms, cephalometric tomograms, etc.), dental models, and clinical evaluations are usually the best diagnostic methods to determine if the growth process is still active.

MRI may show a displaced articular disc on the contra lateral side with mild arthritis (Fig. 6c) and sometimes disc displacement on the ipsilateral side of CH Type 1B. The disc on the ipsilateral side is often thinner than a normal disc, making it sometimes difficult to identify on MRI (Fig. 6a). Occasionally, there can be a posteriorly displaced disc on the ipsilateral side (Fig. 6b).

Treatment Protocol

The treatment options for CH Type 1B are similar to those of CH Type 1A, where confirmed nongrowing patients can be treated with traditional orthognathic surgery. The TMJs only need to be addressed if the articular discs are displaced; a relatively common occurrence in facial asymmetries. If active growth is confirmed, then there are two options for predictable treatment outcomes.

Option 1 Wolford's surgical protocol for active CH Type 1B is as follows: (1) unilateral high condylectomy to arrest the aberrant condylar growth and disc repositioning (Fig. 7); (2) contralateral disc repositioning if the disc is displaced; (3) orthognathic surgical procedures, often requiring double jaw surgery to optimize the functional and esthetic outcome (Fig. 10b); and (4) other ancillary procedures as indicated. This protocol predictably stops ipsilateral mandibular growth and provides highly predictable and stable outcomes with normal jaw function and good esthetics (Figs. 8d–f and 9d–f) [4, 9].

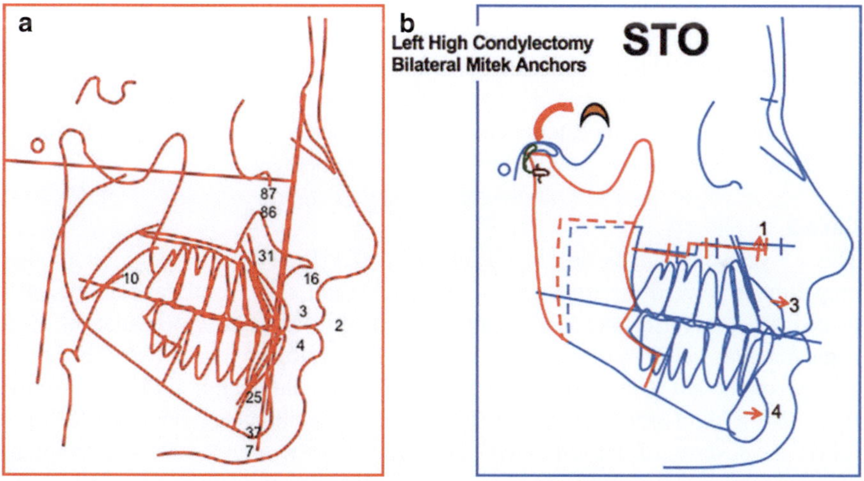

Fig. 10 Case 2, (**a**) A lateral cephalometric analysis does not reflect the severity of her left-sided CH Type 1B as the growth vector is predominantly horizontal with the mandible deviating off to the right side. (**b**) Surgical treatment objective included (1) left high condylectomy, (2) bilateral articular disc repositioning, (3) bilateral mandibular ramus sagittal split osteotomies, and (4) maxillary osteotomies to establish good facial balance with skeletal and occlusal stability

Option 2 Delay surgery until growth is complete which could be in the early to mid-20s; then perform orthognathic surgery only. However, the longer the abnormal growth is allowed to proceed, the worse the facial deformity, asymmetry, occlusion, and dental compensations will become, along with warping of the mandible, and ipsilateral excessive soft tissue development. This will increase the difficulties in obtaining an optimal functional and esthetic result, besides the adverse effects on the occlusion, dental compensations, mastication, speech, and psychosocial development. If the TMJ articular discs are displaced (a common occurrence), these patients may also suffer from TMJ pain, headaches, and myofascial pain. TMJ surgery may still be indicated to stabilize the joints as well as eliminate the pain factors.

Age of Surgery

Surgery for CH Type 1B cases should be deferred until age 15 years for females and 17 to 18 years for males. The severity of the deformity, however, may warrant earlier surgery. If the ipsilateral high condylectomy is done too early (before the age of 15 years in females and 17 to 18 years in males) where normal jaw growth is still occurring, then there is the risk of the unoperated contralateral condyle continuing with normal growth and shifting the mandible toward the ipsilateral side until normal growth cessation. In CH Type 1B, the contralateral TMJ articular disc is commonly displaced. Therefore, disc repositioning with the Mitek anchor technique would be indicated, but without the high condylectomy. However, if surgery is indicated at an earlier age during active growth, then a high condylectomy can also be performed on the contralateral side so that the mandible will not grow and will remain symmetrical.

Case 2

This 15-year-old female developed left-sided CH Type 1B, deviated mandibular prognathism toward the right side (Fig. 8a–c), right side (contralateral side) displaced articular disc, and significant right-sided TMJ pain and headaches. Her occlusion was getting progressively worse with development of a Class III cuspid relation on the left (Class I on the right side), mandibular dental midline shift to the right, and a right-sided cross bite (Fig. 9a–c). Cephalometric analysis does not reflect the severity of her left-sided CH Type 1B as the growth vector is predominantly horizontal with the mandible deviating off to the right side (Fig. 10a). Following orthodontic preparation, she was treated in a single surgical stage with (1) unilateral left high condylectomy, (2) bilateral disc repositioning with Mitek anchors, (3) bilateral ramus osteotomies, (4) multiple maxillary osteotomies (Fig. 10b), (5) nasal partial turbinectomies, and 6) third molar removal x4. At 3 years post-surgery, the patient had good facial balance and stable skeletal and occlusal relationships and was pain-free (Figs. 8d–f and 9d–f).

Research Studies for CH Type 1

We have previously demonstrated that mandibular setback surgery for correction of mandibular prognathism in nongrowing patients without active CH is a very stable procedure [21]. Fourteen nongrowing mandibular prognathic patients (11 females and 3 males) treated with orthognathic surgery only were evaluated with an average age of 24 years and average postsurgical follow-up of 29 months. The results were stable with no statistically significant A-P changes at point B from immediate post-surgical to longest follow-up. This demonstrates that orthognathic surgery for non-growing mandibular prognathic patients is a stable and predictable procedure. However, numerous studies have reported relapse for mandibular setback ranging from 20% to 91% of the amount of posterior surgical movement [22–30]. It is likely that this high percentage of relapse is due to unrecognized and untreated active CH Type 1 patients included in the studies. Understanding the etiology of CH Type 1, nature of the pathology and deformity, clinical presentation, options available for treatment, and timing of treatment is important for achieving optimal treatment outcomes. In 1979, Wolford [31] used a technique to predictably eliminate mandibular growth in CH Type 1 by performing high condylectomies and disc repositioning along with simultaneous orthognathic surgery to correct the associated jaw deformity. The high condylectomy (Fig. 6) arrests the excessive and disproportionate growth of the mandible by surgically removing one of the important mandibular growth centers and the site responsible for the CH Type 1 pathological growth process [2, 7].

Wolford et al. [2] reported on 54 patients diagnosed with active CH Type 1. Group 1 ($n = 12$) was treated with orthognathic surgery only, while Group 2 ($n = 42$) was treated with high condylectomies, articular disc repositioning, and orthognathic surgery. The results showed the average age at surgery for Group 1 was 17.5 years and for Group 2 was16.6 years. The average presurgical follow-up for Group 1 was 12.5 months and for Group 2 was 12.1 months, used to confirm active CH Type 1. The average postsurgical follow-up for Group 1 was 5.6 years and for Group 2 was 5.1 years. Presurgery there were no statistically significant differences ($p > 0.05$) in the two groups for maximal incisal opening (MIO), lateral excursion (LE), and subjective jaw function. Although both groups exhibited active accelerated growth, Group 2 showed a statistically significant ($p < 0.05$) difference with greater presurgical mandibular growth compared to Group 1. At long-term postsurgical follow-up, no differences were found in LE and subjective jaw function. Group 2 showed a statistically significant greater increase in MIO ($p < 0.01$) as well as skeletal and occlusal stability ($p < 0.05$) at long-term follow-up. All of the patients in the Group 1 grew back into skeletal and occlusal Class III relationships requiring secondary intervention. All patients in Group 2 remained stable in a Class I skeletal and occlusal relationship. This study [2] confirms the predictability of this surgical protocol for treating CH Type 1.

Condylar Hyperplasia Type 2

CH Type 2 is a unilateral mandibular condylar enlargement caused by an osteochondroma that vertically lengthens the ipsilateral mandible and face (Fig. 11a–c), can shift it towards the contralateral side, and is not self-limiting relative to growth. The growth rate for this pathology varies from slow to moderate, but some cases can have a more rapid growth rate. Confirmation of the condylar pathology usually requires histological assessment. Osteochondroma is one of the most common benign tumors of bone, representing approximately 35–50% of all benign tumors and 8–15% of all primary bone tumors, and the most common tumor of the mandibular condyle.

CH Type 2 can be subdivided into two primary groups based on tumor morphology. CH Type 2A indicates an enlargement of the condylar head and neck with a predominate vertical growth vector of the osteochondroma without significant exophytic tumor development (Fig. 5g–l). There can be unevenness or lumpiness on the condyle. CH Type 2B indicates exophytic tumor extensions off the condyle, usually

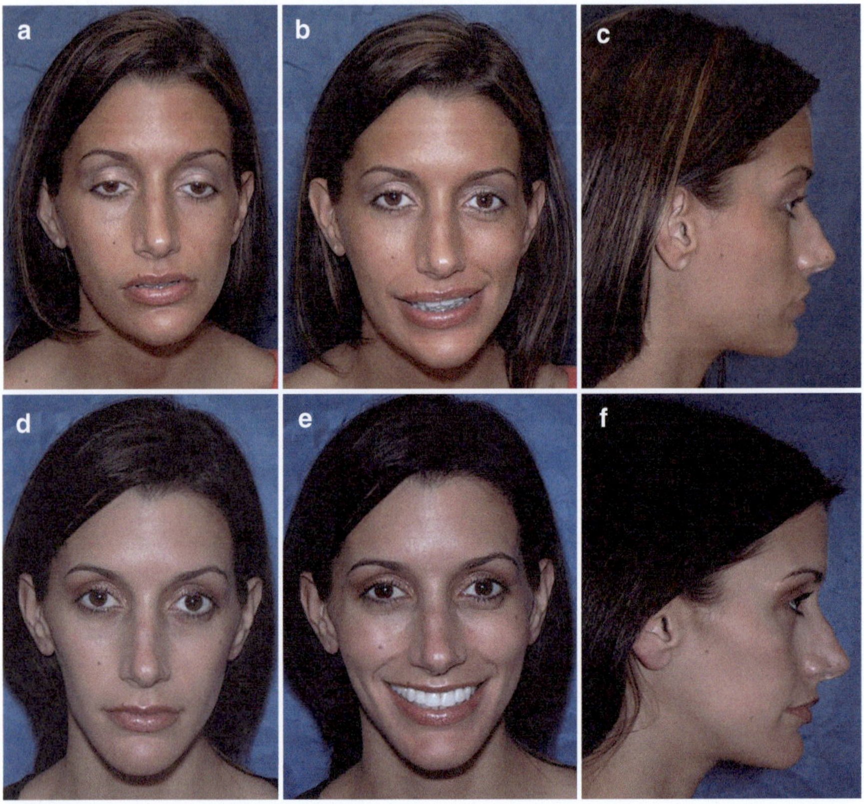

Fig. 11 Case 3, (**a–c**) A 27-year-old female presents with CH Type 2B. She became aware of developing facial asymmetry 4–5 years prior. She developed significant elongation of the right side of the face as well as TMJ pain and headache. Surgical treatment in a single stage included (1) right low condylectomy, (2) right TMJ disc repositioning, (3) bilateral mandibular ramus osteotomies, and (4) multiple maxillary osteotomies. (**d–f**): The patient at 3.5 years post-surgery showed good facial balance as well as a stable skeletal and occlusal result

forward and medially, with the head becoming significantly enlarged and deformed (Fig. 5m–o). The exophytic growth can also occur posterior and lateral, but are less common. These tumors usually have a significant vertical growth vector, but the exophytic growths, when relatively large, can disarticulate the condyle down and out of the fossa creating a greater exaggeration of the ipsilateral increased vertical height of the jaws and face (Fig. 6f). When performing surgery to remove the tumors, the incision for removal of CH Type 2A can usually be smaller compared to a large CH Type 2B that may require greater access and difficulty for removal. CH Type 2B may have a greater risk of intraoperative and postsurgical vascular and neurological complications.

The different growth patterns of the tumors for CH Type 2A and 2B may be related to the anatomical origin of the tumor on the condylar head, rate of growth, and elongation adaptation of the muscles of mastication and other soft tissues on the ipsilateral side. The constraints of the rate of muscular and soft tissue adaptation and elongation compared to the rate of tumor growth may redirect the tumor development in the direction of least resistance: anterior and anteromedial. The roof and posterior wall of the fossa as well as the lateral and medial capsular ligaments may act as barriers, directing the growth forward. However, we have treated cases with the less common development of the exophytic growth extending laterally and posteriorly.

Histology

Osteochondroma (CH Type 2) includes a cartilaginous cap similar to that seen in a normal growth cartilage, endochondral ossification, cartilaginous islands in the subcortical bone, and a marrow space contiguous with the underlying bone (Fig. 4c, d). The cartilaginous cap may be thicker than normal. Gray et al. [32, 33] reported that the bony trabeculae are often thickened and irregular, resulting in a consistently large volume of trabecular bone and a higher than normal percentage of surfaces covered in osteoid. They also point out the presence of an uninterrupted layer of undifferentiated germinating mesenchymal cells, hypertrophic cartilage, and islands of chondrocytes in the subchondral trabecular bone. They made the direct correlation between the scintigraphy activity and the frequency of cartilage islands at depth in the trabecular bone. The cartilage islands are mini growth centers producing bone, causing enlargement of the condyle.

Clinical Characteristics

Common clinical features of CH Type 2 (Figs. 11a–c and 12a–c) include the following: (1) develops at any age, but for most cases, in the second decade (68% of cases); (2) predominately occurs in females (76% of cases); (3) increased unilateral mandibular height involving the condyle, neck, ramus, body, and dentoalveolus of the ipsilateral mandible; (4) increased soft tissue volume on the ipsilateral side of the face including elongation of the muscles of mastication; (5) low mandibular plane angle facial type morphology, particularly on the ipsilateral side; (6) chin asymmetry vertically and transversely, with shifting toward the contralateral side; (7) compensatory downward growth of the ipsilateral maxillary dentoalveolus; (8) lateral open bite on the ipsilateral side particularly in more rapid-growing pathology (Fig. 12a–c); (9) labial tipping of the mandibular ipsilateral posterior teeth and lingual tipping of the contralateral posterior teeth may occur; (10) transverse cant in the occlusal plane with the ipsilateral side vertically lower; (11) mandibular anterior teeth crowns may be tipped toward the ipsilateral side and the long axis of the roots angled toward the contralateral side; and (12) commonly, contralateral TMJ articular disc dislocation (76% of cases) with or without arthritis, accompanied by symptoms such as clicking, popping, TMJ pain, headaches, etc., [8] as a result of the functional overload caused by the ipsilateral pathology.

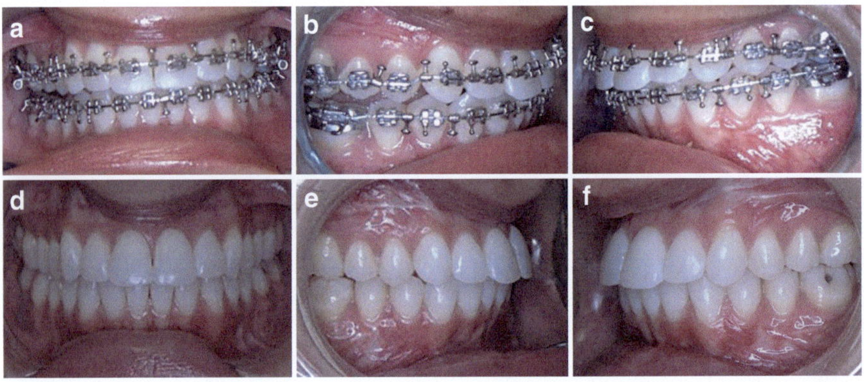

Fig. 12 Case 3, (**a–c**) The patient has a transverse cant in the occlusion with the right side vertically elongated and mandibular dental midline shift to the left 2 mm, and there is a right posterior open bite. (**d–f**) At 3.5 years post-surgery, she had a Class I stable occlusal relationship with a level transverse occlusal plane

Imaging

Radiographic features will include the following: (1) enlarged, elongated, deformed ipsilateral condyle (CH Type 2A) (Fig. 5g–l), and commonly there may be exophytic extensions of the tumor off of the condyle (CH Type 2B) (Fig. 5m–o); (2) increased A-P and mediolateral thickness of the ipsilateral condylar neck; (3) increased vertical height of the ipsilateral mandibular condyle, neck, ramus, body, symphysis, and dentoalveolus (Fig. 13a); (4) increased vertical height of the ipsilateral maxillary dentoalveolus; (5) transverse cant in the occlusal plane with the ipsilateral side vertically lower; (6) facial asymmetry; (7) posterior border of the ipsilateral mandibular ramus may be more vertical than normal; (8) coronoid process is usually normal in size and may be displaced below the zygomatic arch with elongation of the temporalis muscle (Fig. 5i, l, o); (9) loss of antigonial notching with downward bowing of the inferior border on the mandible; (10) the inferior alveolar nerve canal may be positioned adjacent to the apices of the teeth, but more commonly located toward the inferior border of the mandible; and (11) chin vertically longer on the ipsilateral side and may be prominent in profile.

MRI may show a displaced articular disc on the contralateral side (76% of the cases) and associated arthritic condylar changes (Fig. 6c). The disc is commonly in position on the ipsilateral side (Figs. 6d–f and 14) although it can also be displaced. In CH Type 2A, the disc can become posteriorly displaced similar to Fig. 6b. Unless the tumor is very slow growing, bone scintigraphy will usually show increased uptake particularly in the more active tumors (Fig. 15).

Treatment Protocol

There are two basic treatment approaches for managing CH Type 2. Since this pathology is usually progressive and deforming, both options include a condylectomy to remove the tumor.

Option 1 Wolford's surgical protocol (Figs. 13b and 16) for CH Type 2 includes the following: (1) low condylectomy removing the ipsilateral condyle at the condylar base, preserving the condylar neck (Fig. 16); (2) reshaping the condy-

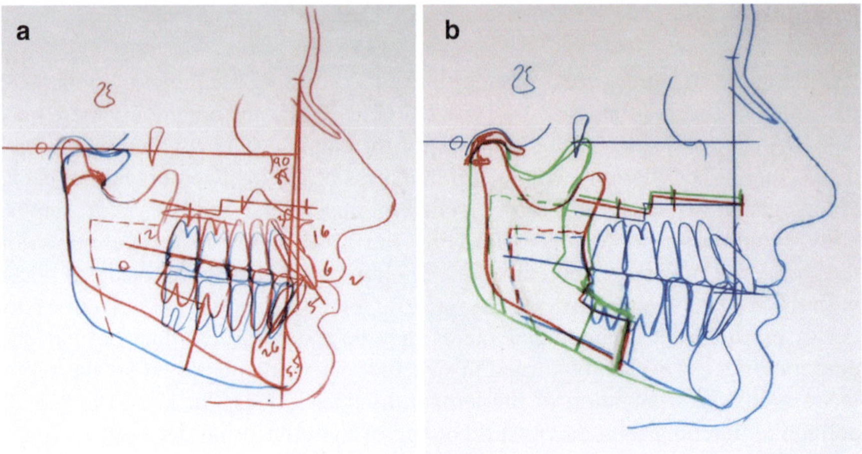

Fig. 13 Case 3, (**a**) Cephalometric analysis shows significant vertical elongation of the right side of the mandible at the inferior border as well as at the occlusal plane. The blue tracing represents the right side and the red the left side. (**b**) Surgical treatment objective includes (1) right low condylectomy, (2) right TMJ articular disc repositioning, (3) bilateral mandibular ramus osteotomies, and (4) multiple maxillary osteotomies to transversely level the occlusion and skeletal structures

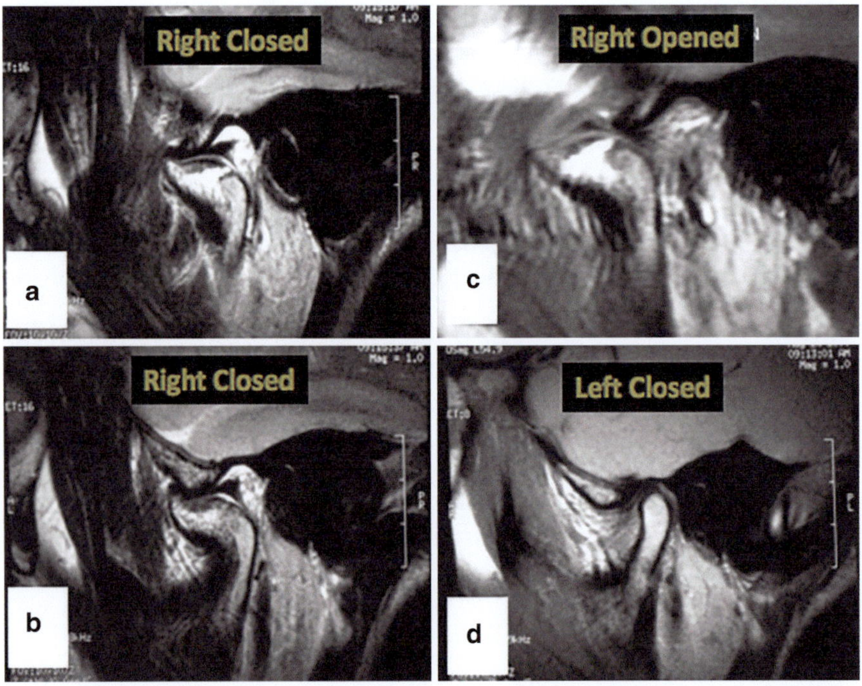

Fig. 14 Case 3, (**a**, **b**) MRI T1 and T2 show the significant enlargement of the right condyle, totally disarticulating the condyle out of the fossa. (**c**) The right mandibular condyle/tumor demonstrates good translation of the condyle upon opening, with the articular disc in position. (**d**) The contralateral TMJ shows the articular disc in position

lar neck to function as the new condyle; (3) repositioning the articular disc over the top of the condylar neck and stabilizing it; (4) repositioning the articular disc on the contralateral side, when displaced; (5) orthognathic surgery (usually double jaw surgery) to correct the associated maxillary and mandibular deformities (Fig. 13b); and (6) inferior border ostectomy on the ipsilateral side to reestablish vertical height balance of the mandibular ramus, body, and symphysis if indicated (Fig. 16). This last procedure will require dissection and preservation of the inferior alveolar nerve if it is located low in the mandible where the ostectomy will be performed. This protocol will provide predictable and stable outcomes as well as optimize the functional and esthetic results (Figs. 11d–f and 12d–f). This treatment approach will allow removal of the tumor yet still use the enlarged condylar neck as the new condyle. The articular disc on the ipsilateral side and frequently on the contralateral side (if that disc is displaced) will require repositioning and stabilization to provide the best treatment outcome relative to function, esthetics, and elimination of any associated pain and dysfunction [34]. If the disc is non-salvageable, then the author prefers a custom-fitted total joint prosthesis to reconstruct the ipsilateral and/or contralateral TMJ.

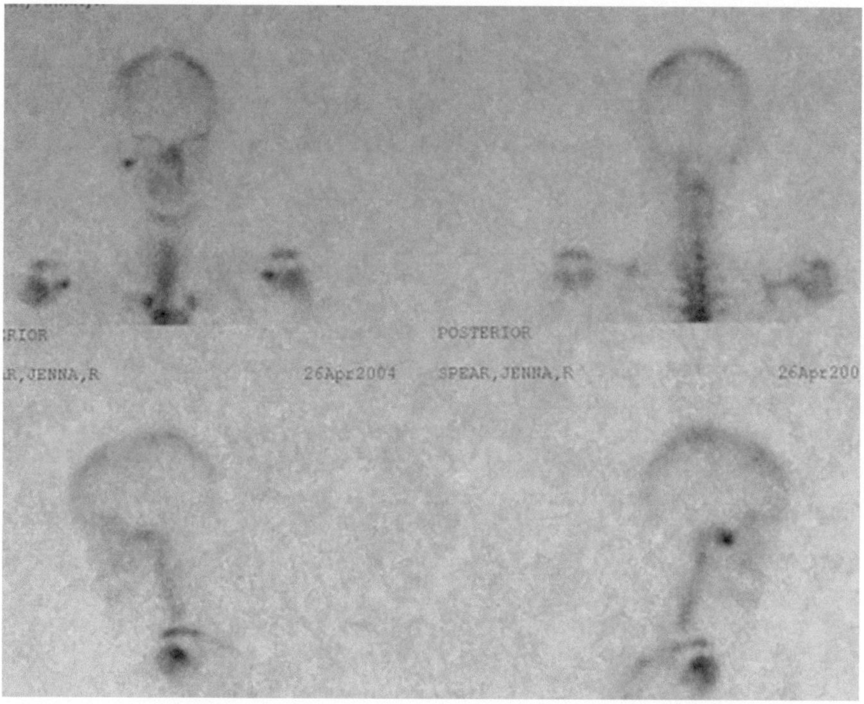

Fig. 15 The bone scan shows activity in the right TMJ compatible with condylar/tumor growth

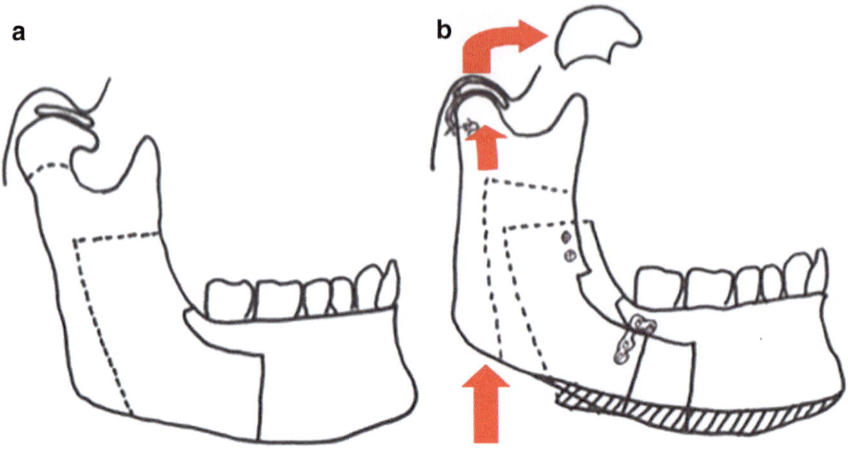

Fig. 16 (**a**) Schematic for the treatment of CH Type 2 includes a low condylectomy to remove the osteochondroma tumor and preserve the condylar neck. (**b**) The usual surgical protocol indicated for optimal functional and esthetic outcomes may include low condylectomy, condylar neck recontoured, articular disc repositioned with a Mitek anchor, mandibular ramus sagittal split osteotomies, maxillary osteotomies, ipsilateral mandibular inferior border ostectomy, and any other indicated ancillary procedures

Option 2 A popular approach for treating CH Type 2 is performing only an ipsilateral condylectomy, either partial or complete without any orthognathic surgery. Proponents of a partial condylectomy recommend no other surgery, but a malocclusion can occur as well as a risk of recurrence since the tumor may not be completely removed. When the condylectomy results in significant functional and occlusal instability, or where the entire condyle and neck have been removed, then condyle reconstruction techniques that have been advocated include the following: TMJ total joint prosthesis, sliding ramus osteotomy, rib graft, sternoclavicular graft, free bone graft, pedicled osseous graft, etc. When only the ipsilateral condyle is addressed with no additional orthognathic surgery included, the patient is often left with a compromised functional and esthetic result since a major component of facial asymmetry will remain as well as a significant malocclusion. This is particularly the case if significant ipsilateral downgrowth of the maxilla and vertical elongation of the ipsilateral mandibular body and ramus occurred as a result of the tumor. These patients may require secondary orthognathic procedures to achieve a functional occlusion and to restore good facial balance and esthetics. Without maintaining a functional ipsilateral articular disc when using the autogenous condylar reconstruction techniques, significant postsurgical TMJ dysfunction may develop.

Age of Surgery

When CH Type 2 is identified during the normal growth years, then surgery should be deferred, if possible, until age 15 years for females and 17–18 years for males after normal jaw growth is relatively complete. The severity of the deformity, however, may warrant earlier surgery. If the ipsilateral low condylectomy is done too early (before the age of 15 years in females and 17–18 years in males) where normal jaw growth is still occurring, then there is the risk of the contralateral condyle continuing with normal growth shifting the mandible toward the ipsilateral side until growth cessation. In CH Type 2, the contralateral TMJ articular disc is commonly displaced (76% of cases) and therefore, disc repositioning would be indicated. However, if surgery is indicated at an earlier age, then a high condylectomy can be performed on the contralateral side so that no further growth will occur and the mandible will remain symmetric. Another option would be to perform the unilateral condylectomy and plan for orthognathic surgery as a second stage after cessation of growth.

Ideal facial balance may be difficult to achieve post-surgery for CH Type 2 patients because of the excessive amount of soft tissue development that occurs with the unilateral elongation and transverse asymmetry that develops presurgery. In addition, the ipsilateral mandibular body becomes more curved and the contralateral body contour is flatter. Thus, with vertically shortening the ipsilateral bony structures and rotation of the chin toward the ipsilateral side, there is excessive soft tissue bulk, including the masseter muscle that will make the ipsilateral side appear fuller, even with the most accurate skeletal correction.

Case 3

This 27-year-old female presents with CH Type 2B. She became aware of developing facial asymmetry 4–5 years prior. She developed significant elongation of the right side of the face (Fig. 11a–c) as well as TMJ pain and headaches. The patient has a transverse cant in the occlusion with the right side vertically elongated and mandibular dental midline shift to the left 2 mm, and there is a right posterior open bite (Fig. 12a–c). Cephalometric analysis shows significant vertical elongation of the right side of the mandible at the inferior border as well as at the occlusal plane. The blue tracing represents the right side and the red the left side (Fig. 13a). Her MRI demonstrated a large exophytic tumor attached to the right mandibular condyle, but her left TMJ articular disc was in position (Fig. 14). Surgical treatment in a single stage included (1) right low condylectomy (Fig. 16), (2) right TMJ disc repositioning, (3) bilateral mandibular ramus osteotomies, and (4) multiple maxillary osteotomies (Fig. 13b). In this case, the ipsilateral inferior border ostectomy was not required. The patient at 3.5 years post-surgery showed good facial balance and stable skeletal and occlusal result, without tumor recurrence (Figs. 11d–f and 12d–f).

Research Studies for CH Type 2

Adams in 1836 and Humphry in 1856 demonstrated that excision of the condyle in a unilateral condylar hyperplasia (these cases were CH Type 2B) would arrest the condylar hyperplastic growth process [8, 36]. Gruca and Meisels (1926) supported this treatment approach and stated: "The earlier the operation is done, the smaller the deformation will develop in the upper jaw and position of the teeth. The early resection is not only advisable, but even absolutely indicated." [35] Rushton (1946) also supported this concept, but emphasized that the deformity must be progressive and that a condylectomy of the affected side at an early age, prior to completion of normal growth, will foreshorten that side of the jaw permanently [13]. This early treatment philosophy for condylar hyperplasia was to remove as much condyle as necessary to correct the bite problem, but not to overcorrect it. During the past 170 years, many surgeons have advocated and demonstrated that condylectomy for CH Type 2 is a predictable method to stop the pathological growth process.

For CH Type 2, there are numerous case reports that have demonstrated successful management with condylectomy. Wolford et al. [36] reported a series of six cases of mandibular condylar osteochondroma treated with the protocol described in this paper including a low condylectomy, recontouring the condylar neck to function as the new condyle, repositioning the articular disc on top of the "new" condyle, and performing the appropriate orthognathic surgery (usually double jaw) to correct the associated dentofacial deformity in a single operation. The average follow-up was 52 months (range 22–108 months) with no tumor recurrence. The six patients had stable outcomes with a Class I occlusion, good facial balance, average incisal opening of 54 mm (range 45–61 mm), good excursion movements with an average of 5.8 mm (range 2–10 mm), average postsurgical pain at 0.3 (range 0–2, where 0 = no pain, 10 = worst pain imaginable), and jaw function at 1.6 (range 0–3, where 0 = normal function, 10 = inability to move jaw, frozen jaw).

Yang et al. [37] presented a study of 17 patients with mandibular condylar osteochondroma treated with a condylectomy at the sigmoid notch and vertical ramus osteotomy to move the posterior border of the mandible into the glenoid fossa fixated with bone plates. The authors did not correct the facial asymmetry as no orthognathic surgery was performed on any of the patients. The articular disc was preserved and there were no reoccurrences of the tumor and all patients reportedly had improved jaw function at longest follow-up.

Ord et al. [38] reported on eight cases threated with sub-sigmoid osteotomy, removal of the tumor and repositioning of the proximal segment in five cases, and a condylectomy with rib graft reconstruction in three cases. No orthognathic surgery procedures were performed to correct the dentofacial deformity. There were no recurrences reported but four cases were only followed for 3–6 months post-surgery. Postsurgical function was not reported. The authors reviewed the literature and showed that 32 of the 57 cases reported were female (56%). This is different from our series where 76% of the cases were female [8].

Wolford et al. [8] reported on a series of 37 patients with CH Type 2. There were 28 females (76%) and 9 males (24%) treated with Wolford's protocol followed for an average of 48 months (range 12–288 months). There was only one case that had a reoccurrence and that patient was initially diagnosed as a CH Type 1 based on his facial morphology, imaging presentation, and growth pattern. He received a high condylectomy (removing the top 4–5 mm of the condyle) along with the disc repositioning and double jaw orthognathic surgery. However, the histologic report revealed an osteochondroma and the tumor continued to grow requiring a repeat surgery 14 months later for a low condylectomy and partial repeat of the orthognathic surgery with a stable outcome at 4 years post-surgery. This case confirms the importance of performing a low condylectomy to eliminate the tumor. In this study, the 37 patients had statistically significant improvement in pain, headaches, jaw function, diet, and disability. Importantly, 76% of the patients had contralateral TMJ arthritis and disc dislocation from the functional overload created from the ipsilateral tumor, requiring contralateral disc repositioning. At longest follow-up, there was a nonsignificant decrease in incisal opening of 2.3 mm (average postsurgical incisal opening was 44.9 mm) and a significant decrease in excursive movements of 2.5 mm on the right and 2.2 mm on the left (average postsurgical excursion to the right 5.3 mm, to the left 5.0 mm).

Condylar Hyperplasia Type 3 and Type 4

CH Type 3 includes rare benign tumors originating in the mandibular condyle such as (1) osteoma, (2) chondroblastoma, (3) osteoid osteoma, (4) osteoblastoma, (5) aneurysmal bone cyst, (6) central giant cell granuloma, etc. CH Type 4 would include malignant tumors originating in the mandibular condyle such as (1) chondrosarcoma, (2) osteosarcoma, (3) metastatic carcinoma, etc.

Clinical Features

Benign and malignant tumors affecting the mandibular condyle may have a relatively slow or more rapid progressive development, firm enlargement, and not typically painful until advanced. If numbness, paralysis, and/or significant pain develop, regardless of whether there is significant facial enlargement, then malignancy must be strongly considered. Unilateral facial enlargement occurs with expansile hard and/or soft tissue tumors: benign or malignant.

Imaging

X-ray will usually show bone destruction or deposition associated with the condyle with expansion when the skeletal structures are involved. MRI, CT scans, and bone scans may show bone and/or soft tissue involvement.

Treatment Considerations

Treatment will be dependent on the nature and extent of the pathology, benign or malignant, structures involved, age of patient, other medical conditions present, etc. Treatment may include removal of the tumor or pathological process with appropriate adjunctive treatment for the specific neoplasia.

Conclusions

This chapter describes a classification for CH conditions, based on occurrence rate and type of pathology, focusing on the two most common benign forms of CH. CH Type 1A is the most common occurring form and CH Type 4 is the rarest. Classifying CH pathology in this manner will help the clinician understand the nature of the pathology, progression if untreated, recommended ages for surgical intervention to minimize an adverse effect on subsequent facial growth and development in younger patients, and the surgical protocols to comprehensively and predictably treat these conditions.

References

1. Hayward JD, Walker RV, Poulton G, Bell WH. Asymmetric mandibular excess. In: Bell WH, Proffitt WB, White RP, editors. Surgical correction of dentofacial deformities. Philadelphia: W. B. Saunders; 1980. p. 947–53.
2. Wolford LM, Morales-Ryan CA, García-Morales P, Perez D. Surgical management of mandibular condylar hyperplasia type 1. Proc (Bayl Univ Med Cent). 2009;22:321–9.
3. Obwegeser HL, Makek MS. Hemimandibular hyperplasia—hemimandibular elongation. J Maxillofac Surg. 1986;14:183–208.
4. Nitzan DW, Katsnelson A, Bermanis I, Brin I, Casap N. The clinical characteristics of condylar hyperplasia: experience with 61 patients. J Oral Maxillofac Surg. 2008;66:312–8.
5. Buschang PH. In: Bell WH, Guerreiro CA, editors. Distraction osteogenesis of the facial skeleton. Hamilton, ON: BC Decker Inc; 2007. p. 141151.
6. Reid RR. Facial skeletal growth and timing of surgical intervention. Clin Plast Surg. 2007;34:357.
7. Wolford LM, Mehra P, Reiche-Fischel O, Morales-Ryan CA, Garcia-Morales P. Efficacy of high condylectomy for management of condylar hyperplasia. Am J Orthod Dentofac Orthop. 2002;121:136–50.
8. Wolford LM, Movahed R, Dhameja A, Allen W. Surgical treatment of condylar hyperplasia type 2: retrospective study of 37 cases of Osteochondroma. J Oral Maxillofac Surg. 2014;72:1704–28.

9. Aufdemorte TB, Van Sickels J, Dolwick FM, et al. Estrogen receptors in the temporomandibular joint of the baboon (Papio cynocephalus): an autoradiographic study. Oral Surg Oral Med Oral Pathol. 1986;61:307–14.
10. Milam SB, Aufdemorte TB, Sheridan PJ, et al. Sexual dimorphism in the distribution of estrogen receptors in the temporomandibular joint complex of the baboon. Oral Surg Oral Med Oral Pathol. 1987;64:527–32.
11. Abubaker AO, Arslan W, Sotereanos GC. Estrogen and progesterone receptors in the temporomandibular joint disc of symptomatic and asymptomatic patients. J Oral Maxillofac Surg. 1993;51:1096–100.
12. Tsai CL, Liu TK, Chen TJ. Estrogen and osteoarthritis: A study of synovial estradiol and estradiol receptor binding in human osteoarthritic knees. Biochem Biophys Res Comm. 1992;83:1287–91.
13. Gottlieb OP. Hyperplasia of the mandibular condyle. J Oral Maxillofac Surg. 1951;9:118.
14. Riolo ML, Moyers RE, McNamara JA, Hunter WS. An atlas of craniofacial growth: cephalometric standards from the university school growth study. Ann Arbor MI: The University of Michigan; 1974. p. 101–6.
15. Lindblom G. On the anatomy and function of the temporomandibular joint. Acta Odont Scand. 1960;17:23.
16. Rushton MA. Unilateral hyperplasia of the mandibular condyle. Proc Roy Soc Med. 1946;39:431–8.
17. Wolford LM, Rodrigues DB. Orthognathic considerations in the young patient and effects on facial growth. In: Preedy VR, editor. Handbook of growth and growth monitoring in health and disease. New York: Springer; 2012. p. 1789–808.
18. Wolford LM, Rodrigues DB. Temporomandibular joint (TMJ) pathologies in growing patients: effects on facial growth and development. In: Preedy VR, editor. Handbook of growth and growth monitoring in health and disease. New York: Springer; 2012. p. 1809–28.
19. Wolford LM, Karras SC, Mehra P. Considerations for orthognathic surgery during growth, part 1: mandibular deformities. Am J Orthod Dentofac Orthop. 2001;119:95–101.
20. Wolford LM, Karras SC, Mehra P. Considerations for orthognathic surgery during growth, part 2: maxillary deformities. Am J Orthod Dentofac Orthop. 2001;119:102–5.
21. Fuselier JC, Freitas RZ, Wolford LM. Mandibular setback procedures with sagittal split osteotomies in non-growing patients. J Oral Maxillofac Surg. 1999;57:94–5.
22. Phillips C, Zaytoun HS Jr, Thomas PM, Terry BC. Skeletal alterations following TOVRO or BSSO procedures. Int J Adult Orthodon Orthognath Surg. 1986;1(3):203–13.
23. Ingervall B, Thüer U, Vuillemin T. Stability and effect on the soft tissue profile of mandibular setback with sagittal split osteotomy and rigid internal fixation. Int J Adult Orthodon Orthognath Surg. 1995;10:15–25.
24. Schatz JP, Tsimas P. Cephalometric evaluation of surgical-orthodontic treatment of skeletal class III malocclusion. Int J Adult Orthodon Orthognath Surg. 1995;10(3):173–80.
25. Proffit WR, Phillips C, Dann C 4th, Turvey TA. Stability after surgical-orthodontic correction of skeletal class III malocclusion. I Mandibular setback. Int J Adult Orthodon Orthognath Surg. 1991;6(1):7–18.
26. Reitzik M. Skeletal and dental changes after surgical correction of mandibular prognathism. J Oral Surg. 1980;38(2):109–16.
27. MacIntosh RB. Experience with the sagittal osteotomy of the mandibular ramus: a 13-year review. J Maxillofac Surg. 1981;9(3):151–65.
28. Komori E, Aigase K, Sugisaki M, Tanabe H. Skeletal fixation versus skeletal relapse. Am J Orthod Dentofac Orthop. 1987;92(5):412–21.
29. Bailey LJ, Duong HL, Proffit WR. Surgical class III treatment: long-term stability and patient perceptions of treatment outcome. Int J Adult Orthodon Orthognath Surg. 1998;13:35–44.
30. Mobarak KA, Krogstad O, Espeland L, Lyberg T. Long-term stability of mandibular setback surgery: a follow-up of 80 bilateral sagittal split osteotomy patients. Int J Adult Orthodon Orthognath Surg. 2000;15:83–95.
31. Wolford LM, LeBanc J. Condylectomy to arrest disproportionate mandibular growth abstract presented at the American cleft palate association meeting, New York, 1986.

32. Gray RJ, Sloan P, Quayle AA, Carter DH. Histopathological and scintigraphic features of condylar hyperplasia. Int J Oral Maxillofac Surg. 1990;19(2):65–71.
33. Gray RJ, Horner K, Testa HJ, Lloyd JJ, Sloan P. Condylar hyperplasia: correlation of histological and scintigraphic features. Dentomaxillofac Radiol. 1994;23(2):103–7.
34. Mehra P, Wolford LM. The Mitek mini anchor for TMJ disc repositioning: surgical technique and results. Int J Oral Maxillofac Surg. 2001;30(6):497–503.
35. Gruca A, Meisels E. Asymmetry of the mandible from unilateral hypertrophy. Ann Surg. 1926;83:755.
36. Wolford LM, Mehra P, Franco P. Use of conservative condylectomy for treatment of osteochondroma of the mandibular condyle. J Oral Maxillofacial Surg. 2002;60:262–8.
37. Yang X, Hu J, Zhu S, Liang X, Li J, Luo E. Computer-assisted surgical planning and simulation for condylar reconstruction in patients with osteochondroma. Br J Oral Maxillofac Surg. 2011;49(3):203–8.
38. Ord RA, Warburton G, Caccamese JF. Osteochondroma of the condyle: review of 8 cases. Int J Oral Maxillofac Surg. 2010;39:523–8.

Management of Facial Asymmetry in TMJ Ankylosis and Degenerative Joint Disease

Daniel E. Perez and David Szalay

Abstract

Temporomandibular joint (TMJ) pathology, particularly ankylosis and degenerative joint disease (DJD), can cause profound morphological changes in the mandible resulting in significant facial asymmetry. These pathologic anatomical changes are especially pronounced when they occur unilaterally and can be significantly worse when the insult occurs during the growing years of the patient's life. The morphological changes caused by both ankylosis and DJD have the potential to disseminate their effects to surrounding facial soft tissues and bones, especially the maxilla, further complicating treatment. Unlike some other pathological causes of facial asymmetry, the cosmetic and asymmetric problems associated with ankylosis and DJD almost always come with debilitating functional problems, the combination of which may lead to malnourishment, depression, and an overall decreased quality of life. Proper management and surgical treatment of these patients must aim to correct both the functional and esthetic sequela associated with these pathologies.

Keywords

TMJ ankylosis · Degenerative joint disease · Gap arthroplasty · TMJ autografts · TMJ Total Joint Reconstruction

D. E. Perez (✉) · D. Szalay
Oral and Maxillofacial Surgery, UT Health San Antonio, San Antonio, TX, USA
e-mail: Perezd5@uthscsa.edu

P. Mehra, L. M. Wolford (eds.), *Management of Facial Asymmetry*,
https://doi.org/10.1007/978-3-030-44971-1_7

Introduction

Temporomandibular joint (TMJ) pathology, particularly ankylosis and degenerative joint disease (DJD), can cause profound morphological changes in the mandible resulting in significant facial asymmetry. These pathologic anatomical changes are especially pronounced when they occur unilaterally and can be significantly worse when the insult occurs during the growing years of the patient's life. The morphological changes caused by both ankylosis and DJD have the potential to disseminate their effects to surrounding facial soft tissues and bones, especially the maxilla, further complicating treatment. Unlike some other pathological causes of facial asymmetry, the cosmetic and asymmetric problems associated with ankylosis and DJD almost always come with debilitating functional problems, the combination of which may lead to malnourishment, depression, and an overall decreased quality of life. Proper management and surgical treatment of these patients must aim to correct both the functional and esthetic sequelae associated with these pathologies. Ideally, these patients should be treated as early as possible to restore the patient's function and prevent any further progression of facial deformity or asymmetry. This is particularly important in children, or growing patients, who are vulnerable to the psychosocial effects of such conditions.

Treatment of patients with TMJ ankylosis or DJD presents a unique challenge to surgeons for multiple reasons. Growth of the patient and the timing of the surgery must be carefully considered as alloplastic solutions do not grow with the patient and autograft techniques usually provide unpredictable growth and may be susceptible to the original disease process causing recurrence. Since both these disease processes often affect the growing patient, the surgeon may decide to proceed with early surgery to restore function and esthetics quickly with the potential drawback of needing future surgical correction of any abnormal growth that compromises the results. Alternatively, the surgeon may decide to wait until growth is complete prior to definitive reconstruction which would secure a stable result but may leave the patient with a dentofacial deformity (DFD), functional limitations, and a decreased quality of life throughout the remainder of the growing years.

There is often an asymmetry or an associated dentofacial deformity present, which may involve the surrounding skeletal and soft tissue structures, necessitating concomitant orthognathic surgery techniques (LeFort I, bilateral mandibular ramus sagittal split osteotomy (BSSO), genioplasty, etc.) with consideration of proper sequencing and sterile technique. Significant malocclusion is often present and must be corrected. Due to the three-dimensional complexity of these two disease processes and their associated asymmetries and dentofacial deformities, virtual surgical planning (VSP) is an indispensable tool to achieve optimal outcomes.

These patients usually present with limited opening, especially in ankylosis, which may require alternative airway techniques such as fiber-optic intubation, submental intubation, or even tracheotomy. Both DJD and especially ankylosis have the ability to significantly distort the normal anatomy of the joint, making surgery more difficult and increasing the risk of complications such as bleeding or damage to surrounding structures.

Asymmetry may or may not be present in either TMJ ankylosis or DJD. In general, unilateral involvement is more likely to cause asymmetry. It is important to note, however, that although bilateral disease may appear more symmetrical, it often leads to striking retrognathia, anterior open bite, and severe dentofacial deformities as well. If there is an asymmetry, the extent to which it develops depends on the age or remaining growth potential of the patient at the time of disease onset, as well as the speed at which the asymmetry develops. Slowly developing asymmetries will allow for compensation by the opposing arch, dentition, and soft tissues, even in the adult patient, which may lead to a more extensive asymmetric problem. In the growing patient, this effect is exaggerated, as there is more plasticity in surrounding tissues to adapt and try to accommodate the asymmetry. If an asymmetry has developed relatively quickly, the opposing arch and dentition do not have adequate time to adapt, which often leads to obvious malocclusions with premature contacts on the affected side, and open bite on the opposing side.

Facial asymmetries and deformities as consequences of ankylosis and DJD are typically signs of severe or progressive disease. Although conservative therapies and medical management have an important role in the treatment of temporomandibular disease, they have a limited ability to restore function and form in patients with ankylosis or DJD severe enough to cause such changes. These patients generally require more extensive surgical intervention or reconstruction, which will be the main focus of this chapter.

TMJ Ankylosis

Pathophysiology

TMJ ankylosis refers to a pathological condition in which the mandible has become fused to the fossa by bony or fibrotic tissues. It is usually confined to the intracapsular condyle, glenoid fossa, and articular eminence region, but can occasionally spread extracapsular to include the coronoid process, zygomatic arch, lateral pterygoid plate, external auditory canal, and even the skull base [1] (Fig. 1). Topazian, Sawhney, and He et al. have all proposed classification systems for TMJ ankylosis [2–4] (Table 1).

Traumas, specifically unilateral and bilateral condyle fractures, are the most common cause of ankylosis throughout the literature, accounting for up to 90% of cases of ankylosis [5–8] (Fig. 2). The second most common etiology is infection, most often suppurative otitis media [9]. Other less common causes include chronic arthritis, rheumatoid arthritis, psoriasis, osteochondromas, ankylosing spondylitis, syndromic, failed previous reconstructions, and idiopathic [5]. Iatrogenic ankylosis may also occur with failed TMJ surgery.

Although the condyle is the second most common anatomical site for mandibular fractures, accounting for approximately 30% of fractures [10], ankylosis is a relatively uncommon outcome of such injuries. Ankylosis tends to occur

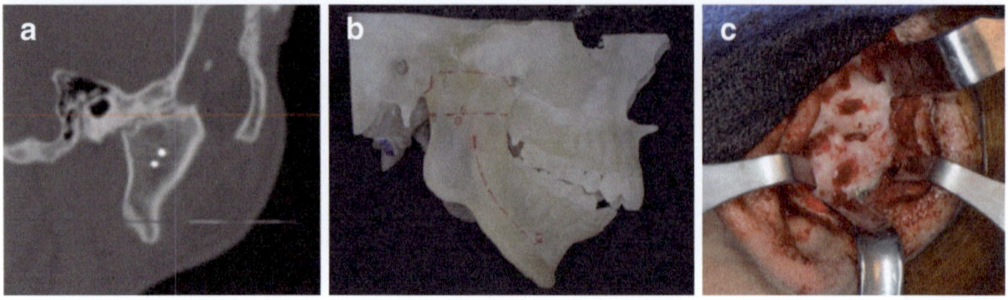

Fig. 1 TMJ ankylosis. (**a**) Sagittal cut from CT scan on patient with severe bony ankylosis of bilateral temporomandibular joints (R side shown here). (**b**) STL model showing pathological bony continuity between the mandibular ramus and the zygoma. (**c**) R-sided bony ankylosis as seen intraoperatively through endaural approach with complete obliteration of normal anatomy

Table 1 Different classification systems for TMJ ankylosis

Topazian (1964)	Sawhney (1986)	He et al (2011)
Stage I: Ankylotic bone limited to condylar process condyle present	**Type 1:** Extensive fibrous adhesions around joint, condyle present	**A1**: Fibrous ankylosis without bony fusion
Stage II: Ankylotic bone extending to sigmoid notch	**Type 2:** Bony fusion, especially at lateral articular surface, no fusion in the medial joint space	**A2**: Bony ankylosis in lateral joint, residual condyle fragment is larger than 50% of contralateral normal condyle
Stage III: Ankylotic Bone extending to coronoid process.	**Type 3:** Bony bridge between ascending ramus of mandibular and temporal bone/zygomatic arch	**A3:** Similar to A2, residual condyle is smaller then 50% of contralateral normal condyle
	Type 4: Joint is replaced by a mass of bone between the ramus and the skull base	**A4**: Complete bony ankylosis

more often in condylar fractures involving children that are not properly managed and do not undergo appropriate physical therapy and monitoring after injury. Condylar fractures that are particularly prone to ankylosis are intracapsular condyle fractures treated with long periods of maxillomandibular fixation (MMF) or laterally displaced subcondylar fractures with mandibular widening, which is not properly reduced, leading to extracapsular healing [11]. Children are thought to be prone to ankylosis due to their higher number of progenitor stem cells, rapid reparative fibroplasia, and predisposition for rapid bone regeneration [11]. The most commonly reported pathophysiological mechanism for ankylosis is TMJ hemarthrosis in the setting of articular surface damage predisposing to heterotopic bone formation [11]. Proper treatment of pediatric condyle fractures with appropriate physical therapy postoperatively may prevent the formation of ankylosis (Fig. 3).

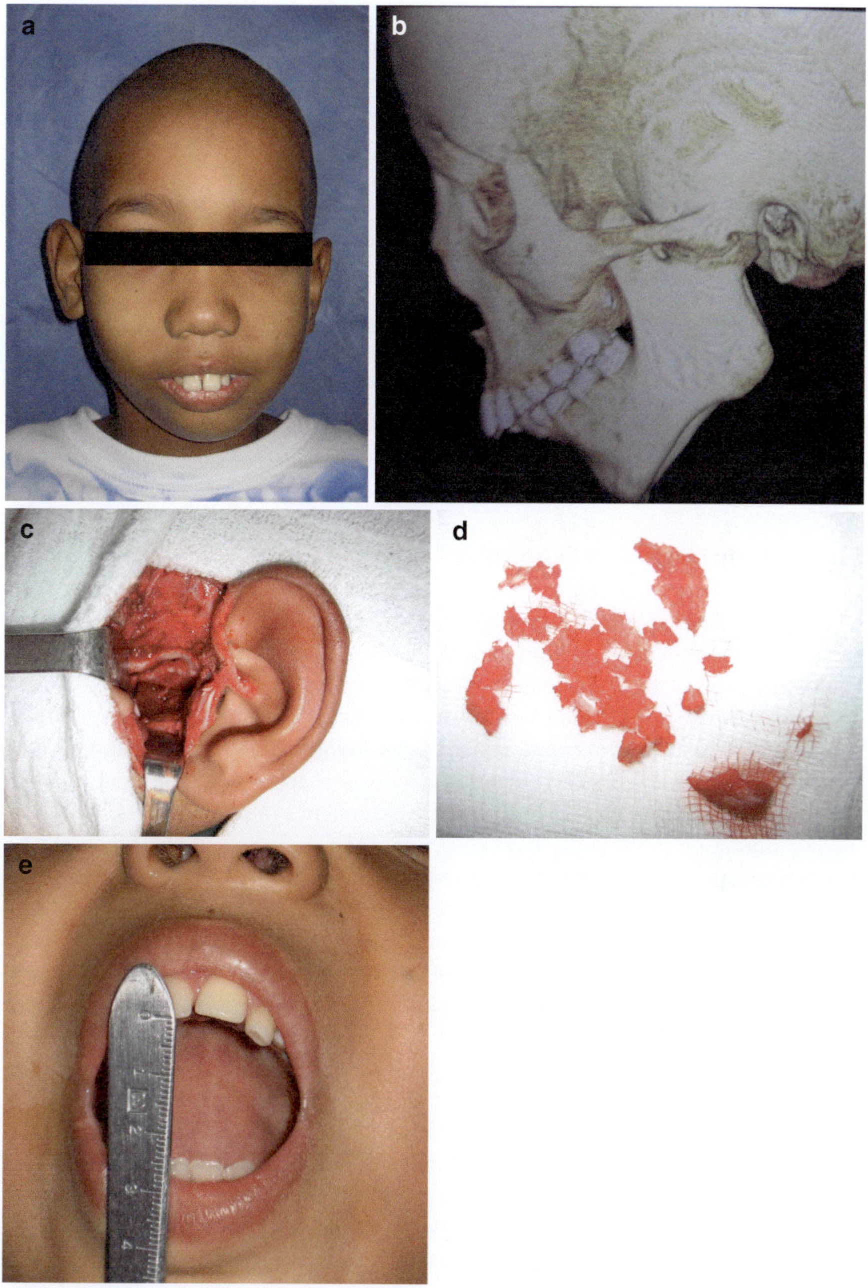

Fig. 2 Ankylosed left temporomandibular joint in a pediatric patient after L-sided condylar fracture. (**a**) Note asymmetry with left-sided chin deviation. (**b**) Note left-sided TMJ ankylosis with retrognathia and short ramus. (**c**) Intraoperative photos of gap arthroplasty showing removal of ankylotic joint. Spacer was placed. (**d**) Pieces of ankylotic mass and condyle that were removed during surgery. (**e**) Postoperative maximum opening with return to function after physical therapy and jaw exercises

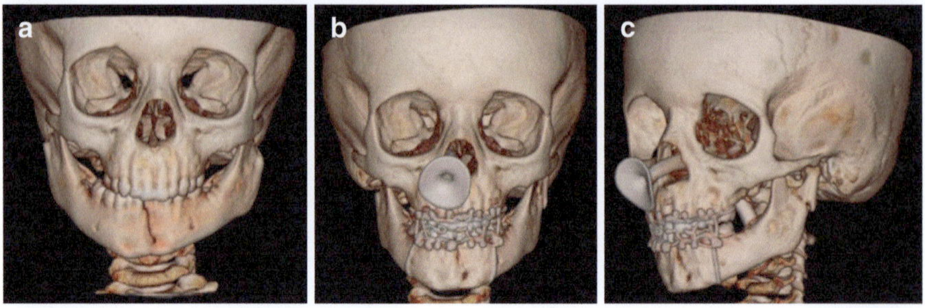

Fig. 3 Properly treated pediatric condyle fracture. (**a**) 5-year-old male with bilateral mandibular subcondylar and symphysis fractures resulting in significant widening and posterior displacement of the mandible, medially displaced condyles, and loss of airway. Note the position of the fractured mandibular ramus directly inferior to zygomatic arch increasing the risk of ankylosis if untreated. (**b**) Properly reduced pediatric mandible fracture with lingual splint, pediatric pelvic reduction forceps used to control transverse dimension intraoperatively, circummandibular wiring to secure lingual splint, and a short period of elastic MMF. (**c**) Note reduced condyle after treatment

Signs, Symptoms, and Diagnosis

Diagnosis of TMJ ankylosis is usually done by clinical exam and imaging studies, such as CT scans, MRI, and three-dimensional reconstructions [12]. These patients commonly present for treatment at a younger age, with studies reporting 68% to 76% under the age of 15 and over half of patients less than 10 years of age [1, 7]; however, ankylosis may occur at any age. It is slightly more common in boys than in girls with a 1.4:1.2 ratio. Unilateral ankylosis is more common than bilateral ankylosis, with a ratio of 1.5:1 [13]. The most frequent symptoms of TMJ ankylosis include limitation of maximal incisal opening (MIO), decreased jaw function, and diet limitations. Other symptoms may include TMJ pain, facial pain, headaches, disability, dentofacial deformity, and facial asymmetries [5]. Many patients have associated psychosocial problems such as anxiety and depression. Severe cases of ankylosis allow only a few millimeters of opening or less, making it nearly impossible for patients to perform daily tasks as simple as eating, brushing their teeth, or in some extreme cases, breathing comfortably. This can ultimately lead to malnutrition and poor oral health. On exam, patients often have severely limited opening, with studies showing an average maximal incisal opening (MIO) of 14.5 mm [5], with a range of 0–20 mm.

Patients with ankylosis may have significant and sometimes striking asymmetries or dentofacial deformities. However, the specific pattern of facial deformity and extent of asymmetry depend on many factors, such as if the ankylosis occurred before or after growth was complete and whether it's unilateral or bilateral.

For example, in the adult nongrowing patient, whose ankylosis occurred after growth is complete, the main finding may simply be severe limitation in jaw opening and function. Even in unilateral disease, dentofacial deformities and asymmetries are not as common, and if present, generally less pronounced because these patients did not have the pathological growth that affects growing ankylosed patients. If unilateral involvement occurs in this patient population, it generally manifests as deviation on opening to the affected side. The ankylosed joint does not allow proper rotational or translational movements leading to deviation on opening to the ankylosed side. Overtime, in long-standing untreated ankylosis, these patients may develop some dental compensation in the opposing arch. Although they may not have the severe dentofacial deformities or asymmetries that plague those patients affected in their growing years, they suffer from the same TMJ pain, facial pain, headaches, limitations in jaw function, decreased maximal incisal opening(MIO), severe diet limitations, and disability and often have psychosocial issues as well (Fig. 4).

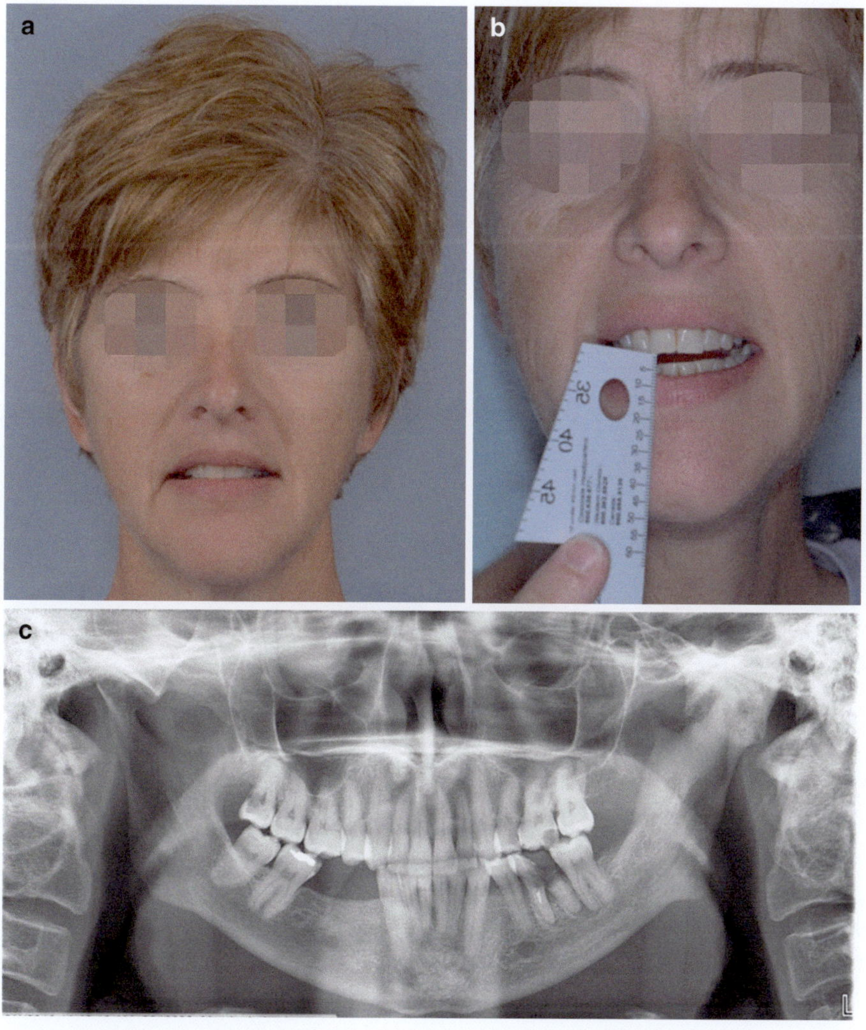

Fig. 4 Unilateral ankylosis in the adult patient. (**a**) Ankylosis occurred after growth was complete. No gross facial asymmetry seen. (**b**) Severe limitation in maximum incisal opening is present, with slight deviation toward ankylosed joint. (**c**) Unilateral L-sided ankylosis seen on Panorex

TMJ ankylosis effectively alters the growth of the involved condyle, while the rest of the face continues to grow and adapt. As the maxilla and the opposing condyle grow, the ankylosed condyle anchors the patient's mandible to that side. Unilateral involvement commonly causes deviation of the mandible to the ipsilateral side of the ankylosis with a class II skeletal and dentofacial deformity and a short ramus, usually more pronounced on the pathological side. Additionally, the surrounding facial skeleton and soft tissues try to adapt as well, spreading the problem to the opposing arch causing a maxillary cant, and continuing to affect the rest of the face complicating future surgical treatment (Fig. 5) Unilateral bony ankylosis may also lead to contralateral fibrous ankylosis further limiting function.

With bilateral ankylosis in the growing patient, the growth of the entire mandible is severely limited, but the rest of the face continues to grow. As the maxilla continues to grow anteriorly and inferiorly, the opposing ankylosed mandible with minimal to no growth falls further behind, leading to a retrognathic small mandible, short ramus height, steep mandibular plane angle, and anterior open bite with significant overjet. This has been referred to as a "bird-beaking" deformity due to the significant facial deformity that can develop. Obstructive sleep apnea (OSA) is common with this anatomy (Fig. 6).

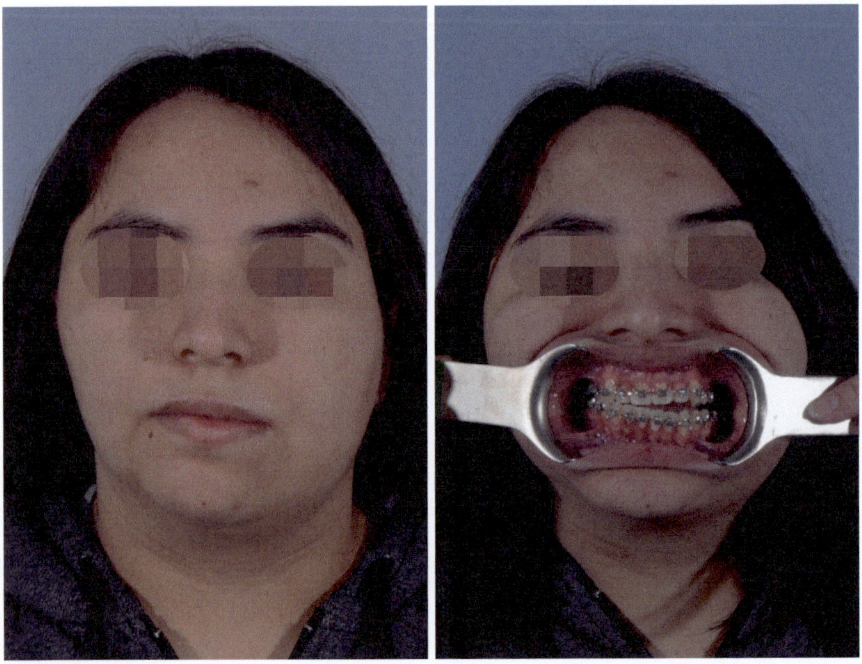

Fig. 5 Unilateral TMJ involvement. In unilateral cases, the surrounding facial skeleton and soft tissues try to adapt as well, spreading the problem to the opposing arch causing a maxillary cant, and continuing to affect the rest of the face complicating future surgical treatment

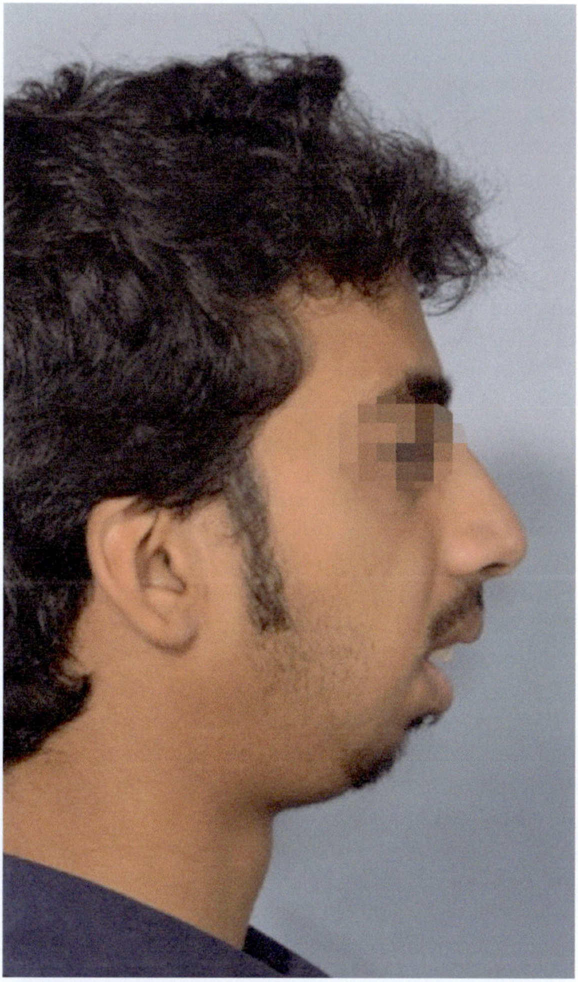

Fig. 6 Bilateral ankylosis in the growing patient. Retrognathic small mandible, short ramus height, steep mandibular plan angle, with significant overjet causing "bird-beaking" deformity. Anterior open bite present

The ankylosed patient may present as a child or an adult with unilateral or bilateral joint involvement, but proper treatment with quick return to function and correction of associated dentofacial deformities, while preventing recurrence or relapse, is essential to improve the quality of life in these patients.

Treatment Options and Staging for Facial Asymmetry in Ankylosis

Treatment of ankylosis is one of the greatest challenges in TMJ surgery, and although a variety of techniques for treatment in adults and children have been reported, no single method has been proven to be consistently successful and predictable in all situations [9, 14]. The main treatment goals of TMJ ankylosis are to increase the patient's mandibular function with stable results, correct associated facial deformities, decrease pain, and prevent re-ankylosis [5, 12].

Gap Arthroplasty and Interpositional Gap Arthroplasty

Gap arthroplasty is the simplest treatment with the shortest operating time. It essentially consists of aggressive excision of the ankylotic mass, ipsilateral and/or contralateral coronoidectomy, and leaving a gap of significant width between the ascending ramus and the temporal bone. Unfortunately, this technique has many disadvantages including failure to remove all bony pathology, an unacceptably high risk of re-ankylosis (up to 53%) [15], unsatisfactory range of motion, inadequate restoration of function, creation of a pseudo-articulation, anterior open bite in bilateral cases, and premature contact on the affected side with open bite on the contralateral side in unilateral cases.

With interpositional gap arthroplasty, alloplastic or autogenous materials are placed in the gap or ostectomy site in the hopes of preventing re-ankylosis. Various interpositional materials have been used including autogenous (temporalis myofascial flap, auricular cartilage, articular disc, dermis) and alloplastic (silicone blocks, silastic materials, acrylic ball) materials. No ideal interpositional material has been found. The temporalis muscle is the most commonly autogenous solution, but it is susceptible to problems such as muscle fibrosis or calcification leading to scar contracture and trismus and also comes with donor site morbidity. Studies comparing interpositional to gap arthroplasty have found increased maximal incisal opening and approximately three times less recurrence of ankylosis with interpositional grafting [13].

Unfortunately, interpositional grafting does not restore the joint's proper form and function; autogenous materials for interpositional grafting are susceptible to wear, fibrosis, or calcification, while alloplastic graft may cause foreign body reactions. Re-ankylosis may still occur even with interpositional grafting. Additionally, those who receive interpositional gap arthroplasty tend to have more pain than those who get total joint replacements [13]. Gap arthroplasty with interpositional grafting can, however, provide an adequate temporary solution in patients until a more definitive reconstruction can be completed (Fig. 7). Some

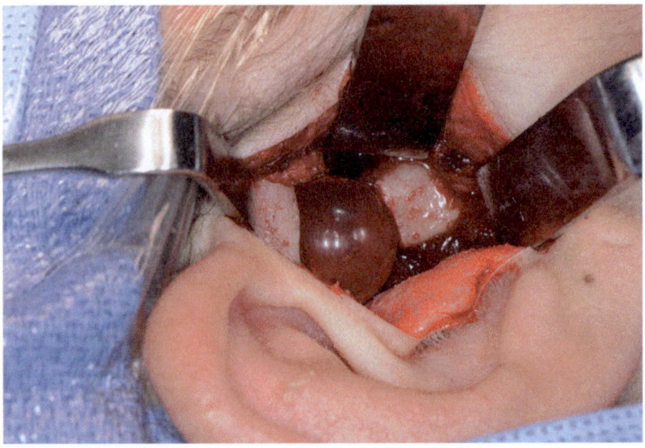

Fig. 7 Interpositional gap arthroplasty. Nonporous PMMA (polymethylmethacrylate) sterile eye sphere used as a spacer after gap arthroplasty

patients may do well with gap arthroplasty with or without interpositional grafting, and if no DFD or asymmetry is present, it may be used as a long-term solution with close monitoring.

Autografts Reconstruction in TMJ Ankylosis

Prior to the advances in total joint prosthesis and 3D imaging technology, autografts were considered the "gold standard" for TMJ ankylosis. The benefit of these reconstructions with costochondral grafts (CCG) and sternoclavicular grafts, in theory, is the graft can grow with the patient. Kaban and colleagues have defined a protocol for the management of TMJ ankylosis in children that centers on aggressive excision of the ankylotic mass, ipsilateral and sometimes contralateral coronoidectomy, lining of the fossa with the native disc or a temporalis myofascial flap, joint reconstruction with distraction osteogenesis (DO) or a costochondral graft, early mobilization, and aggressive physical therapy [15]. Unfortunately, costochondral grafting in the setting of ankylosis produces inconsistent and unsatisfactory results. Two major problems have come to light regarding the costochondral graft. First, growth of the grafts is unpredictable with decreased, or more often, increased, growth on the ipsilateral side ultimately leading to asymmetry. Long-term reports of mandibular growth in children whose TMJs were reconstructed with CCG show that excessive growth on the treated side occurred in 54% of the 72 cases examined and growth equal to that on the opposite side occurred in only 38% of the cases[1] [16]. Recent studies seem to suggest that the cartilaginous component of these grafts may not even be necessary to restore and maintain mandibular growth [17] (Fig. 8).

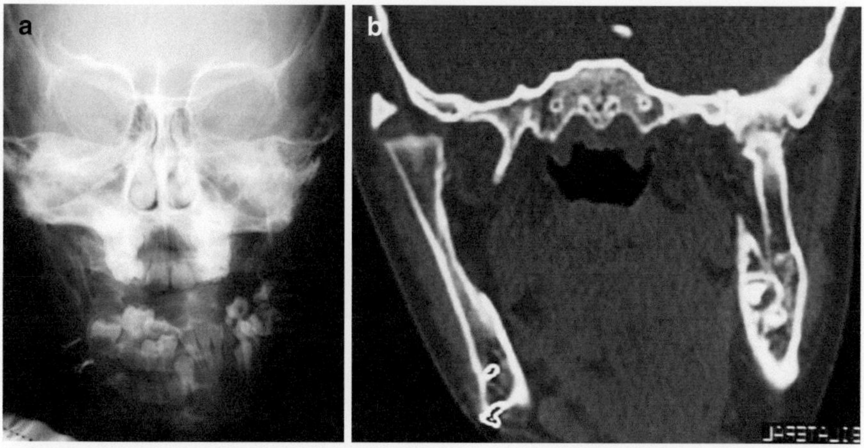

Fig. 8 Re-ankylosis of a joint 3 years after costochondral grafting for treatment of ankylosis resulting in asymmetry. (**a**) Note left-sided mandibular deviation with overgrowth on the right side. (**b**) Note overgrowth of costochondral graft on the right side with mandibular deviation on this coronal slice of CT scan

The second problem seen in autografts used in ankylosis cases is that they are susceptible to re-ankylosis. Unfortunately, patients who had ankylosis previously and undergo autogenous costochondral grafting have a high incidence of re-ankylosis. It is logical that autogenous tissues placed in an area with reactive and heterotopic bone formation may be susceptible to the same pathological process that affected the original joint. In these cases, the chance of re-ankylosis may be further increased as a result of autograft fixation failure or the uncooperative nature of the young patient with physical therapy after reconstruction [16] Additionally, graft mobility during healing may compromise blood supply and incorporation of the graft leading to failure [18]. Of note, orthopedic surgeons typically choose alloplastic reconstruction in similar situations involving other joints [19, 20]. Caution is advised when using autogenous materials in sites of previous ankylosis, with outcomes favoring alloplastic reconstruction [20] (Fig. 8).

Alloplastic Reconstruction in TMJ Ankylosis

With recent improvements in technology, alloplastic TMJ reconstruction is gaining popularity. Advantages include mimicking the normal anatomy, restoring vertical dimension, avoiding donor site morbidity, reduction in operative time, reduction in joint pain, reduced risk of re-ankylosis, improved esthetic result, and immediate physiotherapy as well as the possibility of associated DFD correction [21–23].

The success of alloplastic TJR has been repeatedly shown in literature. Notably, in 2016, Wolford et al. specifically addressed TMJ ankylosis treated with alloplastic TJR with the TMJ Concepts system and fat grafting in 48 ankylosed joints with a mean follow-up period of 68 months and found statistically significant improvement in pain, headache, jaw function, diet, disability, MIO, and lateral excursion [5]. When compared directly to costochondral grafting, TJR with alloplastic materials also seems to provide the greatest benefit in regard to pain reduction [13]. Several studies have compared alloplastic joint reconstruction with autogenous costochondral or sternoclavicular grafts in the presence of ankylosis, generally favoring alloplastic TJR.

The poor functional outcomes of gap arthroplasty and interpositional grafts, along with the unpredictable outcomes of autogenous grafts, have ultimately led to alloplastic total joint replacement becoming the treatment of choice in most cases of ankylosis. Alloplastic total joint replacement, either with custom-made TMJ Concepts total joint prosthesis or stock joint prosthesis, is our preference for the following ankylosis situations.

Treatment Considerations and Staging in TMJ Ankylosis

There are four major categories that patients with TMJ ankylosis fit into, with each group having their own unique treatment considerations. They are separated based on remaining growth potential and presence of an additional dentofacial deformity. Unilateral and bilateral disease must also be considered (Fig. 9).

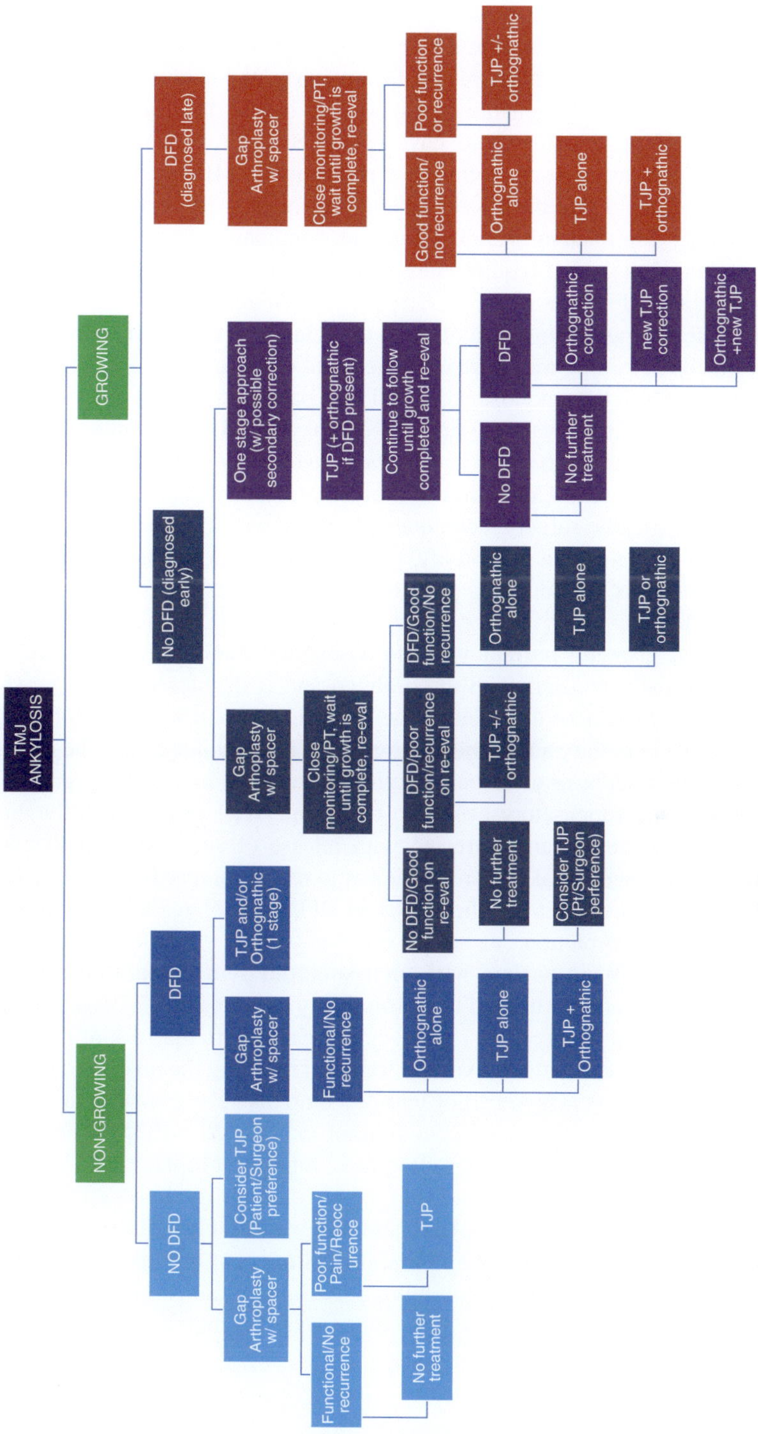

Fig. 9 Treatment flowchart for TMJ ankylosis. DFD – dentofacial deformity. TJP – total joint prosthesis. PT – physical therapy. GA w/ spacer – gap arthroplasty with spacer

1. The **ankylosed nongrowing patient with no associated dentofacial deformity**. This patient usually develops the ankylosis after his or her growth is complete, and there is no underlying malocclusion or skeletal abnormality prior to the ankylosis event. They generally present early before dental compensation has occurred. If these patients do have asymmetry, it's generally minimal. Clinically, they usually present with severe restriction in MIO, functional problems, and deviation toward the ankylosed joint on opening. Treatment is predictable and stable. Contralateral mandibular ramus osteotomy may need to be done even in unilateral disease if required movement is not easily accommodated by the opposing joint (Fig. 10a-d).
2. The **ankylosed nongrowing patient with associated dentofacial deformity.** The dentofacial deformity may have been the result of the ankylosis or may have been present prior to the ankylosing event. These patients are often retrognathic and may have deviation toward the side of their ankylosis. Long-standing unilateral ankylosis may lead to dental compensations in the opposing arch and maxillary cant may be present. Correction of the dentofacial deformity may require traditional orthognathic surgery techniques combined with TJR such as LeFort I osteotomy, unilateral ramus osteotomy, genioplasty, or additional procedures. Since the patient has no remaining growth potential, the results are likely to be stable (Fig. 11a–c).
3. The **ankylosed growing patient with no associated dentofacial deformity**. This patient usually presents with the problem and is diagnosed before gross facial asymmetry has time to develop. The challenge is to restore function and promote normal maxillary and mandibular growth. These children must be monitored on a consistent basis after their ankylosis is released to detect any growth abnormalities or compensatory events to try to intervene and mitigate larger changes. These patients can be treated with release of ankylosis and spacer placement or may need total joint replacement to restore proper form and function. Despite intervention, they often develop DFD as they age and may need secondary surgical correction.
4. The **ankylosed growing patient with an associated dentofacial deformity.** These patients are usually treated late or multiply operated and have an associated dentofacial deformity that is now complicated with the lack of mobility. This is the most challenging patient because removing the ankylotic mass first and restoring function does not lead to compensatory growth and symmetry, and they frequently need concomitant or delayed orthognathic surgery procedures in addition to their alloplastic total joint replacement. Since these patients commonly have poor quality of life and psychosocial issues, release of ankylosis with spacer placement and waiting for definitive reconstruction after growth is complete is not always the best option. Alloplastic total joint prosthesis even with remaining growth potential can be done with the understanding that secondary procedures may be required later in life (Fig. 12).

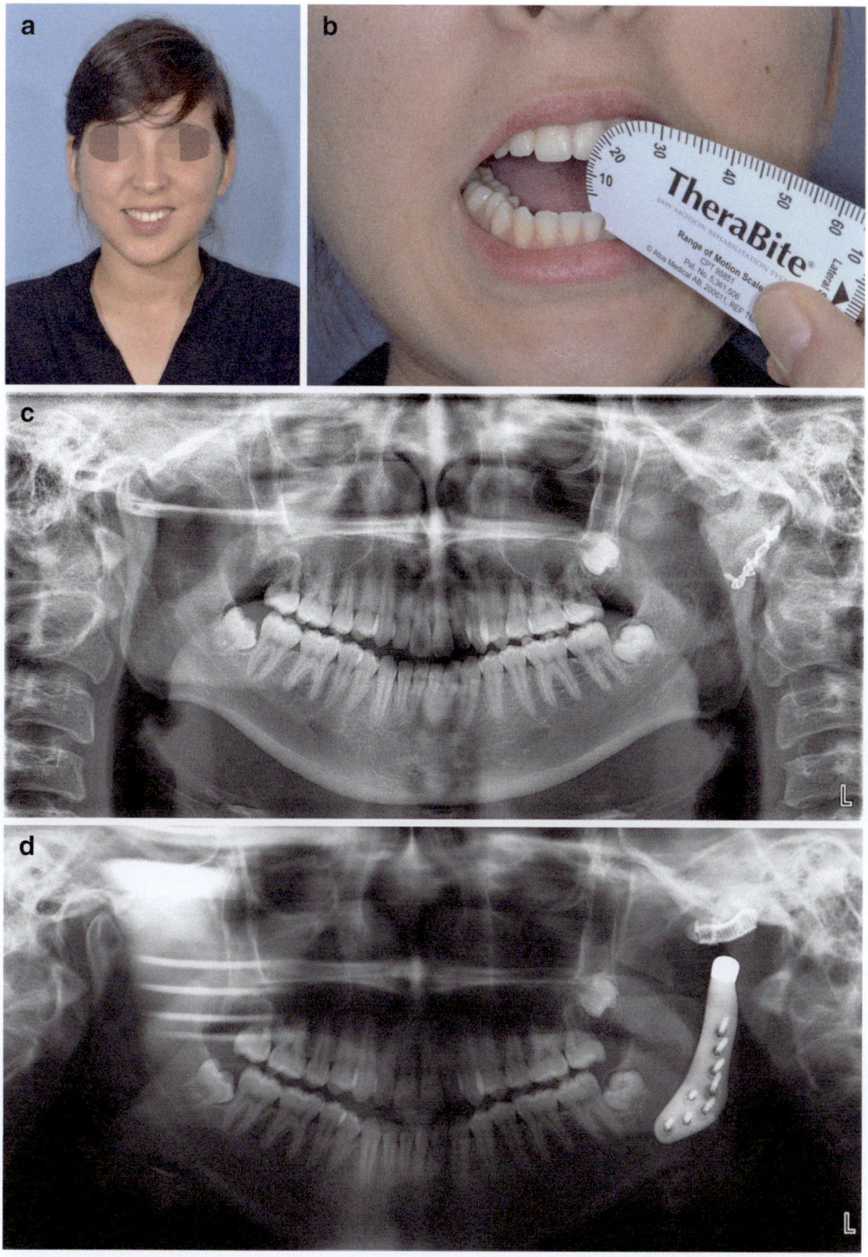

Fig. 10 Nongrowing, unilaterally ankylosed patient with no associated DFD. (**a**) No gross asymmetry noted. (**b**) Note limitation in function with left-sided deviation on opening. (**c**) Panorex showing left-sided ankylosis. (**d**) Postoperative Panorex after unilateral total joint prosthesis

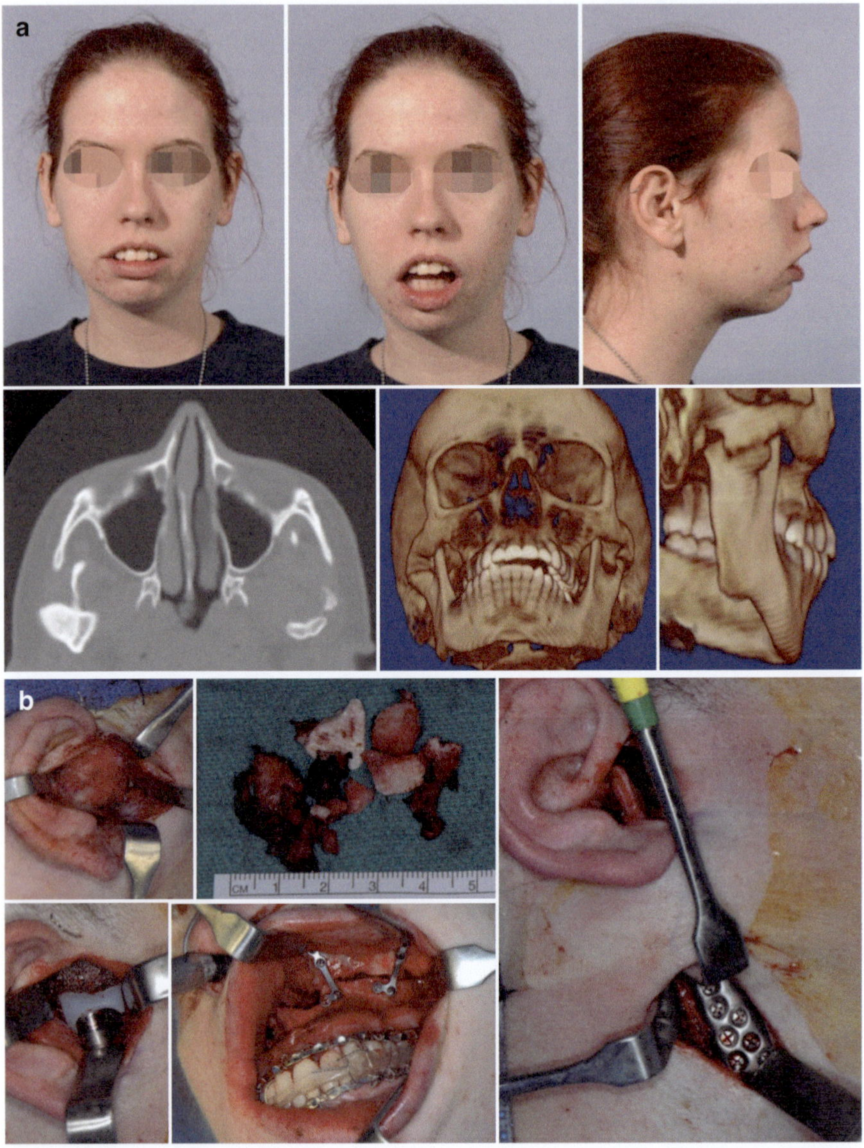

Fig. 11 Ankylosed nongrowing patient with associated DFD. (**a**) On presentation, dentofacial deformity with R-sided chin deviation and retrognathia with compensations present in the maxilla. (**b**) Surgery completed in one stage, with release on ankylosis, BL TJR through submandibular and endaural incisions, combined with LeFort I osteotomy. (**c**) Postoperative result with correction of DFD and asymmetry with good occlusion and function

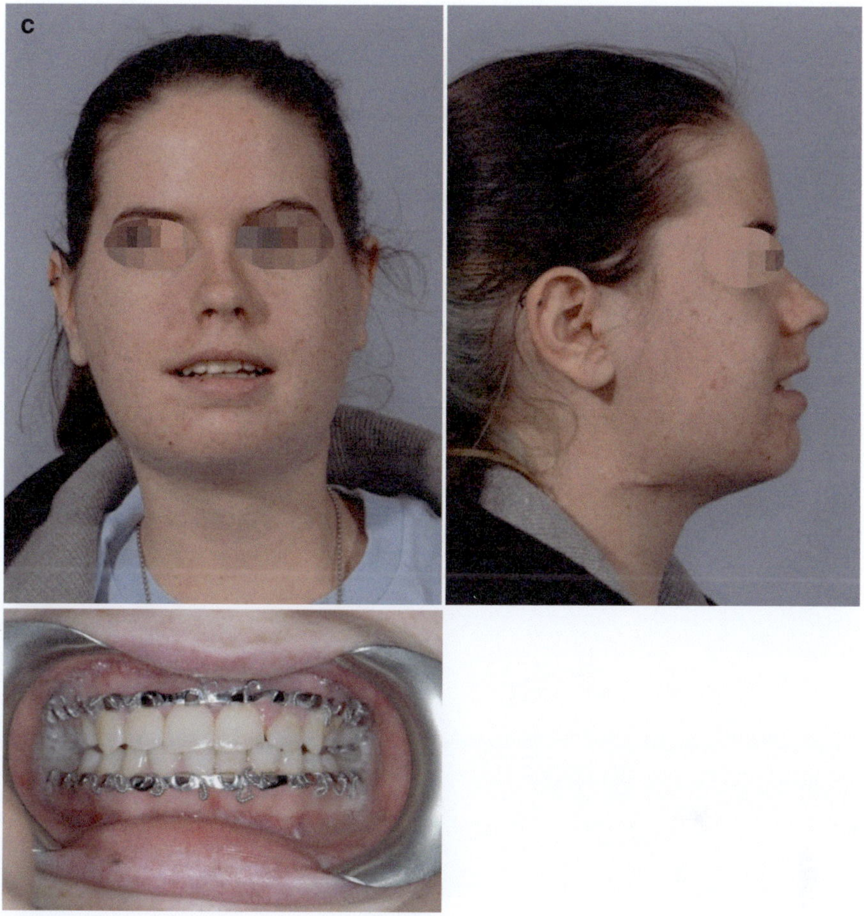

Fig. 11 (continued)

There are two general approaches to restore an ankylosed patient to function and correct associated asymmetries and facial deformities. You may plan to use either a one-stage or two-stage/multi-staged approach.

For both approaches, planning for the TJR often begins with a CT scan which is used to generate a stereolithic (STL) model from which the surgery is planned, and the custom-fitted TMJ TJR components are designed and manufactured, with dimensional accuracy estimated at approximately 97.9 [12]. Virtual surgical planning is also used and can be helpful to plan any concomitant orthognathic surgery that needs to be completed.

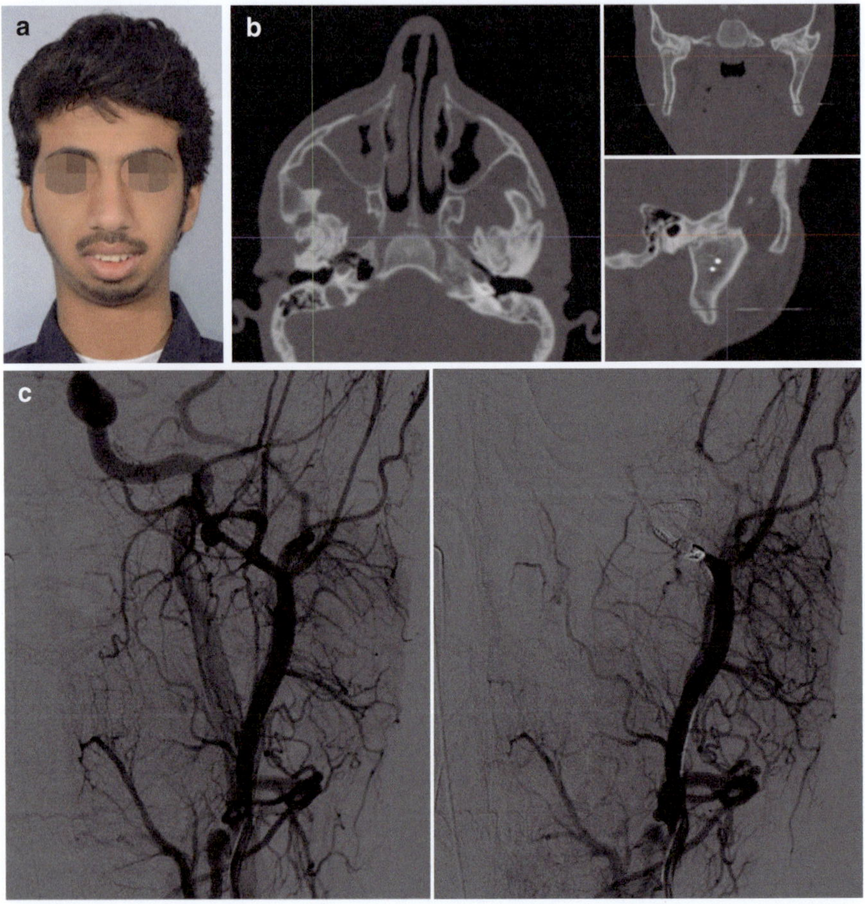

Fig. 12 Ankylosed growing patient with associated dentofacial deformity. One-stage approach with secondary correction. (**a**) Note DFD, retrognathia, and "bird-beaking" associated with BL TMJ ankylosis. (**b**) BL ankylosis as seen on CT scan. (**c**) Before and after internal maxillary artery embolization. Note decreased blood flow to surgical field. (**d**) Release of ankylosis and surgery completed on STL model and reproduced in the patient. BL TJR was completed with fat grafting at this same time. (**e**) Immediate postoperative return of form and function with improved quality of life. Posterior open bite left to be corrected later when growth is complete with traditional orthognathic surgery. (**f**) CT scan showing bilateral total joint prosthesis. Patient will require secondary surgery once growth is complete for a functional and esthetic outcome with good occlusion

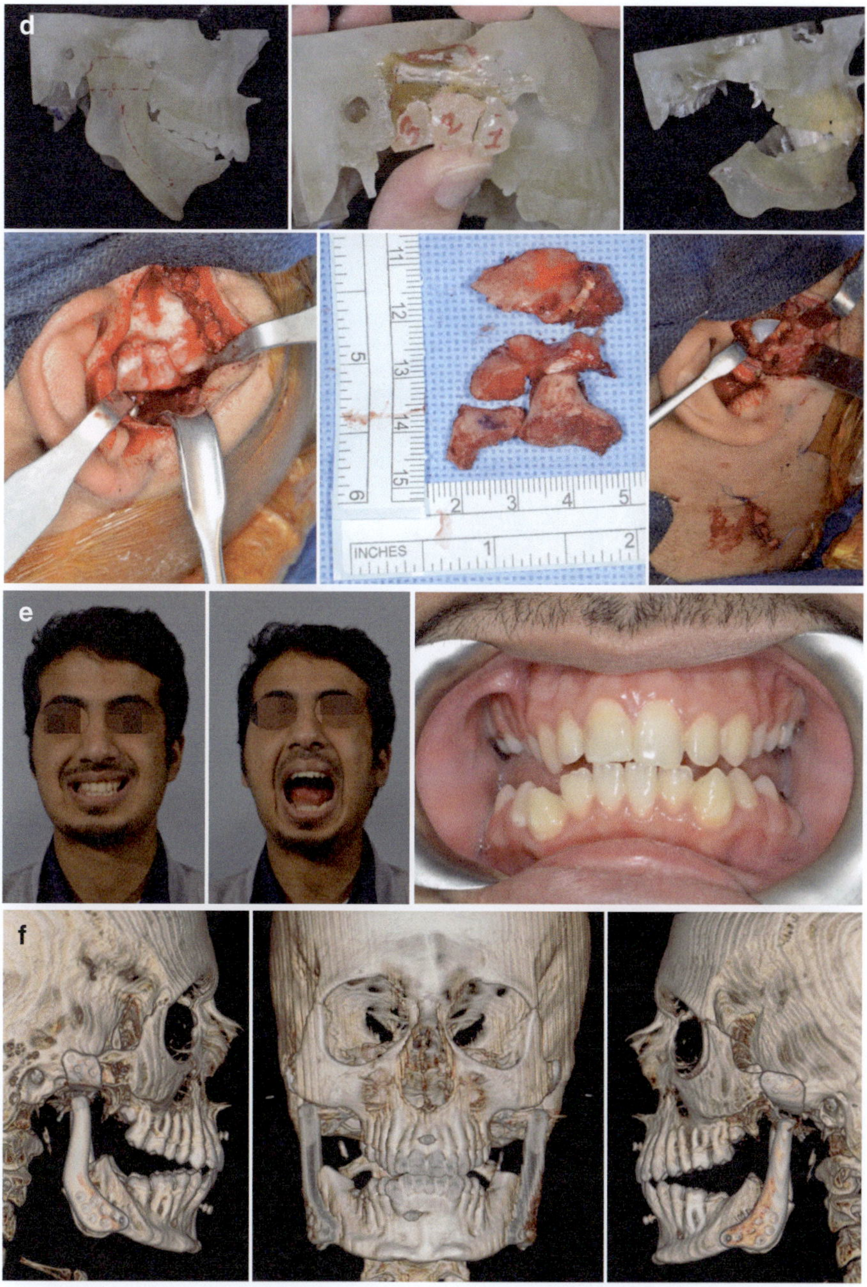

Fig. 12 (continued)

Two-Stage/Multi-stage Approach

At stage 1 surgery – the surgeon must remove the ankylotic bone, create an adequate gap of approximately 2–2.5 cm, and place a material spacer to prevent the reformation of tissue and or/bone (silastic, acrylic, or bone cement). A postoperative CT scan can be completed for future virtual surgical planning and to help generate a custom TMJ prosthesis (Fig. 13).

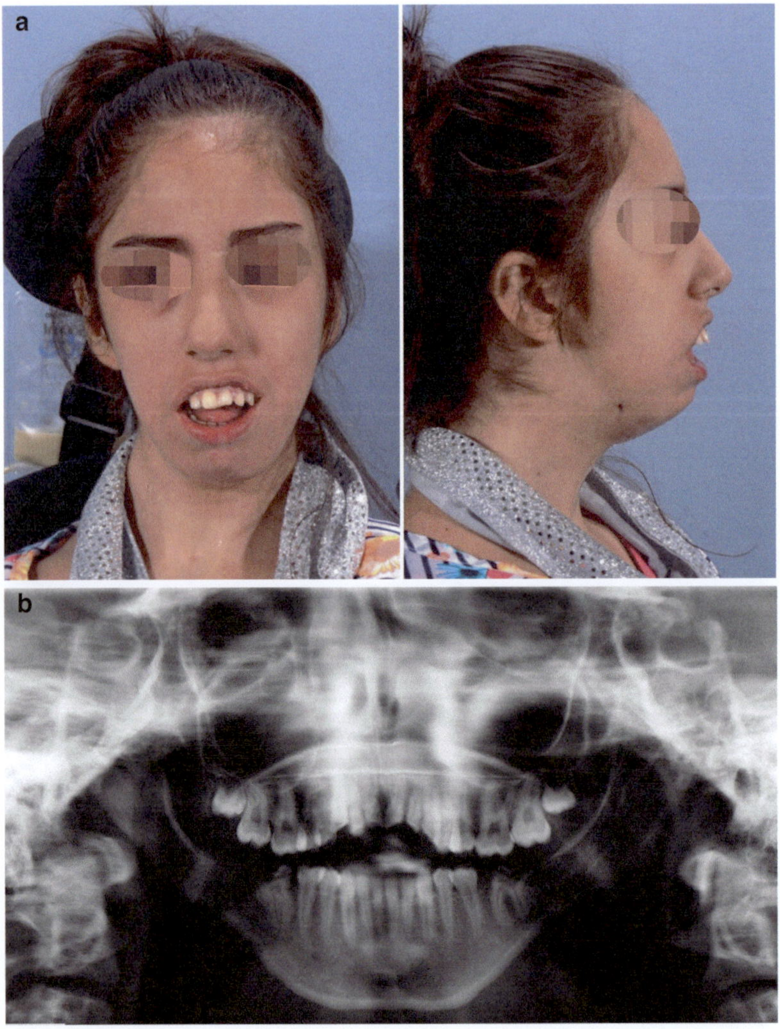

Fig. 13 Ankylosed growing patient with associated dentofacial deformity. Multi-staged approach. (**a**) Note gross underlying DFD worsened by BL ankylosis with anterior open bite and retrognathia. (**b**) Bilateral ankylosis present on Panorex. (**c**) Ankylosis release with placement of spacer and immediate return to function. (**d**) Patient returned for total joint replacement to improve function

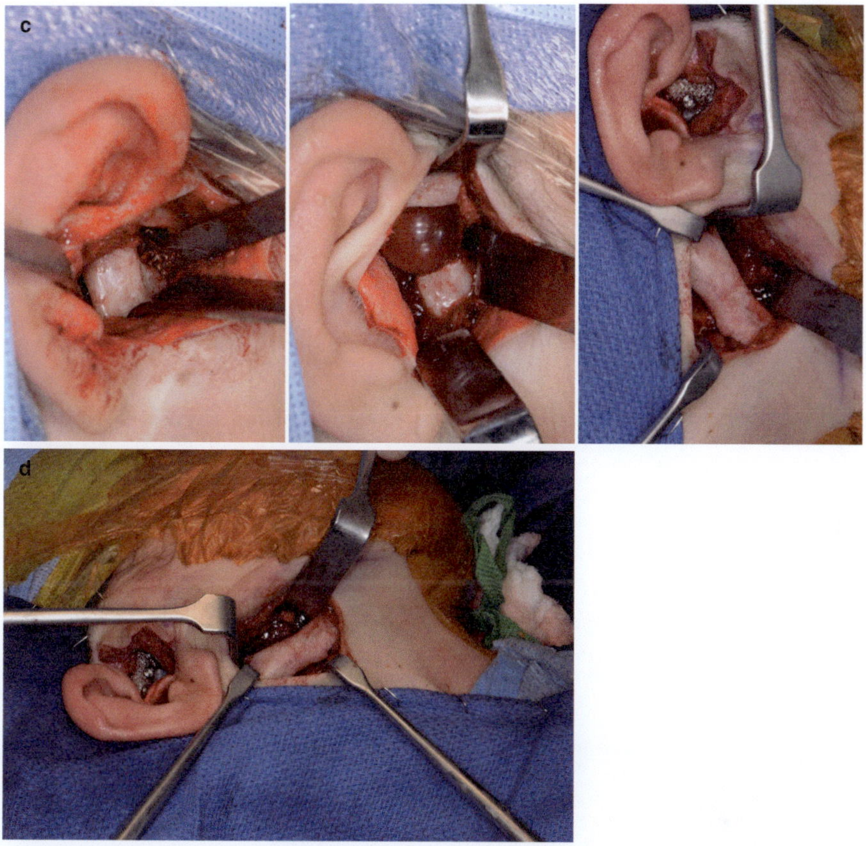

Fig. 13 (continued)

At stage 2 surgery – the spacer is removed, and the patient is fitted with the TMJ TJR components. An autogenous fat graft is placed around the articulation to inhibit formation of heterotopic bone and development of re-ankylosis. The patient can begin immediately with post-op physical therapy. In the nongrowing patient, any dentofacial deformities can be corrected with traditional orthognathic techniques at this stage, in the same surgery. This is often required for gross asymmetries. If the patient has remaining growth potential, combining orthognathic surgery at this stage may lead to unpredictable results and need for future secondary surgery. It may be decided to wait until growth is complete and finalize any DFD correction at that point in a multi-stage approach (Fig. 14).

The major benefit of the two-stage or multi-stage approach is that a postoperative CT scan taken after the first-stage surgery can be used to generate a new stereolithic model which can then be used to create a custom TJP that fits the specific anatomical circumstance of the case. Since the virtual surgical plan is based on a CT scan that is taken once all heterotopic bone has been reduced, placement of the prosthesis during the second stage is easier and quicker. The other obvious advantage is that

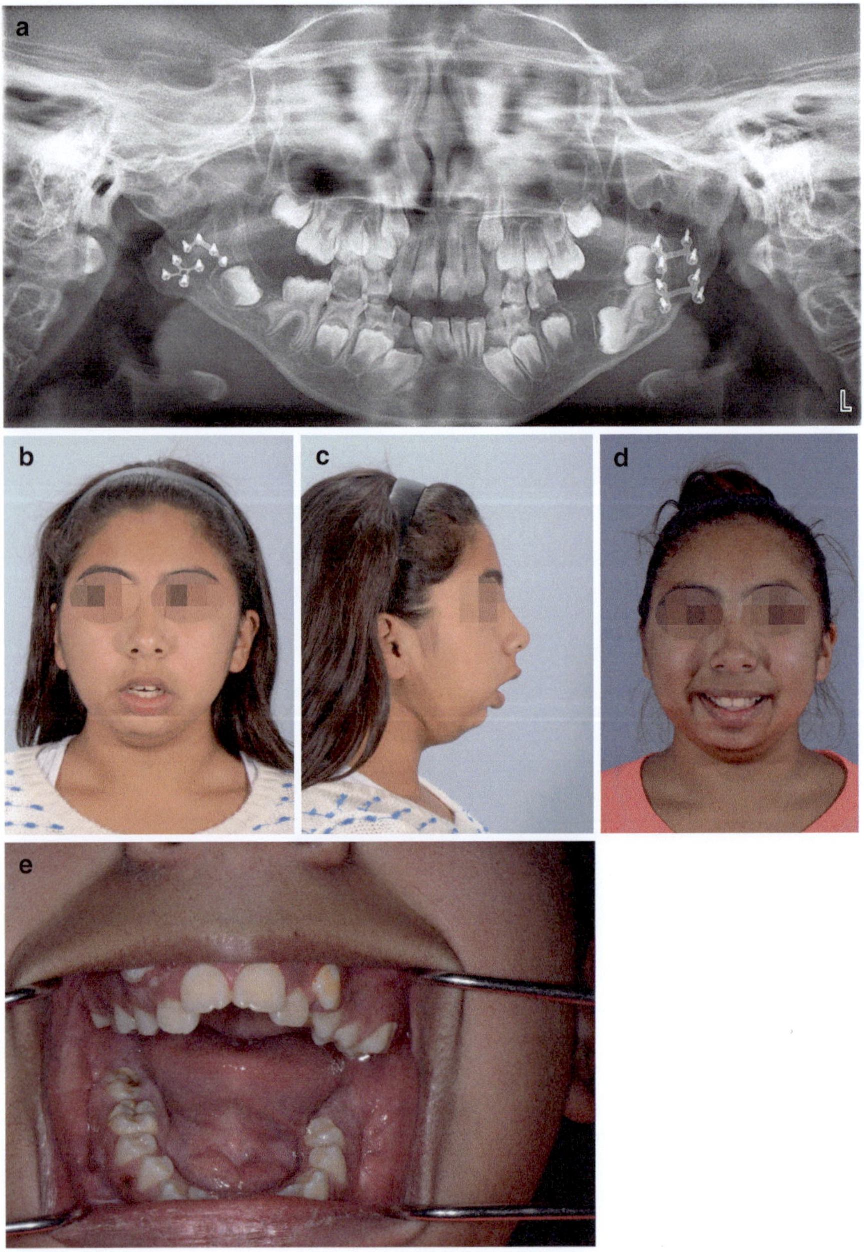

Fig. 14 BL TMJ ankylosis after failed distraction with original onset at age 5 years old. (**a**) Patients' Panorex showing bilateral ankylosis. (**b**) Patient at maximal incisal opening. (**c**) Note severely class II retrognathic appearance. (**d**) Patient after BL gap arthroplasty with spacer placement doing well. Patient is awaiting further growth at which point BL TJP and any indicated orthognathic surgery will be performed. (**e**) Post-op maximal incisal opening

the early release of the ankylosis with a spacer can improve a patient's function quickly. This can significantly improve the patient's quality of life as they wait for their final total joint prosthesis to be made, if they are waiting until the orthodontic therapy is complete, or even while they wait for their facial growth to stop so their final surgery can be more predictable with less risk and faster operative time.

The One-Stage Approach

A one-stage protocol can be considered in most nongrowing patient with ankylosis, with or without significant dentofacial deformity. The obvious benefit is immediate restoration of function and cosmetics in one surgery without needing additional procedures later. Total joint prosthesis placement and orthognathic techniques for correction of dentofacial deformities may all be done in one surgery. This approach is best done by experienced surgeons, as recreating the ankylosis release done on the STL model in the actual patient at the time of surgery, with accurate placement of the prosthesis, may be difficult.

Although a growing patient may be better treated with a two-stage approach to allow for facial growth to complete and achieve more predictable results, in cases where the patient has severe functional deficits, decreased quality of life, or psychosocial issues, they may benefit from completing the ankylosis release and total joint replacement in one stage. If alloplastic TJR with or without orthognathic surgery is completed with remaining growth potential, it is important that the patient and family understand that secondary surgeries after growth is completed will likely be needed to finalize the results. For example, the mandibular position may be planned in the final location with the total joint prosthesis, with secondary traditional orthognathic surgery completed after growth is complete (Fig. 12).

Fat Grafting

The importance of fat grafting to prevent the formation of heterotopic bone has been described in the literature. The rationale for placing autologous fat grafts around the TMJ TJR is to obliterate the dead space around the joint prosthesis, thus preventing the formation and subsequent organization of a blood clot. Creating this physical barrier serves to minimize the presence of pluripotential cells and prevents the formation of extensive fibrosis and heterotopic calcification. The fat grafts may be inhibitory to heterotopic bone formation. It may also isolate any residual reactive tissue from previous alloplastic failure or disease to the periphery of the region, minimizing its formation around the joint components.

Wolford and Karras published the first study evaluating fat grafts placed around the prosthesis after TJR with TMJ Concepts in 22 joints and showed no radiographic or clinical evidence of heterotopic calcifications in any of the fat graft group but found seven control patients (35%) developing heterotopic bone and ultimately requiring reoperation [22].

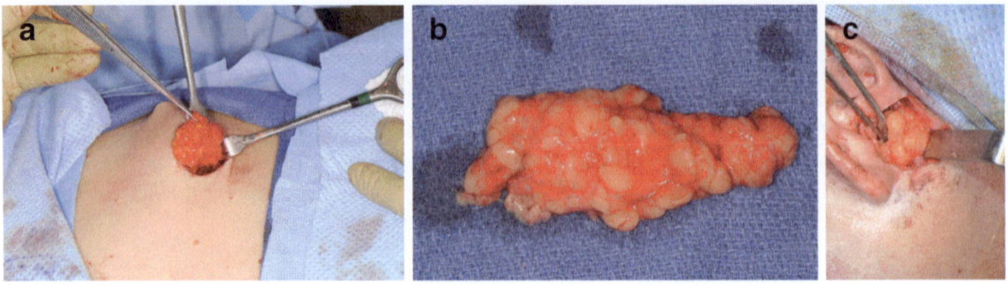

Fig. 15 Abdominal fat graft harvesting. (**a**) Fat is harvested through a small periumbilical incision. (**b**) Adequate amount of harvest fat on table ready to be placed into TMJ site. (**c**) Insertion around TMJ prosthesis through endaural incision obliterating dead space

Mercuri and colleagues evaluated 20 patients with 33 ankylosed TMJs managed with patient fitted-TMJ TJR devices and placement of periarticular autogenous abdominal fat grafts. Mean follow-up was 50.4 months. Results showed 52% reduction in pain, and improvement in jaw function (76%), diet (72%), and maximum incisal opening (MIO) (140%) from 11.75 mm to 32.9 mm, whereas 17 of 20 patients (85%) reported improvement in quality-of-life scores [23].

We generally harvest the fat graft through a small periumbilical incision. The incision can be hidden at the umbilicus and fat is easily harvested in sufficient quantity to obliterate all dead space around the joint. It is important to remember to prep the abdomen at the beginning of the case and maintain sterility throughout the procedure (Fig. 15).

Internal Maxillary Artery Embolization

In cases with severe distortion of normal TMJ anatomy or large amount of heterotopic bone formation near the internal maxillary artery, prophylactic embolization may be considered 24 hours before surgery. Decreasing blood flow to the area makes excision of the ankylosis easier and quicker. It has also been shown to decrease average surgical blood loss (Fig. 12c).

Degenerative Joint Disease

Degenerative joint disease (DJD) is a term encompassing a wide range of conditions that can generally be split into two main categories. The first is low-inflammatory arthritic disorders, including osteoarthritis, degenerative joint disease, post-traumatic arthritis, and idiopathic condylar resorption, and the second is high-inflammatory arthritic disorders, such as infectious arthritis, rheumatoid arthritis conditions (adult and juvenile), gouty arthritis, psoriatic arthritis, lupus erythematosus, ankylosing spondylitis, Reiter syndrome, and arthritis associated with ulcerative colitis [24]. Although a comprehensive review of all these conditions is beyond the scope of this chapter, some of the more prevalent conditions leading to end-stage degenerative joint disease and asymmetry, requiring surgical treatment, are briefly discussed here. The surgical management of many of these conditions is similar and can be applied to many of the pathologies described above.

The classic low-inflammatory arthritic disorder causing degenerative changes of the TMJ is primary osteoarthritis. The condition originates at the articular surface of the joint with eventual involvement of the subcondylar bone and joint capsule [24]. Functional overloading is thought to result in degenerative changes of the articular cartilage, leading to further degeneration and bony changes. In the elderly population, degenerative changes can be found in 50% of patient without a disk problem, and 80% of subjects with a disk problem, indicating that osteoarthritis is highly correlated with internal derangement [25].

The most common symptom of patients with osteoarthritic DJD is painful joints, but patients may also complain of joint crepitus, loss of joint function, and joint instability. Patients with unilateral DJD typically present with premature occlusion on the affected side, anterior open bite and/or open bite on the contralateral side, and loss of facial height on the affected side (Fig. 16). Long-standing disease may lead to dental compensation complicating treatment.

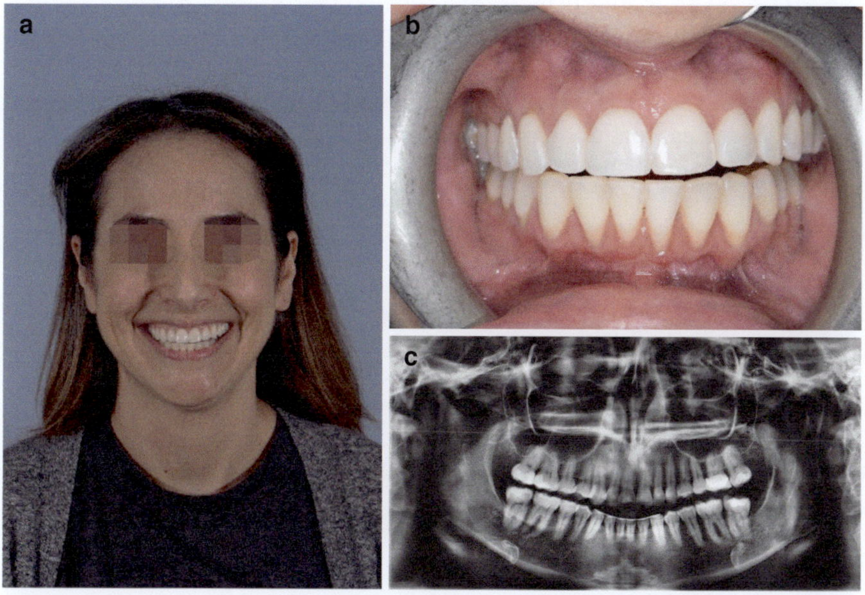

Fig. 16 Female patient with recent onset of R-sided DJD. (**a**) Note there is no gross facial asymmetry seen on full smile, but only slight mandibular deviation to the right side. (**b**) On closer inspection, changes in occlusion are noted, including premature contact on the effected side, anterior open bite, and open bite on the contralateral side. (**c**) Panorex showing right-sided condylar degeneration

Diagnosis of degenerative disease is generally made with a combination of history, clinical exam, and imaging. A history of parafunctional habits such as bruxism, clenching, excessive gum chewing, etc. may be helpful. Clinical examination of early low-inflammatory DJD may simply manifest as joint pain, crepitus, decreased function, or slight changes in occlusion such as in Fig. 16. If unilateral DJD is allowed to progress and is long-standing, maxillary compensation may occur with the development of a cant and worsening facial asymmetry, further complicating future treatment (Fig. 17).

Bilateral joint involvement is generally more common, and although it does not produce the pronounced facial asymmetries that may be seen in unilateral cases, it often leads to a severe class II skeletal profile, worsening anterior open bite, lip incompetence, mentalis strain, difficulty chewing, and occasional asymmetry if one side is more significantly affected than the other (Fig. 18). Additionally, bilateral involvement commonly leads to decreased airway space and obstructive sleep apnea.

Although a Panorex can be used for screening, the CT scan gives a more detailed view of the condyles and surrounding structures. It is particularly useful if ankylosis or heterotrophic bone is suspected. If surgical correction of an asymmetry or ankylosis is being considered, a detailed CT scan can be instrumental in surgical planning and also for creation of an STL model, for virtual surgical planning, or for custom-made total joint prosthesis.

MRI has emerged as the gold standard in these cases, being consistently sensitive for evaluation of arthritic involvement of the TMJ. MRI has the advantage of differentiating between acute disease (synovial enhancement, synovial effusion, synovial thickening, bone marrow edema) and chronic changes (TMJ arthritis, pannus, condylar flattening, bone erosion, articular disc changes, and displacement changes) [26]. Many classification systems have been proposed for DJD, including osteoarthritis as well as rheumatoid arthritis and related disorders (Table 2).

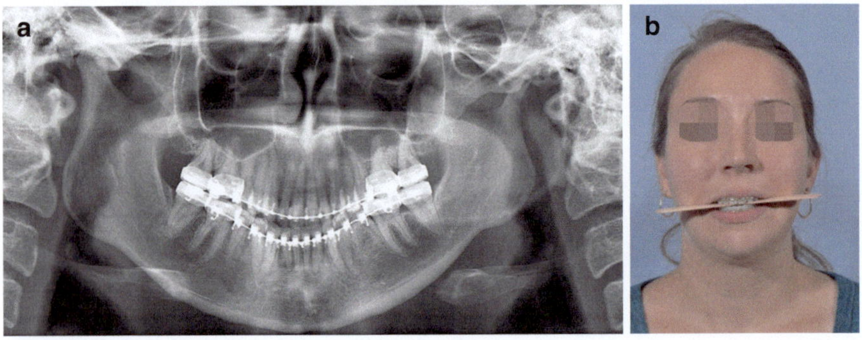

Fig. 17 Female patient with long standing L sided degenerative joint disease. (**a**) Note L sided condyle degeneration on the Panorex. These atrophic changes in the condyle are typically seen in high-inflammatory types of DJD, in her case juvenile idiopathic arthritis. (**b**) Note dental compensation and maxillary cant, further exaggerating her facial asymmetry

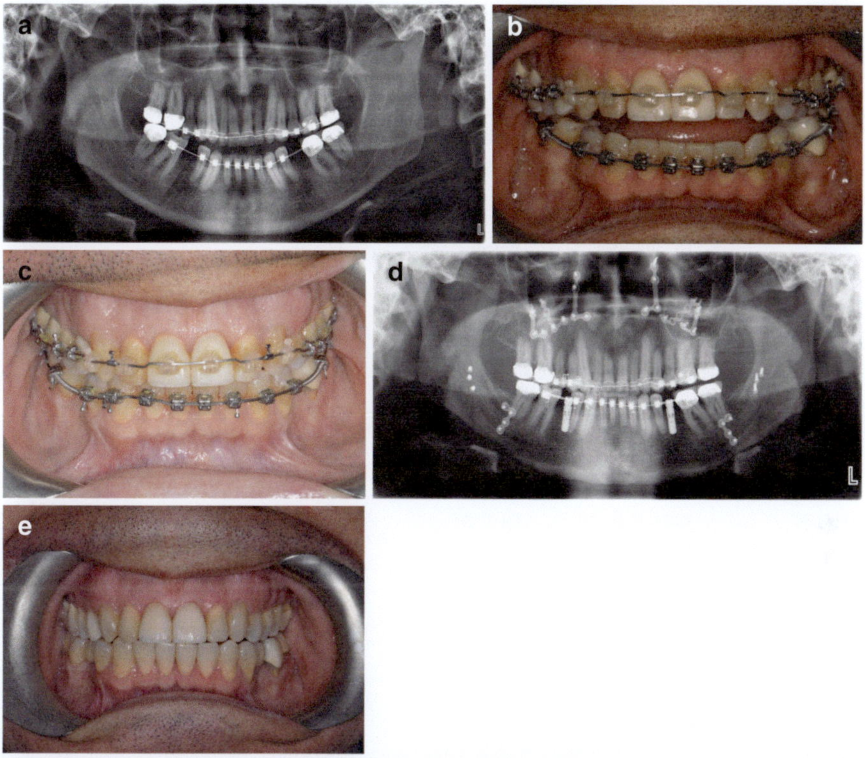

Fig. 18 Male patient with bilateral osteoarthritic low-inflammatory degenerative joint disease. (**a**) Note bilateral, left greater than right DJD. Note classic hypertrophic changes typically seen in low-inflammatory DJD, in his case osteoarthritis, with focal degeneration, osteophyte formation, flattening of the condyle, subchondral sclerosis, and condylar beaking. (**b**) Note development of anterior open bite and midline shift toward the more effected condyle. (**c**) Patients' occlusion after treatment with traditional orthognathic surgery. Note immediate improvement in occlusion and function. (**d**) Panorex after treatment. (**e**) 1 year later patient has some relapse, likely due to further condylar degeneration. This is the risk of using traditional orthognathic surgery in DJD; the disease process may continue

Treatment Options in Degenerative Joint Disease

A wide variety of treatments have been proposed for DJD which vary based on disease severity and pathophysiology. The main treatment goals remain the same and include decreasing joint and muscle pain, restoring or increasing joint function, restoring mandibular form and function, correction of gross facial deformities or asymmetries, preventing further progression, and preventing disability or associated morbidity.

Noninvasive modalities, such as medications, oral appliances/splints, and physical therapy are important tools in the management of degenerative joint disease. Common medications in DJD, especially osteoarthritis and low-inflammatory

Table 2 Classification of TMJ degenerative joint disease and related disorders

Type	Symptoms	Radiographic findings	Clinical findings	Treatment
I- early disease	– Joint/ muscle pain – Crepitus – Mild limitations in function	– Mild to moderate erosive changes to condyle, eminence, or fossa	– Minimal to no esthetic facial changes	Non-invasive or medical
II-arrested disease	– Generally no pain – crepitus – Joint dysfunction – Muscle pain	– Flattened condyle or eminence	– Class II malocclusion – Anterior open bite – Mild facial asymmetry may be present	Non-invasive medical, plus surgical or reconstructive
III- advanced disease	– Joint/ muscle pain – Crepitus – Severe functional limitations or loss of function	– Severe erosive changes – Loss of condylar height – Loss of eminence height – Ankylosis	– Severe class II malocclusion – High mandibular plane angle – Ankylosis – Coronoid hypertrophy – Significant facial asymmetry may be present.	Reconstructive

Adapted from Kent JN, Carlton DM, Zide MF. Rheumatoid disease and related arthropathies. II. Surgical rehabilitation of the temporomandibular joint. Oral Surg 1986;61:423–39 and Mercuri, Louis. "Osteoarthritis, Osteoarthrosis, and Idiopathic Condylar Resorption". Oral and Maxillofacial Surgery Clinics of North America. 20(208) 169–183

arthropathies, include NSAIDS, short courses of oral corticosteroids, and muscle relaxants to control reflex muscle contractions and pain. These medications are also used in high-inflammatory arthritides, such as juvenile idiopathic arthritis (JIA), often with the addition of disease-modifying antirheumatic drugs (DMARDS) under the care of a rheumatologist [27].

Minimally invasive therapies including arthrocentesis and arthroscopy have both been shown to decrease pain and improve function in DJD, even in patients who have failed to respond to other conservative therapies. These procedures remove inflammatory agents and cytokines from the joint and may break up adhesions/fibrosis [28]. These procedures may be used adjunctively prior to correction of DFD or asymmetries. Arthroscopy is not only therapeutic but also diagnostic and may help the surgeon decide the condition of the joint, and whether disc plication is an option, discectomy is needed, or if the joint is unsalvageable and may require a total joint prosthesis. For example, if arthroscopy shows mild early DJD and a salvageable disc with internal derangement, then one may decide to proceed with disc repositioning and correct DFD and asymmetry with traditional orthognathic surgery. Alternatively, if arthroscopy shows an unsalvageable joint, discectomy may be indicated, or if it shows severe and active DJD, one may decide to treat the DFD and asymmetry with a total joint prosthesis in combination with any indicated traditional orthognathic techniques.

Disc plication/repositioning, with or without an anchor, may have a role in early DJD when the articular disc is intact but internal derangement is present. The association between internal derangement and DJD has been previously discussed. Patients who underwent Mitek anchor disc repositioning within 4 years of disease onset have decrease in pain and improvement in function in the 90% range, while those that presented after 4 years had a success rate of approximately 68%, which may indicate that surgical disc repositioning may stop progression of osteoarthritis or disc degeneration [29], although this is controversial. Disc plication, with Mitek anchors, combined with traditional orthognathic surgery techniques has also been shown to significantly reduce pain with stable skeletal and occlusal results [30]. In the setting of early DJD and DFD, Mitek anchors may be used in combination with traditional orthognathic techniques to achieve stable results (Figs. 19 and 20).

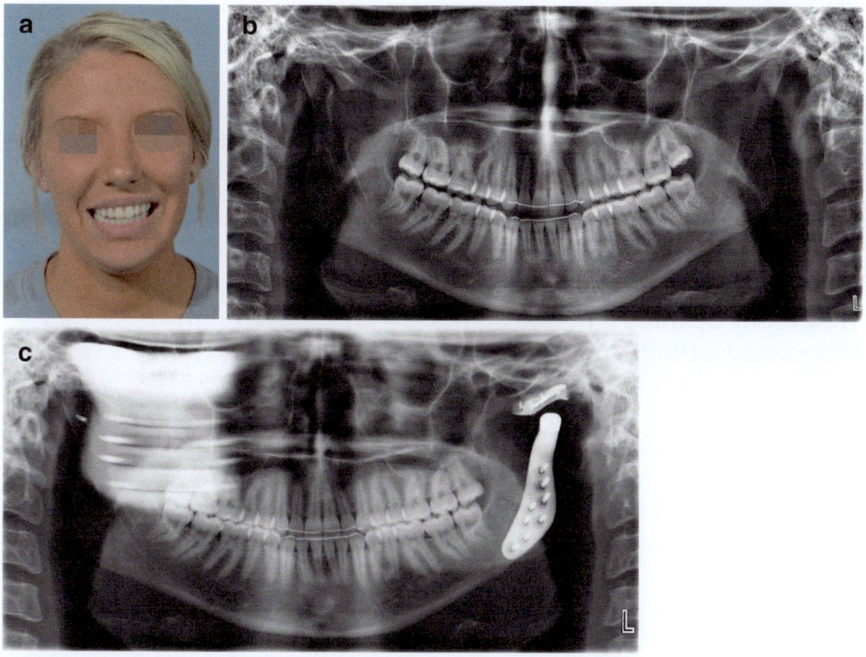

Fig. 19 Female patient with severe left-sided DJD and early R-sided DJD with anterior disc displacement diagnosed with MRI and CT scan. (**a**) Note R-sided chin deviation and malocclusion, as well as malocclusion and midline deviation. (**b**) Panorex showing early R-sided condylar degeneration and L-sided DJD with focal degeneration. (**c**) Patient was treated with R-sided disc repositioning with Mitek anchor and L-sided TJR, with stable results and arrested growth. Note midlines corrected

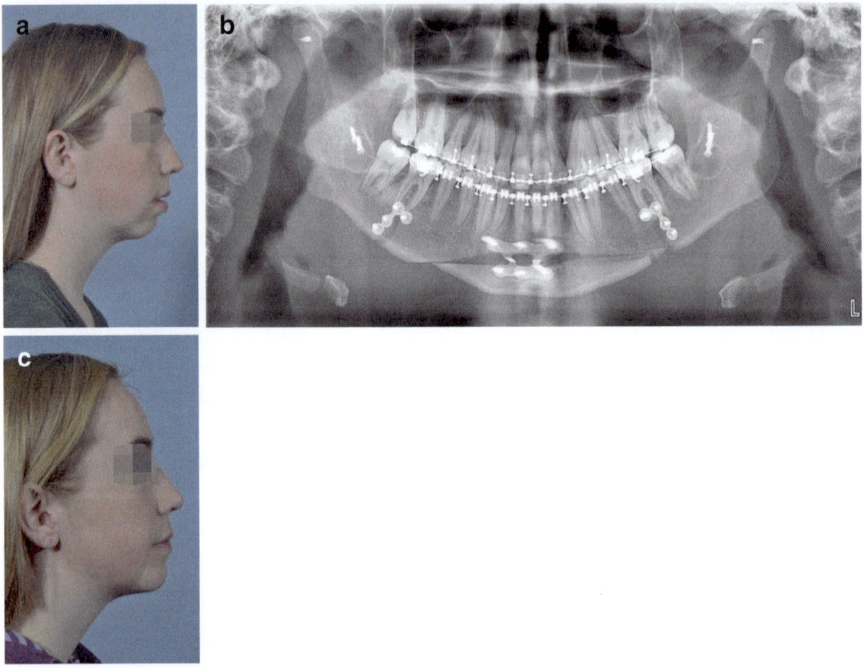

Fig. 20 Female with medically controlled JIA and mild involvement of bilateral TMJ, anterior disc displacement bilateral, and associated retrognathic dentofacial deformity. (**a**) Note retrognathia secondary to bilateral condylar degeneration. (**b**) Patient had JIA medically controlled and disease was stable, but anterior disc displacement was found bilaterally. Patient was treated with disc repositioning with Mitek anchors and BSSO advancement with genioplasty for correction of DFD. (**c**) Postoperative profile

Treatment Options and Consideration for Severe Progressive DJD Associated with Asymmetry or Dentofacial Deformity (Fig. 21)

Although DJD most often responds to conservative management or minimally invasive techniques, it may continue to progress. Once DJD has caused significant dentofacial deformities or asymmetry, it has often progressed too far for conservative therapies alone, and definitive joint reconstruction is required to restore form and function. Autogenous joint replacement, i.e., costochondral grafting, has been reported in the literature with some success, especially in quiescent disease, but continues to be susceptible to the arthritic and degenerative processes of the original joint. This problem is especially pronounced in high-inflammatory arthropathies and ankylosis, and thus it is contraindicated in these conditions. Indeed, no recent orthopedic publications advocate or describe the use of autogenous bone for reconstruction of any joint affected by low- or high-inflammatory arthritis disease [24].

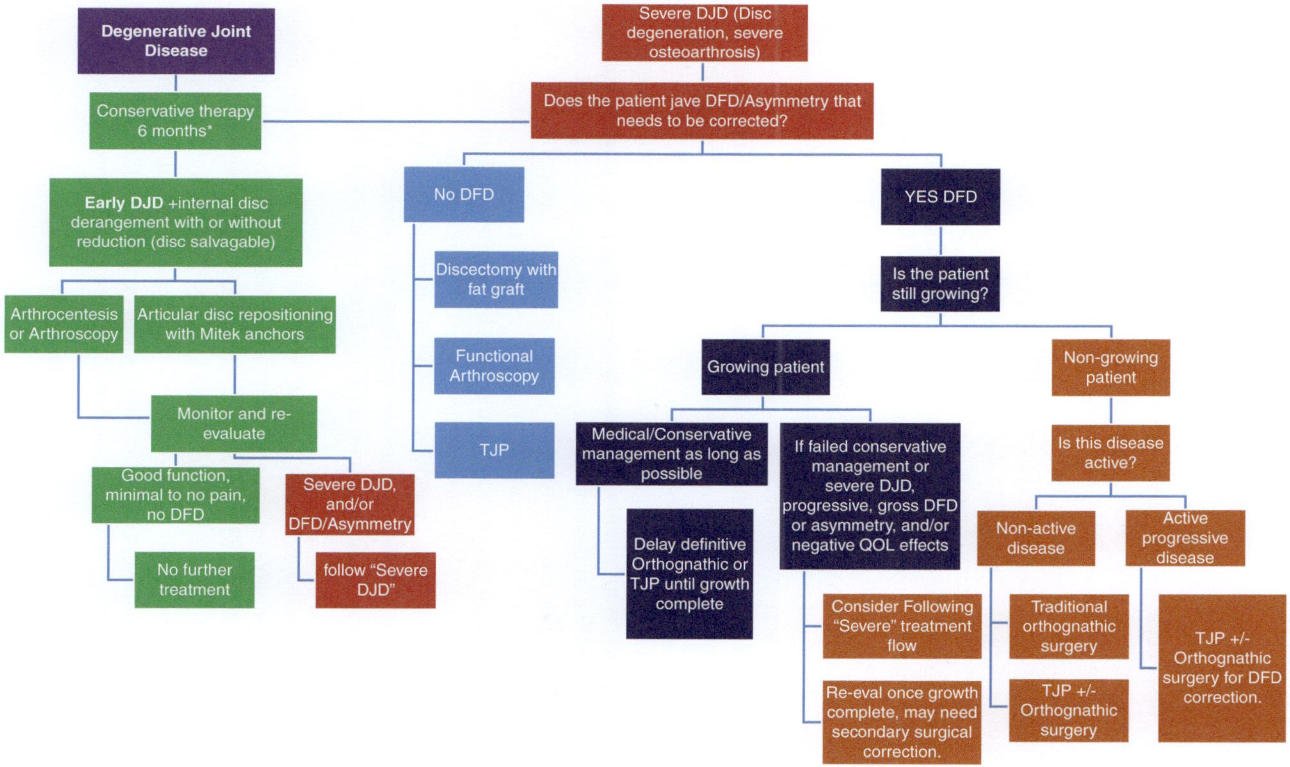

Fig. 21 Degenerative joint disease treatment algorithm. *Conservative therapy is initially tried, but if severe progressive disease is present or patients would like DFD or asymmetry corrected, they may decide to proceed directly to surgery. Conservative therapy, arthroscopy, arthrocentesis, disc repositioning, discectomy, or function arthroscopy may all be used in conjunction with orthognathic surgery or total joint replacement. Arthroscopy is diagnostic as well as therapeutic and may help determine which treatment to proceed with. Key: DJD – degenerative joint disease. DFD – dentofacial deformity

Alloplastic reconstruction of severe DJD has several advantages including immediate return to function, significant decrease in pain, restoration of proper form and function, total arrest of the disease process, no susceptibility to recurrence of original disease process, no donor site morbidity, stable and reproducible results, literature supported improvement in pain and function, and generally improved outcomes compared to autogenous replacement.

One of the first decisions that needs to be made is whether the degenerative joint disease causing the asymmetry is active or inactive. Conventional orthognathic surgery in the setting of active DJD should be used very cautiously, as any result obtained may be unstable and susceptible to further degeneration of the joint with relapse of facial asymmetry and dysfunction (Fig. 18) Arthroscopy, arthrocentesis, and disc repositioning may be used to stabilize the joint in preparation for orthognathic surgery in early degenerative joint disease.

Before deciding that the disease is inactive, the disease must be quiescent for at least a year by either serial cephalometric analysis or contrast-enhanced MRI in JIA or technetium-99 bone scan in ICR. Close follow-up and repeat examinations, serial panogram, cephalometric x-rays and/or CT scans, diagnostic casts and models, and even MRI can all be used to follow the progression of the disease to determine if the degenerative disease is active or inactive.

If it is determined that the degenerative joint disease continued to progress and has caused significant dysfunction and/or gross facial asymmetry, the disease process can be stopped, and the facial deformity corrected with a total joint prosthesis with or without concomitant orthognathic surgery. If the degenerative disease is of recent onset, occlusion is minimally deviated, and maxillary cant or dental compensations have not had time to develop, it may be possible to treat the patient with a unilateral TJP alone (Fig. 22) If only one joint is involved, but correction of the mandibular deformity with unilateral TJR would overload or alter the contralateral joint position too much, or proper occlusion cannot be obtained with unilateral TJP alone, contralateral sagittal split osteotomy or even TJR may be required (Fig. 23). In cases with bilateral DJD and condylar degeneration, patients will present with worsening class II malocclusion and anterior open bite, and if noted to be active and progressive, can be treated with bilateral TJR to establish a good functional and stable result (Fig. 24).

Depending on the pathogenesis of the degenerative joint disease, the disease process may stop without any intervention with increased age, with medications in inflammatory conditions, and with adjunctive procedures (arthroscopy, disc repositioning, condylectomy) or cease with decreased loading of the condyle. If it is determined that the degenerative joint disease has ceased, usually with serial cephalograms, conventional orthognathic surgery can be used to obtain a functional and cosmetic result, unless there is gross deficits in the condyle precluding traditional osteotomy techniques (Fig. 20).

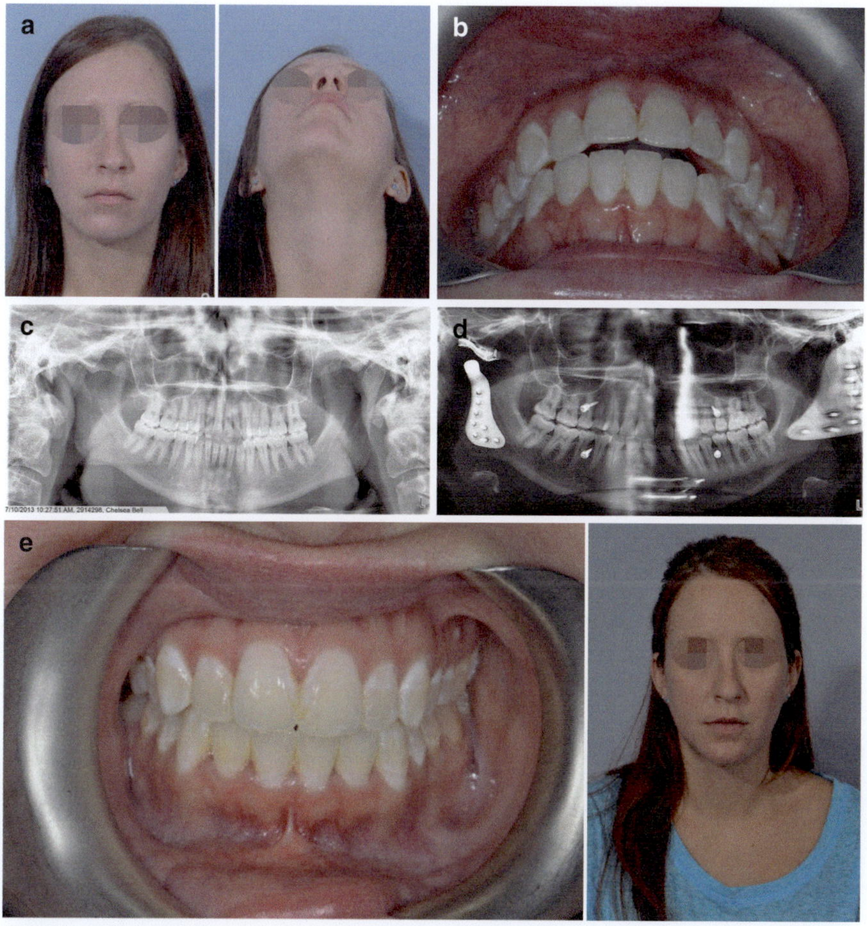

Fig. 22 Female with juvenile idiopathic arthritis on R side treated with unilateral TJR and genioplasty. (**a**) R-sided DJD with vertical shortening of mandibular dimension on the R side. (**b**) Note R-sided deviation in midline and anterior open bite preoperatively. Her malocclusion is minimal allowing for unilateral TJR without the need for L-sided BSSO or TJR.* (**c**) Preoperative Panorex showing severe R-sided condylar degeneration and flattening of condyle. (**d**) Postoperative Panorex. (**e**) Postoperative result with corrected facial asymmetry and occlusion

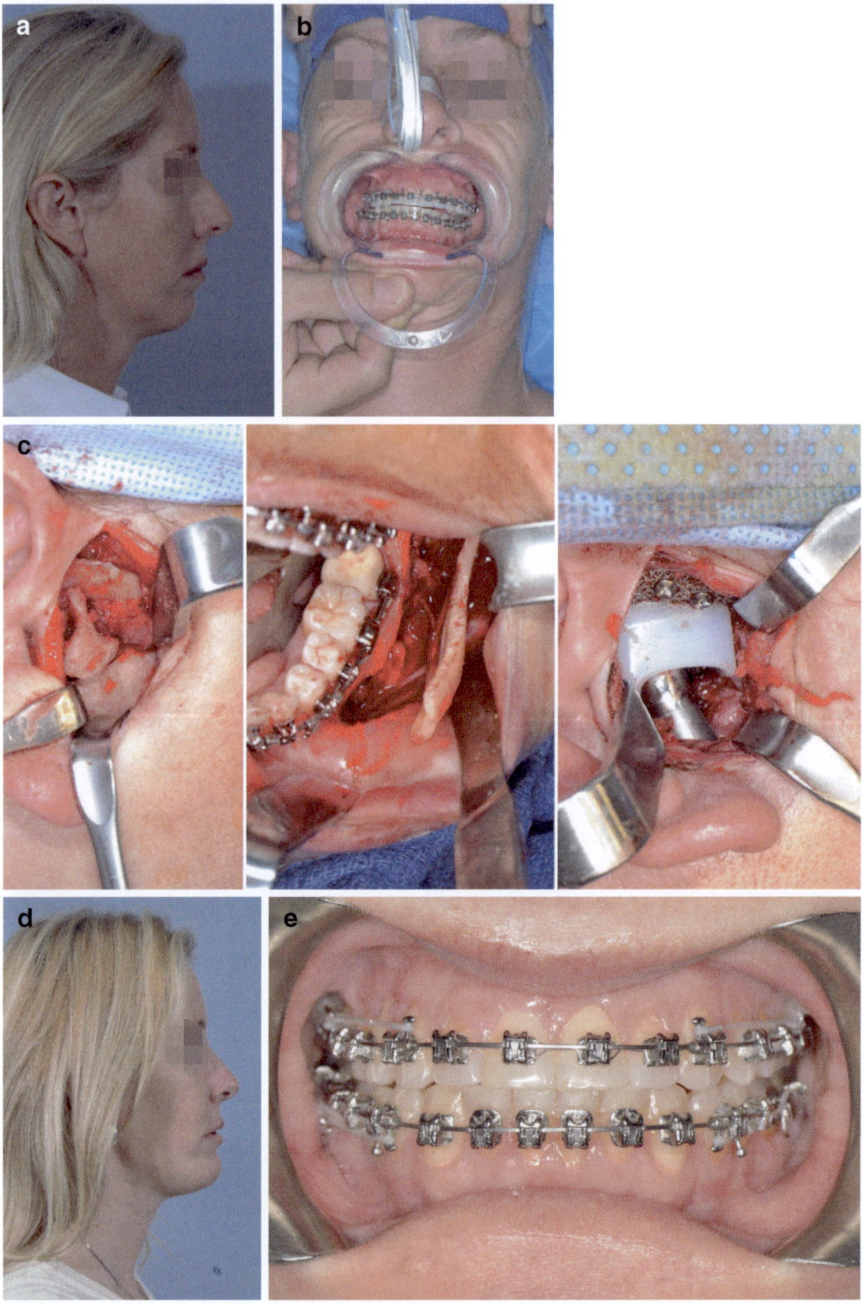

Fig. 23 Female with R-sided DJD, retrognathic dentofacial deformity, and R-sided mandibular deviation. (**a**) Retrognathic class II profile noted on preoperative exam. (**b**) Occlusion on the table with R-sided deviation, anterior open bite, and open bite on L side, typical of R-sided condylar degeneration. (**c**) Intraoperative photos. Note severely degenerated condyle, contralateral sagittal split osteotomy, and R-sided total joint replacement. Correction of this deviation and placement into proper occlusion was only possible with concomitant L-sided sagittal split osteotomy. (**d**) Corrected facial profile post-op. (**e**) Corrected occlusion post-op

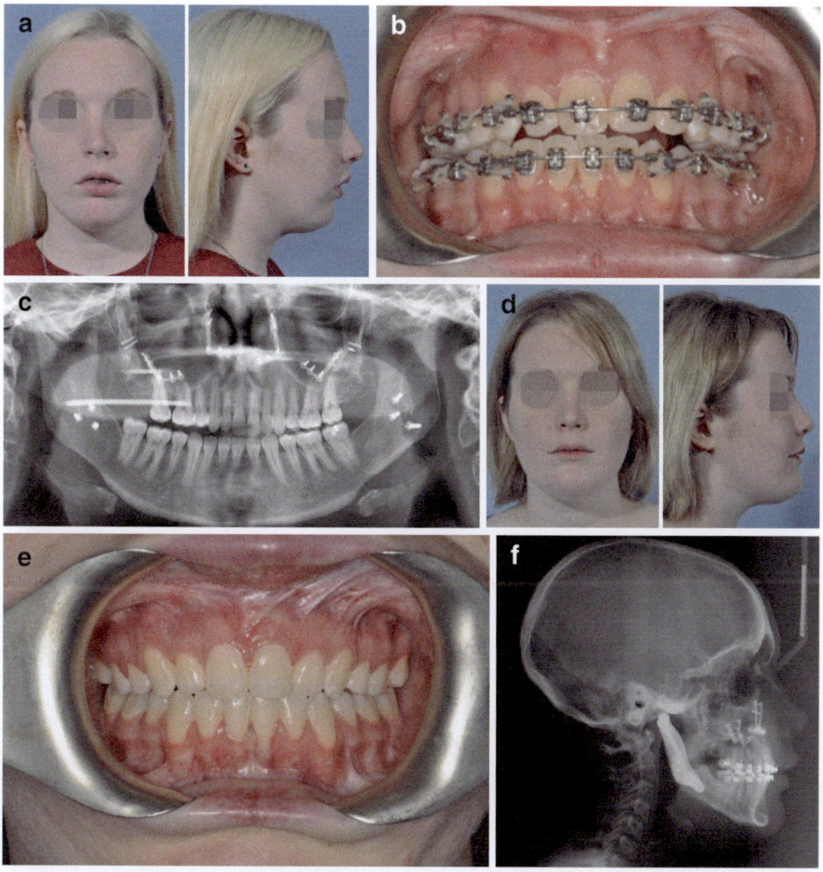

Fig. 24 Female patient with progressive BL DJD after orthognathic surgery. (**a**) Note retrognathic profile. (**b**) R-sided deviation with anterior and L-sided open bite. (**c**) Preoperative Panorex showing BL condylar degeneration and previous history of orthognathic surgery. (**d**) Postoperative results after BL TJR and LeFort I osteotomy. (**e**) Postoperative occlusion after BL TJR. (**f**) Lateral ceph showing BL TJR and redo of LeFort I

Growing Patients

Just like in ankylosis, the remaining growth potential of the patient must be considered before treatment. Patients with onset of unilateral DJD during the growing years are likely to grow and adapt to the mandibular asymmetry, leading to more pronounced facial asymmetries and maxillary cant. Medical management and conservative management in an attempt to cease or limit disease progression is the best initial management during growth, with definitive alloplastic total joint replacement or orthognathic surgery reserved for patients with little to no growth remaining. Exceptions can be made in severe disease causing decreased quality of life with the understanding that secondary procedures may be needed later in life for correction of any discrepancies created by growth (Fig. 25).

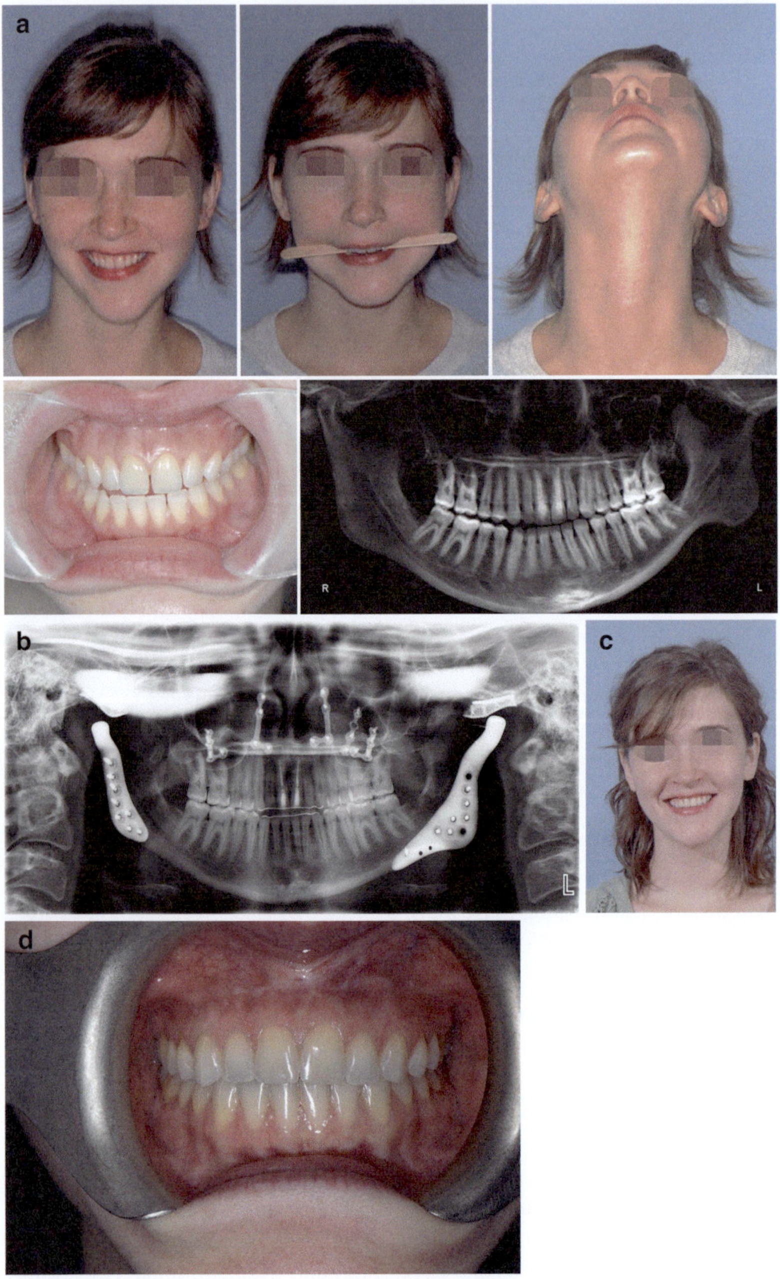

Fig. 25 Teenage female presenting with severe L-sided TMJ degeneration with onset during growth. (**a**) Note L-sided chin deviation, maxillary cant, and malocclusion on preoperative photographs. Note Panorex showing L-sided degeneration. (**b**) Patient was treated with BL TJR to cease degenerative process in combination with LeFort 1 for correction of cant. (**c**) Note correction of asymmetry. (**d**) Occlusion at 8-year follow-up

Surgical Sequence Considerations

When combining procedures to correct these complex cases, especially alloplastic total joint replacement with traditional orthognathic surgery, sequencing must be carefully considered. Procedure which may change or alter the condylar position of the joint, such as disc repositioning, should be done prior to the mandibular osteotomy. In general, doing the sterile procedure first, before doing intraoral orthognathic surgery, saves time as the patient doesn't need to be re-prepped and there is no need for a second set of surgical instruments. For example, if treatment includes bilateral TJP with LeFort, it would be best to complete the bilateral TJP first, close and isolate the incision sites of the joints, and then proceed with the non-sterile LeFort I osteotomy procedure. If a unilateral joint prosthesis is planned, two sets of instruments are needed to maintain sterility. The preferred option is to operate on the joint and prepare the site followed by the intraoral mandibular osteotomy without mixing the instruments. The patient is then placed in MMF in the intermediate position and the joint is placed and closed after changing gowns and drapes. Then the surgeons return to the mouth and rigidly fixate the mandible and then finish with the maxillary osteotomy. Checking the occlusion in every step is necessary to make sure that the plan is executed adequately.

Conclusion

In conclusion, temporomandibular joint ankylosis and degenerative joint disease both have the potential to cause significant dentofacial deformities as well as asymmetries. Both disease processes can have significant effects on the patient's function and quality of life, especially TMJ ankylosis. When considering treatment, the surgeon must consider any remaining growth potential, and when applicable, stage the surgery or incorporate the remaining growth into the surgical plan. Although a variety of treatment options are present for both pathologies, alloplastic total joint prosthesis has the benefit of immediate return to function, decreased pain, and resistance to the original pathological process with no potential for recurrence, which makes this surgical option very predictable. Traditional orthognathic surgeries, especially LeFort I osteotomies, are often required to correct the concomitant asymmetries or dentofacial deformities that are often present in these patients. In the hands of an experienced surgeon, these surgical techniques in combination with careful surgical planning can lead to stable and reproducible outcomes and, ultimately, profound improvements in the patient's quality of life.

References

1. Lello G. Surgical correction of temporomandibular joint Ankylosis. J Cranio-Max-Fac Surg. 1990;18:19–26.
2. Sawhney CP. Bony ankylosis of the temporomandibular joint: follow-up of 70 patients treated with arthroplasty and acrylic spacer interposition. Plast Reconstr Surg. 1986;77:29–38.

3. He D, Yang C, Chen M, Zhang X, Qiu Y, Yang X, et al. Traumatic temporomandibular joint ankylosis: our classification and treatment experience. J Oral Maxillofac Surg. 2011;69(6):1600–7.
4. Topazian RG. Etiology of Ankylosis of temporomandibular joint: analysis of 44 cases. J Oral Surg Anesth Hosp Dent Serv. 1964;22:227–33.
5. Wolford L, Movahed R, Teschke M, Fimmers R, Havard D, Schneiderman E. Temporomandibular joint ankylosis can be successfully treated with TMJ concepts patient-fitted total joint prosthesis and autogenous fat grafts. J Oral Maxillofac Surg [Internet]. 2016;74(6):1215–27. https://doi.org/10.1016/j.joms.2016.01.017.
6. Zhi K, Ren W, Zhou H, Gao L, Zhao L, Hou C, et al. Management of temporomandibular joint ankylosis: 11 years' clinical experience. Oral Surg Oral Med Oral Pathol Oral Radiol Endodontol [Internet]. 2009;108(5):687–92. https://doi.org/10.1016/j.tripleo.2009.06.041.
7. Jain G, Kumar S, Rana AS, Bansal V, Sharma P, Vikram A. Temporomandibular joint ankylosis: a review of 44 cases. Oral Maxillofac Surg. 2008;12(2):61–6.
8. Roychoudhury A, Parkash H, Trikha A. Functional restoration by gap arthroplasty in temporomandibular joint ankylosis. Oral Surgery, Oral Med Oral Pathol Oral Radiol Endodontology [Internet]. 1999;87(2):166–9. Available from: http://www.sciencedirect.com/science/article/pii/S1079210499702672
9. Güven O. A clinical study on temporomandibular joint ankylosis in children. J Craniofac Surg. 2008;19(5):1263–9.
10. Ellis E, Moos KF, El-Attar A. Ten years of mandibular fractures: an analysis of 2,137 cases. Oral Surgery, Oral Med Oral Pathol. 1985;59(2):120–9.
11. Bae SS, Aronovich S. Trauma to the pediatric temporomandibular joint. Oral Maxillofac Surg Clin North Am [Internet]. 2018;30(1):47–60. https://doi.org/10.1016/j.coms.2017.08.004.
12. Movahed R, Mercuri LG. Management of Temporomandibular Joint Ankylosis. Oral Maxillofac Surg Clin North Am. 2015;27(1):27–35.
13. Al-Moraissi EA, El-Sharkawy TM, Mounair RM, El-Ghareeb TI. A systematic review and meta-analysis of the clinical outcomes for various surgical modalities in the management of temporomandibular joint ankylosis. Int J Oral Maxillofac Surg [Internet]. 2015;44(4):470–82. https://doi.org/10.1016/j.ijom.2014.10.017.
14. Resnick CM. Temporomandibular joint reconstruction in the growing child. Oral Maxillofac Surg Clin North Am [Internet]. 2018;30(1):109–21. https://doi.org/10.1016/j.coms.2017.08.006.
15. Kaban LB, Bouchard C, Troulis MJ. A protocol for Management of Temporomandibular Joint Ankylosis in children. J Oral Maxillofac Surg [Internet]. 2009;67(9):1966–78. https://doi.org/10.1016/j.joms.2009.03.071.
16. Cascone P, Basile E, Angeletti D, Vellone V, Ramieri V, Giancotti A, et al. TMJ replacement utilizing patient-fitted TMJ TJR devices in a re-ankylosis child. J Cranio-Maxillofacial Surg [Internet]. 2016;44(4):493–9. https://doi.org/10.1016/j.jcms.2015.06.018.
17. Ellis E, Schneiderman ED, Carlson DS. Growth of the mandible after replacement of the mandibular condyle: an experimental investigation in Macaca mulatta. J Oral Maxillofac Surg. 2002;60(12):1461–70.
18. Mercuri LG. Alloplastic temporomandibular joint reconstruction Oral Surgery, Oral Med Oral Pathol Oral Radiol Endodontology [Internet]. 1998;85(6):631–7. Available from: http://linkinghub.elsevier.com/retrieve/pii/S1079210498900282
19. Mercuri LG. Total joint reconstruction-autologous or alloplastic. Oral Maxillofac Surg Clin North Am. 2006;18(3):399–410.
20. Saeed NR, Kent JN. A retrospective study of the costochondral graft in TMJ reconstruction. Int J Oral Maxillofac Surg. 2003;32(6):606–9.
21. Mercuri Dds LG. The use of alloplastic prostheses for temporomandibular joint reconstruction indications for alloplastic joint reconstruction. J Orat Maxillofac Surg. 2000;58:70–5.
22. Wolford LM, Karras SC. Autologous fat transplantation around temporomandibular joint total joint prostheses: preliminary treatment outcomes. J Oral Maxillofac Surg. 1997;55(3):245–52.

23. Mercuri LG, Ali FA, Woolson R. Outcomes of Total alloplastic replacement with periarticular autogenous fat grafting for Management of Reankylosis of the temporomandibular joint. J Oral Maxillofac Surg. 2008;66(9):1794–803.
24. Mercuri LG. Osteoarthritis, osteoarthrosis, and idiopathic condylar resorption. Oral Maxillofac Surg Clin North Am. 2008;20(2):169–83.
25. de Bont LGM, Stegenga B. Pathology of temporomandibular joint internal derangement and osteoarthrosis. Int J Oral Maxillofac Surg. 1993;22(2):71–4.
26. Vaid YN, Dunnavant FD, Royal SA, Beukelman T, Stoll ML, Cron RQ. Imaging of the temporomandibular joint in juvenile idiopathic arthritis. Arthritis Care Res (Hoboken) [Internet]. 2014;66(1):47–54. Available from: http://doi.wiley.com/10.1002/acr.22177
27. Carrasco R. Juvenile idiopathic arthritis overview and involvement of the temporomandibular joint. Prevalence, systemic therapy. Oral Maxillofac Surg Clin North Am [Internet]. 2015;27(1):1–10. https://doi.org/10.1016/j.coms.2014.09.001.
28. Gynther GW, Holmlund AB. Efficacy of arthroscopic lysis and lavage in patients with temporomandibular joint symptoms associated with generalized osteoarthritis or rheumatoid arthritis. J Oral Maxillofac Surg. 1998;56(2):147–51.
29. Mehra P, Wolford LM. Use of the Mitek anchor in temporomandibular joint disc-repositioning surgery. Proc (Bayl Univ med cent) [Internet]. 2001;14(1):22–6. Available from: http://www.ncbi.nlm.nih.gov/pubmed/16369582%0Ahttp://www.pubmedcentral.nih.gov/articlerender.fcgi?artid=PMC1291307
30. Wolford LM, Cardenas L. Idiopathic condylar resorption: diagnosis, treatment protocol, and outcomes. Am J Orthod Dentofac Orthop. 1999;116(6):667–77.

Intraoral Distraction Osteogenesis in Facial Asymmetries

Cesar A. Guerrero, Marianela Gonzalez Carranza, and Elena V. Mujica

Abstract

This chapter gives an overview about the indications, biology and biomechanics of intraoral distraction osteogenesis as its relates to the surgical management of facial and jaw asymmetry patients. It includes examples of clinical cases where predictable outcomes have been achieved with interdisciplinary collaboration. Historical perspective, surgical protocol, recent advances and future trends are discussed.

Keywords

Distraction osteogenesis · Osteodistraction · Micrognathia · Intraoral distraction devices · Bone transport

The aim of this chapter is to review the indications, biology, and biomechanics of intraoral distraction osteogenesis focusing on the clinical outcomes, stability, morbidity, and innovations utilizing intraoral distraction for patients with facial asymmetries. This can be accomplished through a myriad of osteotomies, newer internal distraction devices, and collaboration between orthodontics and prosthodontics with craniofacial surgery.

Historically, problems with osteodistraction were related to controlling the vector of distraction, determination of the ideal distraction site, selection of the proper

C. A. Guerrero (✉)
Private Practice in Houston, TX, USA

M. G. Carranza
Department of Oral and Maxillofacial Surgery, Texas A&M, Dallas, TX, USA

E. V. Mujica
Sta Rosa Maxillofacial Surgery Center, Caracas, Venezuela, South America

P. Mehra, L. M. Wolford (eds.), *Management of Facial Asymmetry*,
https://doi.org/10.1007/978-3-030-44971-1_8

device, quality of the regenerate, management of postoperative occlusion, and avoiding possible damage to nerves, muscles, and teeth, during surgery and following the intervention. Clinical outcomes and long-term follow-up of these surgical interventions permit clinicians to perform a predictable, stable, and set surgical protocols for patients with craniofacial malformations or deformations with severe asymmetries.

Mandibular Lengthening

Distraction osteogenesis is indicated for patients needing long mandibular advancements (over 10 mm), syndromic mandibles with inadequate anatomy, secondary interventions following surgical advancement relapse, and particular sleep apnea patients [1–6].

Today's technology allows all surgical interventions to be performed intraorally, but many clinical situations may require the use of a trocar to fix the plate with transcutaneous screws. Once the surgeon selects the ideal distraction site, an incomplete osteotomy is performed, and the distractor is fixated with the mandible still in one piece and bicortical screws are recommended for stability, then the bone fracture is completed. The ideal distraction chamber is completely surrounded by the periosteal layer, as it is in the long bones with external devices. The surgeon can close the surgical wounds after the incomplete osteotomy is performed, leaving a small opening to place a chisel and finalize the osteotomy. This method permits a closed chamber, all surrounded by an intact periosteal layer, creating the ideal environment for bone formation. Once the osteotomy is completed during surgery, the small gap used to place the chisel is closed, ensuring a primary closure [7–11] (see Figs. 1 and 2).

Important points to consider while lengthening the mandible [8–13]:

1. Avoid damage to the inferior alveolar and mental nerves. Selecting the sites above the nerve in the ramus or anterior to the mental nerve in the body is ideal. An alternative is to perform a sagittal split osteotomy to secure the nerve in the distal segment and continue advancing with the distraction device.
2. Prevent damage to the teeth while performing the osteotomy under abundant irrigation and leaving 2 mm of intact bone next to the adjacent teeth.
3. Protect the temporomandibular joint structures from reciprocal forces while activating and consolidating the bone regenerate. This is obtained by the Class II intermaxillary elastics utilization, after the surgery and for at least 4 months after surgery. This action maintains the mandible projected anteriorly, with no pressure against the temporomandibular joint discs.
4. Place the distractor device in a position that is comfortable for the patient through all phases of distraction. We want to maintain the distractors in place as long as needed to obtain adequate mineralization of the distraction chamber. This mineralization process may take months. Positioning the devices in a comfortable position would benefit the patient's well-being, but also it is more tolerable for

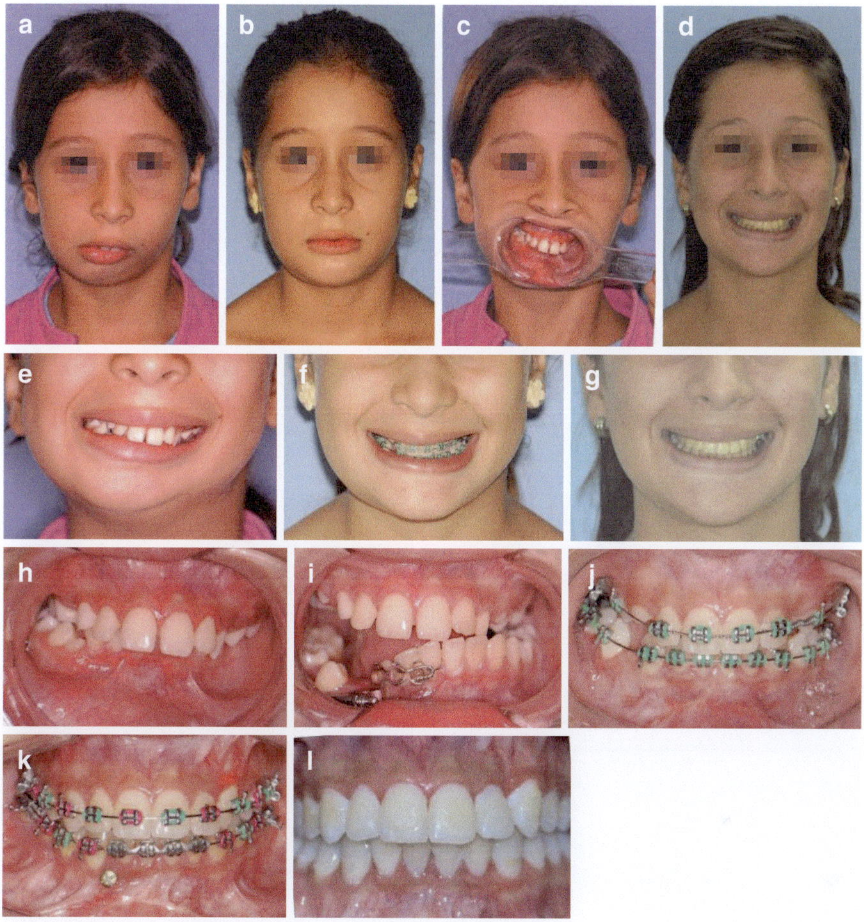

Fig. 1 7-year-old child with a sub-condylar fracture, severe mandibular deficiency, and hypomobility. Distraction osteogenesis was performed by lengthening the right mandibular ramus and body. (**a–d**) Frontal view before and after. (**h–l**) Intraoral views: arch bars were used during 12 weeks to control occlusion and guide the physiotherapy, distractor removal and genioplasty were performed, and orthodontics is continued after removal, (**k**) microscrews used to close the distraction chamber by advancing the right mandibular molars into an ideal Class I. (**l**) Ten-year follow-up. (Orthodontist Dr. Gisela Contasti Bocco)

the postoperative period, and the patient would not complain and request to have the devices removed before ideal consolidation.

Distraction osteogenesis to lengthen the mandible may be limited when the osteotomy is performed where the inferior alveolar nerve is involved, because the biology behind nerve lengthening does not support movement over 20% of the original nerve length [14, 15]. Ilizarov first demonstrated this concept during leg lengthening procedures, where he showed limb paralysis and paresthesia in those patients

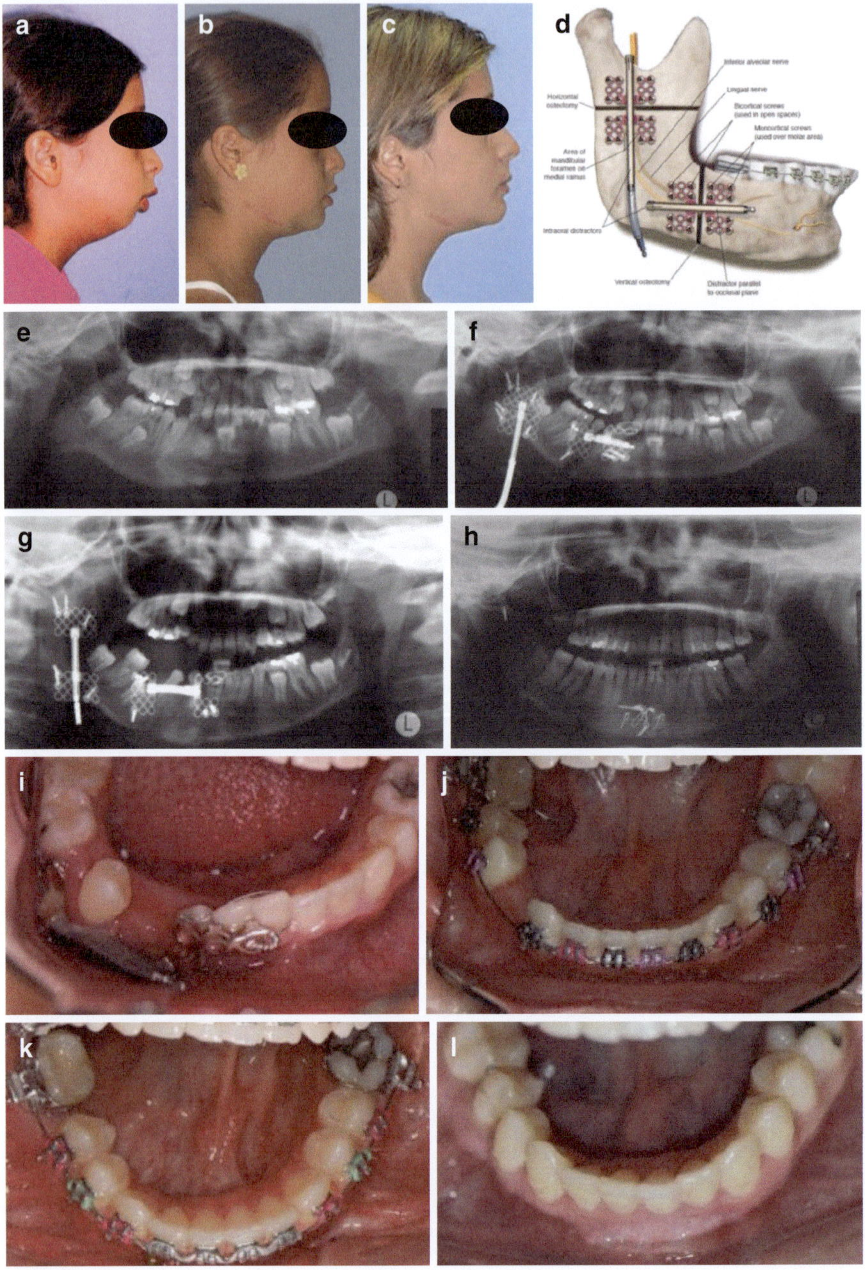

Fig. 2 (**a**–**d**) Same patient before and after profile views. (**e**–**h**) Panoramic radiographs: preoperative, 7 days after surgery, during distraction protocol, and 10 years of follow-up. (**i**–**l**) Occlusal views: during distraction protocol, orthodontics movements, and final results. (Orthodontist Dr. Gisela Contasti Bocco)

where the distraction limits were exceeded [16]. There are three basic indications for the early treatment of micrognathia: Pierre Robin sequence, sleep apnea, and certain craniofacial microsomias. Treating patients this early, sometimes only days or weeks old as neonates, forces the surgeon to perform this surgery in life-threating situations with the understanding that major nerve elongation and cutting of the mandibular angle may eventually lead to nerve dysesthesias and may damage the developing tooth buds resulting in their absence or deformation [14–18]. In the author's experience, patients treated during the first years of life with a 16-year follow-up, who underwent large movements to secure the upper way, did not complain of paresthesia. This may be due to the nerve injury occurring before they could realize the normal anterior mandibular and lip sensation [19–23]. The teeth in the line of fracture could be damaged while performing the mandibular osteotomy; we found molars that are missing or deformed requiring crowns or dental implant restorations, when the patients were treated early in life. Mandibular distraction in the neonate is only acceptable in life-threating situations; otherwise, the surgery should be postponed until anatomic growth and development is advanced, even though not completed, according to the different variables involved in indicating the surgery [19–24].

The same patient with micrognathia, presenting no life-threating airway obstruction, may benefit from receiving the surgery in a later stage of growth and tooth development; there are alternatives to avoid the mandibular nerve and teeth morbidity. The sagittal split ramus osteotomy could leave the nerve in the distal fragment and, with the aid of a large intraoral distractor, permit a large movement (15–30 mm) without injuring the inferior alveolar nerve [19–24]. The osteotomy could be performed anterior to the mental nerve between the roots of premolars, unilaterally or bilaterally, and create a bone regenerate of 20–30 mm without nerve damage (see Figs. 1, 2, and 4). The orthodontist can work preoperatively to create a bony gap between the premolars, therefore avoiding damage to the teeth. Postoperatively, micro-implants are used to allow teeth movement to close major interdental spaces secondary to the distraction chamber and moving the posterior teeth anteriorly as desired. There are indications to perform bidirectional distraction, one distractor is placed intraorally on the ramus, fixed with transcutaneous screws utilizing a trocar, and the osteotomy is performed superior to the lingula, just before the nerve travels intra-osseously avoiding nerve damage. A second distractor is used on the body of the mandible, anterior to the mental nerve between the premolars. These maneuvers allow major bidirectional lengthening (25–30 mm vertically and 20 or 25 anteroposteriorly), creating an excellent mandibular angle and avoiding damage to the nerve [19–24] (see Figs. 1, 2, and 4).

The orthodontist needs to have a thorough biomechanics knowledge, the desire to play a major role in treating these challenging patients, an excellent understanding of growth and development, experience in using orthodontic implants to move teeth through large regenerated bony spaces, and the patience to embark into long surgical-orthodontic treatments, and three-dimensional tooth movement orthodontic mechanics is required [25, 26].

There are several distraction appliances to create curves or change the straight-line chamber. However, the biological and mechanical principles dictate that the osteotomy site is progressively separated and collagen fibers bridge the bony segments [26], the collagen fibers act as elastic fibers attached to the two bony walls; even though the maturation process starts soon after activation occurs, it takes weeks to months to finalize the mineralization period and the collagen fibers are oriented in a straight-line fashion from one wall to the other. Once the activation is finalized, the minerals are deposited into the collagen net, from point A to point B, in a straight line. That is why it is impossible to create a new mandibular angle with a single distractor, since the mineralization will always be in a straight manner, after finalizing the activation period [14, 17, 26] (Fig. 3).

The distraction chamber should be closed, with no saliva or food contamination in the postsurgical phase, throughout the entire healing process. The osteotomy must be completed, wounds closed, and the distraction device placed transmucosal to obtain a watertight distraction chamber. If the chamber has an incomplete periosteal layer due to a lack of meticulous surgery or wound breakdown, there will be bony defects in the contaminated area and the possibility of chamber infection. Major distraction chambers undergo vertical contraction, mostly at the middle of the chamber; this is called "hourglass deformity." The consolidation process depends on the bone stock (quality and quantity), the length of distraction, and the age of the patient. The final distraction osteogenesis phase is the remodeling process, when the mineralized bony chamber has changes secondary to function and movement. The five stages of distraction osteogenesis are listed below [26–30].

First stage: Osteotomy (complete)
Second stage: Latency period (5 to 7 days for collagen fibers to develop)
Third stage: Activation (1 mm a day every 24 h or half every 12 h)
Fourth stage: Mineralization (60 days for every centimeter of distraction)
Fifth stage: Remodeling (up to 3 years after surgery, based on function)

The vector of distraction has been a source of controversy since distraction osteogenesis began. Performing an osteotomy, placing a distractor, and hoping to get the ideal final position after completing the activation is not always realistic. There are many variables when delivering a major distraction movement; removing the distraction appliance during consolidation and hoping to obtain an ideal occlusion utilizing elastics are also not realistic, because different amounts of relapse and fibrous union can occur. Utilizing a single distractor appliance to advance the mandible, close an anterior open bite, and form an appropriate mandibular angle is even less realistic. These issues have forced the surgeons to change the vector of distraction either during activation or just finalizing the activation period, maintaining the ideal bone position until complete mineralization occurs. The mineralization process is monitored with radiographs evaluating adequate distraction chamber radioopacity; this will avoid fibrous union or relapse. The need for multiple distractors to obtain a mandible with ideal architecture is also fundamental [14, 26–30].

Another consideration is secondary damage to the temporomandibular joints by compressing the articular disc and causing reactive subchondral bony changes and

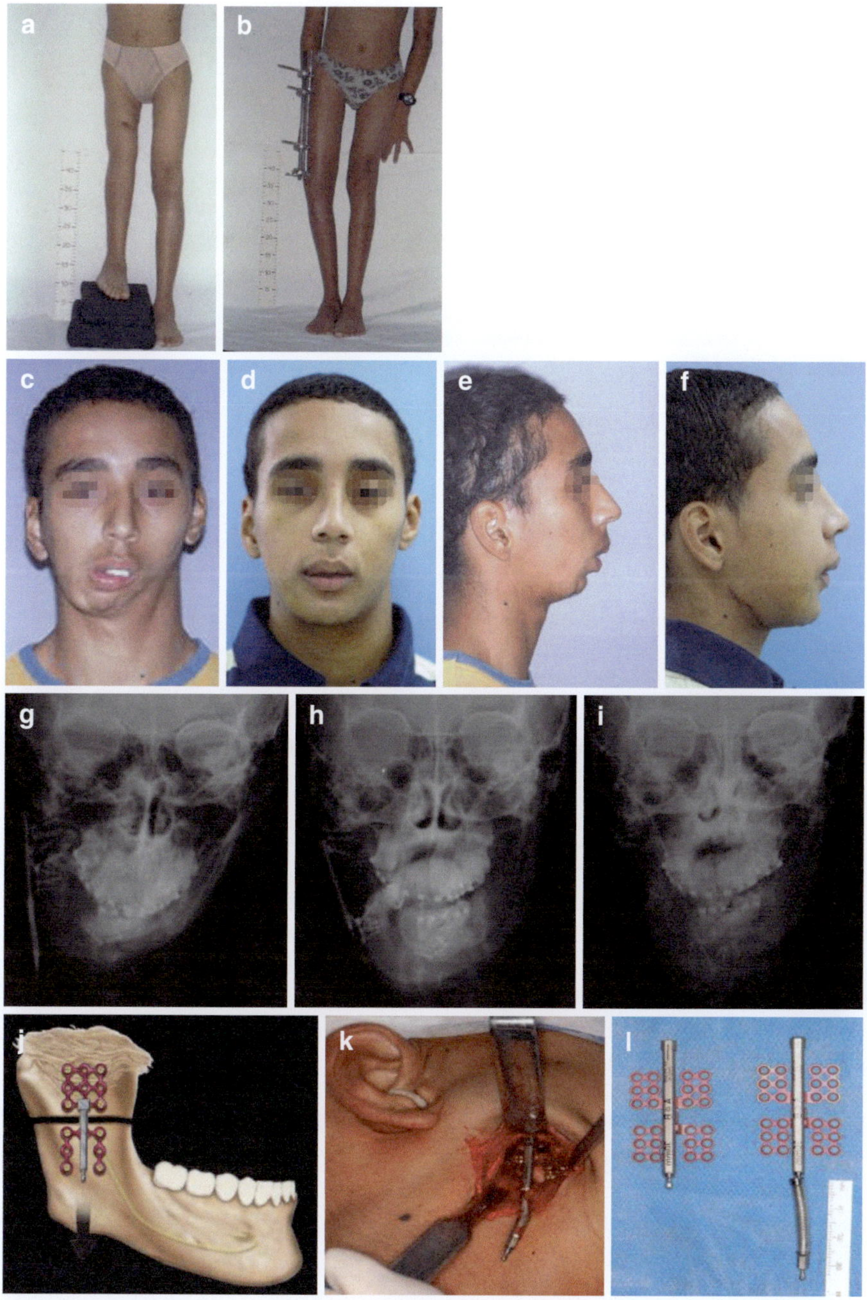

Fig. 3 (**a–i**) 17-year-old teen underwent simultaneous right femur lengthening and right mandibular ramus distraction after neonate sepsis producing right TMJ ankylosis. (**j–p**) Intraoperative view: First stage with mandibular ramus approach and appliances on position, second-stage distractor removal, genioplasty, and TMJ arthroplasty performed after adequate consolidation and Le Fort I osteotomy to correct maxillary canting and lateral open bite, third surgical stage for dental implant insertion. (**q–t**) The mandibular hypomobility was progressively improved from 0 to 30 mm. Panoramic views: right TMJ ankylosis and ramus appliances in position

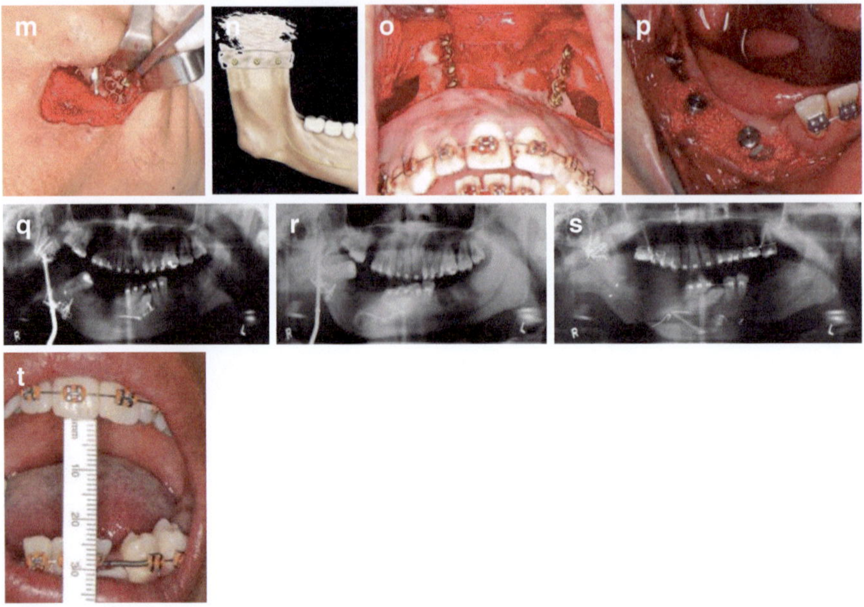

Fig. 3 (continued)

disc perforations; this should be avoided by releasing the forces from the joints and utilizing interdental elastics from the moment the activation starts until the distraction chamber is well mineralized and mandibular muscles are adapted to the new length [12–14, 26–30].

In addition, the distraction vector must be parallel to the two distractors to avoid lateral condylar displacement secondary to the reciprocal forces. As the mandible is advanced, the condyles would be displaced laterally if the distractor were lying flat against the mandible. A 5–8 mm transverse step must be built between the anterior and posterior portions of the distractor, making the distractor forces parallel to the mandibular advancing vector [12–14, 26–30].

The actual intraoral distraction technique is based on a small distractor fixed to the mandible with bicortical screws and/or wires to the teeth. The device is placed intraorally, but the activation arm is projected outside of the mucosa at the level of the occlusal plane for easier activation. An ideal intraoral distraction device permits a closed chamber and is easily placed and removed (Figs. 1, 2, and 4). The surgeon also needs to have the opportunity to change the final position of the device during the course of activation, to ensure an ideal positioning of the bony segments before the consolidation period; this helps to provide the best occlusion and position of the fragments. This distractor repositioning is to be done under IV sedation in the clinic by changing the anterior-superior or inferior bi-cortical screws, the proper occlusion is obtained through digital manipulation, and the removed single screws are replaced to continue with the mineralization period. Performing this mandibular relocation reduces treatment time, avoids long unstable orthodontic treatment, and ensures long-term skeletal stability [26–30].

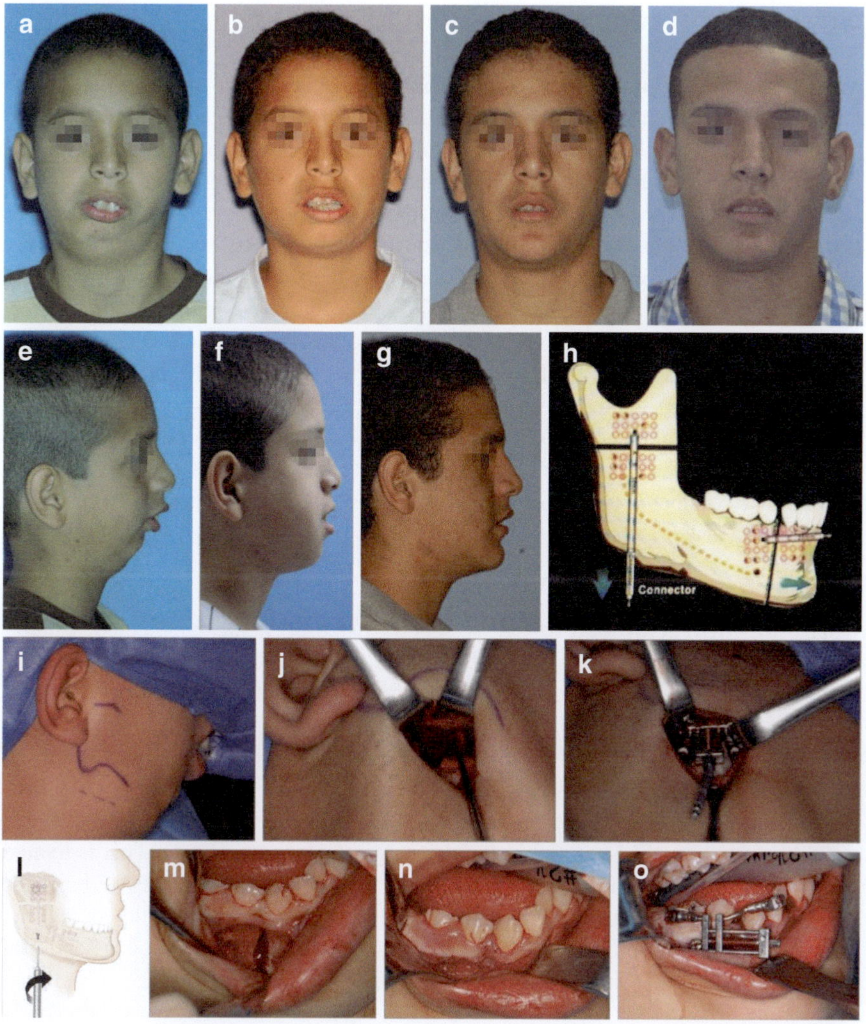

Fig. 4 (**a–d**) An 8-year-old male patient with TMJ ankylosis treated with unilateral mandibular ramus and body lengthening. Immediate post-op, 14-year follow up. (**e–h**) Profile view: Preoperative, after distraction osteogenesis and TMJ arthroplasty, and final view after advancement genioplasty. (**i–l**) Mandibular ramus approach and appliances on position. (**m–o**) Intraoral approach for body osteotomy and the appliances is fixed transmucosally

Combining body and ramus distraction osteogenesis allows the formation of the mandibular angle, a true vertical ramus, and creates bony regenerate to provide space for dental crowding alignment. These patients often need to have an increase in mandibular ramus height, body length, and space to treat severe dental crowding [19–23, 26–30] (Figs. 1, 2, and 4).

Intraoral Bidirectional Distraction Osteogenesis

Vertical distractor placement A 2 cm incision is made in the anterior mandibular ramus area. The lateral mandibular ramus soft tissues are elevated all the way to the posterior mandibular border, and then a tunnel dissection is performed on the medial mandibular ramus superior to the mandibular lingula and a periosteal elevator is placed medially to protect the mandibular nerve. The osteotomy is performed superior to the lingula, but as low as possible, starting from the posterior and progressing anteriorly without completing the bony cut. The distraction device is then placed intraorally and a trocar is used to fixate the upper and lower plates of the device. Once the distractor is in place, the activation head is to be fixed to an adequate connector, which is extended to the inferior border of the mandible through a 2 mm incision on the skin. Once the distractor ideal position is obtained and it is well fixed, the horizontal osteotomy is completed. The wound is then closed in two layers leaving the distraction appliance completely buried [19–23, 26–30]. The distractor external connector is disengaged once the activation is completed, utilizing a special screwdriver (see Fig. 3).

Horizontal distractor placement A second osteotomy site is selected, usually anterior to the mental nerve, between the premolars and anterior to the mental nerve. The reciprocating saw is used from the inferior border of the mandible, carefully elevating the soft tissues to visualize the dental roots or space between the premolars. The osteotomy is not completed, but the wound is partially closed leaving a little gap to exert rotational force with a chisel to complete the osteotomy after placing the distractor. The second distraction device is chosen, bent, and adapted (this should be done on a 3-D model in the pre-surgical planning phase). This is fixated with bicortical screws in the inferior arms and usually interdental wires with acrylic for re-enforcement at the superior arms level, the osteotomy is completed, and the remaining incision is closed. The activation rod must be at the level of the occlusal plane, for easier activation [19–23, 26–30] (see Figs. 1,2, and 4).

This bidirectional surgical technique has two different objectives, one is to obtain equal mandibular ramus heights and the other is to correct the severe anterior-posterior deficiency, therefore allowing the orthodontist to align the teeth and correct the dental midline. Most patients with these combined deficiencies would benefit from this approach. However, the chin deformity and maxillary vertical issue needs to be addressed at the time of distraction device removal. When treating children in active growth period, the orthodontist may use mechanics and orthopedics appliances to treat major discrepancies between the maxilla and mandible and move the teeth through the distraction chamber in the required direction. The created vertical maxilla-mandibular unilateral open bite in adults requires a maxillary Le Fort I osteotomy, unilateral inferior repositioning, fixation with four titanium plates, and interpositional bone grafts to predictably treat the major vertical maxillary discrepancy [19–23, 26–30] (see Figs. 1, 2, 4, and 5).

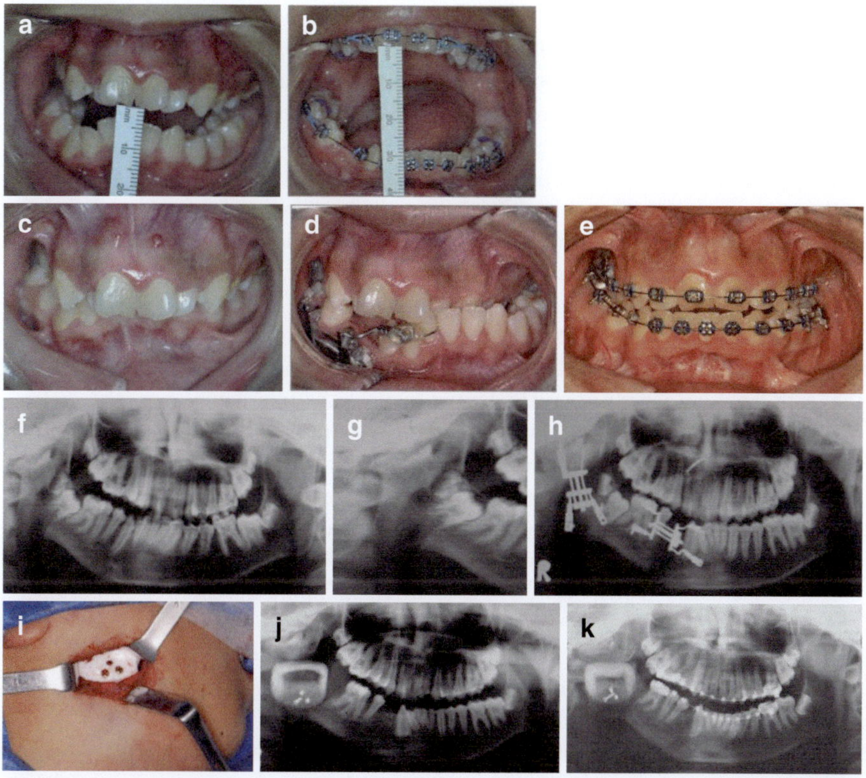

Fig. 5 Same patient case as Fig. 3. (**a–b**) Preoperative ankylosis open mouth and after treatment 30 mm gaining was obtained. (**c–e**) Intraoral views preoperative, during distraction osteogenesis, orthodontics treatment during consolidation phase. (**f–k**) Panoramic views: right TMJ ankylosis, ramus and body appliances on position. Mandibular opening after right TMJ arthroplasty

The consolidation period for large movements varies widely. The body osteotomy heals much faster than the mandibular ramus distraction, and the mineralization process is much slower and incomplete since bone quality and quantity (bone stock) is different. Mandibular physiotherapy is advisable since it increases the range of mandibular motion, enhances muscle power, and indirectly helps mineralize the ramus. Lengthening the ramus requires a much longer mineralization period. Our average time for a neonate is 6 months and up to 18 months in adults. It is important that the appliance be comfortable and allows the patient to go to school or work while consolidation is taking place. Patients with extraoral devices often request to have them removed before the mineralization is completed, therefore reducing the final stability, and resulting in varying degrees of relapse. Distraction osteogenesis is a very stable surgical technique if the complete consolidation period has elapsed before the distraction devices are removed [14–19, 26–30]. Most patients would benefit from bone extra correction since the original musculature underdevelopment secondary to the deficiency needs to be compensated, and overcorrection is advisable in many patients with soft tissue deficiencies.

Two important issues are to be considered: first is the vector of distraction. The surgeon needs to have the ability to change the final position of the distal segment once the activation phase is completed. Large mandibular disharmonies should not be treated by orthodontics means since this dental movement can result in inadvertent relapse, periodontal defects, and tooth loss. Planning to change the vector during activation or early consolidation period is a safe and easy way to close an anterior or posterior open bite. Once the activation phase is completed and the patient is in Class I position with an adequate mandibular projection, the occlusion is carefully evaluated, and a decision to change the medial fragment positioning is taken. The patient is placed under IV sedation and local anesthetics is used to reposition the distraction device. Most patient would benefit from having a larger movement at the inferior border of the mandible for esthetics and a much shorter one at the teeth level, easier for the orthodontist to close the interdental gap. The distraction chamber would have a "truncated pyramid" shape. This is obtained by releasing selected screws bilaterally disconnecting the distractor's superior anterosuperior arms, maintaining one single bicortical screw on either side of the inferior arms; following screw removal, the mandible is digitally rotated around the inferior screw, changing the distal segment inclination. As the segment rotates, the distraction chamber decreases in size between the teeth, maintaining the inferior border of the mandible's distraction chamber distance. The anterior open bite closes and projects Pogonion's position and the 1MPA changes. Finally, the dental midline can be ideally positioned by activating one of the distractors either right or left until upper and lower dental midlines coincide [14–19, 25–30].

The second issue is resuming orthodontics treatment; 3 to 5 months after surgery is the ideal time, since a large distraction chamber requires longer consolidation time. Quite frequently, orthodontic micro-implants are needed to provide anchorage for large anterior movement of the molars. This avoids reciprocal forces between anterior and posterior teeth that can cause an increase in the over jet, poor dental inclination, or Class II canines. Once the interdental space is closed, the orthodontist should start working on finishing the occlusion [25–30]. These distraction techniques are predictable and stable and carry a very low morbidity rate allowing major combined movements of 20–30 mm in each direction; orthodontics mechanics permit teeth to go through soft bone distraction chamber in shorter treatment times. Distraction osteogenesis is indicated for those clinical situations where orthognathic surgery would offer limited outcomes, relapse, instability, or failures [26–30].

Bone Transport by Intraoral Distraction Osteogenesis

The bone transport is based on the concept of creating bone and soft tissues following the biological principles of distraction osteogenesis. Osteotomies are made and distraction devices applied, following the distraction osteogenesis protocol. Depending on the number of surgical sites for the reconstruction, it could be classified as bifocal, trifocal, tetrafocal, and pentafocal. Planning several segments to create an ideal mandibular shape is key to reduce treatment time, obtain ideal height and width, and create the best host to receive the dental implants. Today's technology allows not only to replace the mandibular bone and soft tissues deficiencies but also to predictably permit dental implant insertion to anchor a dental rehabilitation, bringing function and esthetics [28, 29, 31].

In order to obtain bone continuity between the traveling and receiving bones, a docking site surgery is required, the surgeon must eliminate the tissue in between the two bone segments, activate the distractor until the segments touch and add bovine bone grafting and blood morphogenetic proteins. An adequate time is required for consolidation and final bone remodeling around 60 days for every centimeter of distraction is awaited [31].

Indications [28, 29, 31]:

- Patients medically compromised where major bone grafts are not indicated
- As an alternative for re-intervention after an unsuccessful bone graft reconstruction.
- Following removal of benign tumors or malignancies not requiring radiation.
- Reconstructing gunshot wound defects
- Managing osteomyelitis
- Treating malunions/non-unions

The mandible is basically a five different straight-line structure; two rami, two bodies, and one symphysis. Multi-segment bone transport allows the creation of curves and angles, but still maintaining height and width for dental implant insertion [26, 31–34].

The bone transport concept is based on blood supply and careful vector management; understanding bone biology and biomechanics helps in making the surgery easy and predictable, with minimal morbidity and avoiding complications. Radiographs are very useful to visualize bone formation and mineralization and to remove the distraction appliances and insert dental implants to anchorage the dental rehabilitation [26, 31–37].

Pre-surgical Preparation

Stereolithographic models, CT scans' panoramic view, and cephalometric X-rays are used for surgical planning and prediction. The 3-D model is very useful for obtaining large reconstructions and the anatomical model of the defect with the exact measurements for pre-bending of the reconstruction plate, the devices, distraction vector, and location and lengths of screws prior to surgery [31–37].

Principles

Ilizarov studied the biology of distraction histogenesis finding periosteal and endosteal preservation as the most important biological foundation; abundant irrigation and small incisions are mandatory; other variables are age of the patient, quantity and quality of bone, degree of movement, precision in surgery, soft tissue coverage, and protocol of distraction [16, 37].

1. Because the distraction will occur in a linear plane, from point A to point B, the distraction chamber will form bone in a straight line. The stretched collagen elastic fibers will progressively mineralize in the months after surgery to finally convert into calcified bone.
2. The size of the transport disc plays an important role in large reconstructions, especially when the symphysis is involved. Multiple discs could be activated simultaneously or continuous distraction stages could be performed, having the initial disc subdivided, to be transported in a different direction.
3. The hourglass deformity effect will be formed if a single bone disc is traveling a long distance, or if the original thickness is not enough to recreate good bone. The disc must have the following minimal measurements: 0.8 × 1.0 × 2.0 cm in height, width, and length, respectively, to permit implant insertion.
4. The soft tissues will also advance along and recreate soft tissues while the bone is being transported. This is very important in major reconstructions because it includes all the musculature and other soft tissues. Also to be considered in dental implants, where keratinized thick and resistant gingiva around the dental implants is needed, the adjacent gingival tissues are re-created.
5. Most patients after mandibular symphyseal Distraction Osteogenesis would benefit of a horizontal genioplasty to obtain ideal mandibular symmetry.

Multifocal Distraction

The concept is based on the use of as several bone discs as needed for the distraction to repair the defect and rigid fixation to maintain the segments' stability in place [31–38] (Figs. 6 and 7).

The reconstruction plate is placed holding the remaining bone segments in the correct position with at least three bicortical screws on each segment. For defects including the body and half or all of the symphyseal area, a complete side-to-side reconstruction plate is indicated. The appliance travels on top of the plate for vector control, and it is placed supra-periosteally in order to prevent distraction chamber contamination with food and saliva, thereby preventing infections and chamber contraction and maintaining the biological principles of distraction osteogenesis of periosteal nutrition to the area [31–38] (Figs. 6 and 7).

First Stage The tumor is resected after fixating the reconstruction plate, to avoid segment displacement, and distraction devices are fixated to the different transport discs; ideally, 15 mm in length size disc must be obtained and a 2 mm intraoperative activation is performed. The first disc will travel transversely to create a new symphysis, while the second disc will travel anteroposteriorly to reach and create the new mandibular angle. To avoid plate exposure in the angle area, secondary to muscle contraction, an angle silicon prosthesis is placed temporarily fixed to the most posterior aspect of the plate while the second distraction disc is traveling posteriorly, bringing all the soft tissues [38].

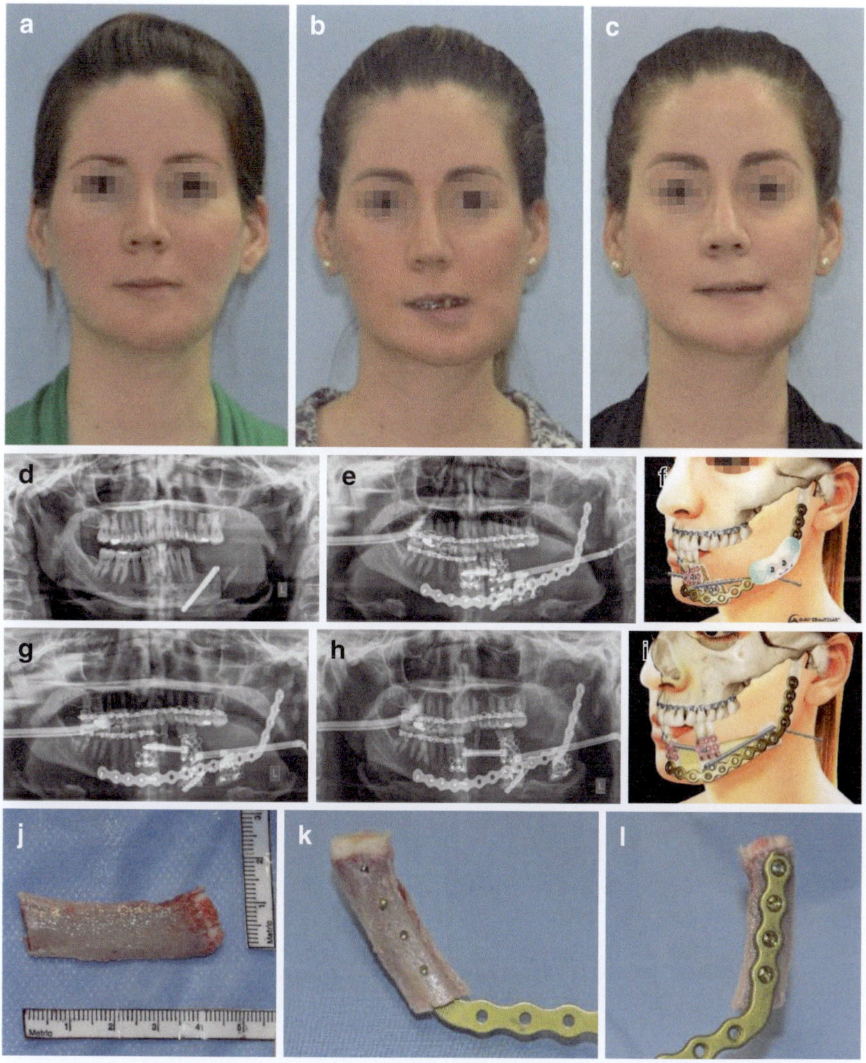

Fig. 6 (**a**–**c**) A 30-year-old female patient with a surgical history of a plexiform ameloblastoma resection. Three-dimensional mandibular reconstruction by multifocal bone transport distraction was performed. All incisions were made intraorally, noticed mild edema in the postoperative photograph. (**d**, **e**, **g**, **h**) Panoramic radiograph preoperative, during latency period, and during bone transport. (**i**) Each segment was distracted 20 mm on symphysis and 30 mm on mandibular body area. (**f**) A Porex implant was fixed to the mandibular angle plate to prevent soft tissue contraction during activation. (**j**–**l**) For condyle and mandibular ramus reconstruction, a rib graft was fixed to the plate with four screws

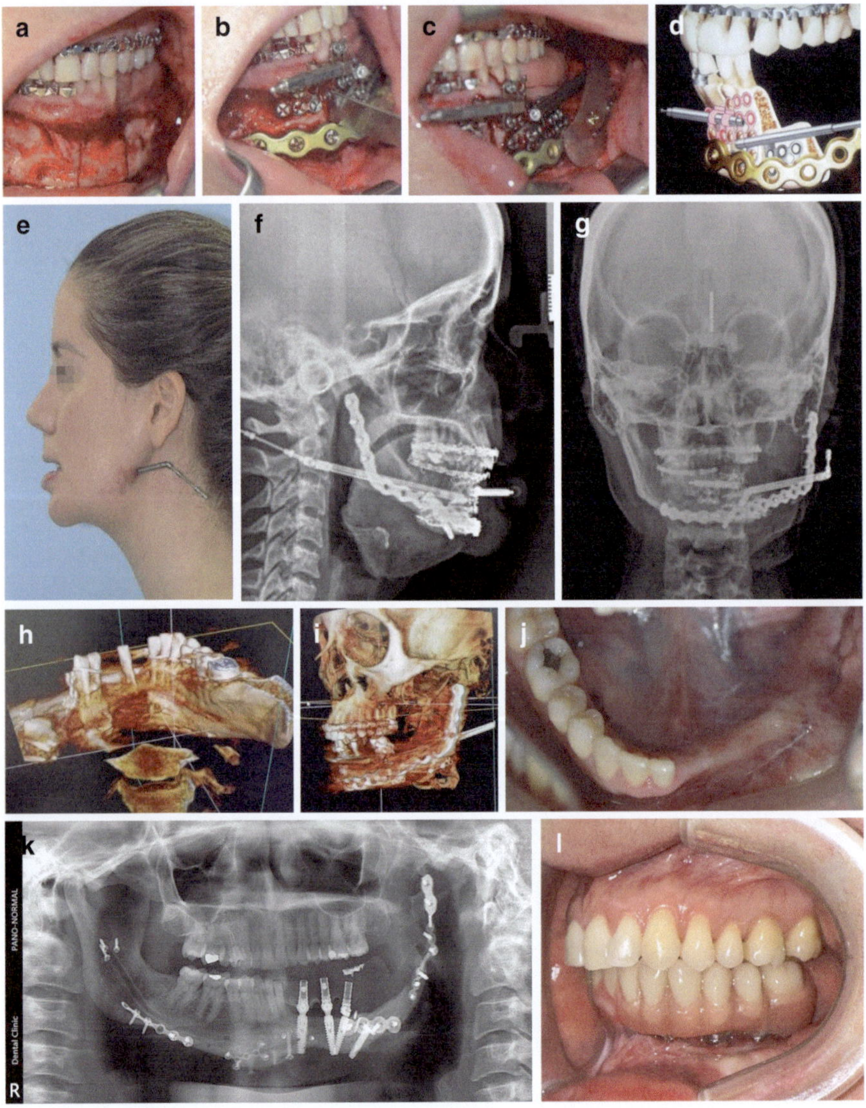

Fig. 7 (**a–d**) Same patient case: arch bars were used for the stability, first two disc osteotomies were performed, and the reconstruction plate is placed holding the remaining bone segments in the correct position with three bicortical screws. The two appliances travel on top of the plate for vector control. (**e**) Profile view preoperative and during activation: notice the appliances' extension arm. (**f–g**) Postoperative lateral and PA X-rays. After consolidation period, the distractor and Porex prosthesis were removed, notice (**h–i**) tridimensional TC during consolidation period and (**j**) intraorally view after docking site surgery, the patient is ready for dental implants

Second Stage The angle prosthesis is removed once the segment is fixated with screws to the reconstruction plate, and the distractor is removed to await for mineralization [31]. Both distraction devices are removed and discs are fixated to the reconstruction plate. A minimal exposure is performed and the lingual aspect is left untouched, since the blood supply is fundamental for healing and maintaining bone volume as distraction chamber heals. The consolidation period for major movements is prolonged for many months [31–38].

Third Stage At the end of the distraction mineralization, docking site surgery is indicated to promote healing between the two docking segments at the angle site. Dental implant insertion is performed at the same surgical stage. This is a short and simple procedure to be done under IV sedation [31–38].

Distraction Protocol [26, 28–38]

Seven days of latency period (no activation) followed by a 1 mm or ½ mm activation once a day, until distraction is completed (the activation will be performed by the patient, family member, or office staff). The distractors remain in place for 2 months per centimeter during the consolidation period as a fixation system, until they are exchanged for bicortical screws from the reconstruction plate to the bone.

Docking Site Surgery [26, 28, 39]

Docking site is the area where the two bone segments meet. At the end of treatment, the edges of these two bones are usually hypotrophic and sclerotic, covered by fibrous tissue as a result of lack of irrigation. To close this gap at the end of the distraction, a docking site surgery needs to be performed. The two edges should be as closed as possible and the non-vital bone needs to be removed. A mucoperiosteal incision with minimal periosteal elevation is used to expose both ends; it is necessary to obtain a network of neoangiogenesis from the bone marrow and periosteum to enhance healing and promote better bone consolidation. The bone edges are prepared by making multiple perforations with a #701 bur into the cortical and medullary bone, the distractor is activated until the two segments closely meet, and the bone graft obtained either from the chin, and tuberosity, or bone trap is placed over the joining bones, possibly combined with additional osteoinductive material (e.g., rh-BMP2). Rigid fixation is used to keep the two bone segments united either by the reconstruction plate or by two miniplates depending on the bone stability and amount of reconstruction.

Physiotherapy

The patient must be on a soft and liquid diet, for a long period of time and the masticatory function is diminished; this leads to mandibular hypomobility secondary to masticatory muscles and TMJ fibrosis, with the consequence of inter-incisal opening reduction at the end of the treatment. The patient needs to start functional and physiologic exercises three times a day for 20 min, to stimulate masticatory muscles and improve function [31–39].

Dental Implants in Bone Transport

Today, new implant technology allows the use of inclined dental implants and converted to parallel utilizing multi-unit abutments, where good quality and quantity of bone is available permitting the location of those implants away to the ideal situation but the implant base is placed where the prosthodontist can fabricate a fixed or hybrid dental rehabilitation. Most patients would have excellent bone in the symphysis area where implants could be inserted and abutment base located at the level of mandibular canines or premolars. Most patients are dentally rehabilitated with at least three dental implants (tripod concept) [39–45].

Future of Distraction Osteogenesis

Research studies have improved the biology knowledge, and there have been new developments in technology especially in the area of miniaturizing and trans-oral distraction devices, e.g., the use of BMP-2 to improve and speed up the healing process. There have been enough data for long-term evaluation, making these procedures available to the patients predictably and safe. Different research studies are trying to diminish the consolidation period using morphogenetic proteins, platelet-enriched plasma, calcium, and other catalysts for the healing process. There are fewer indications for external devices. Education plays a major role in selecting the patients, applying the biological principles, and using the best technology available. Long-term studies are published more frequently and the variables are better identified; this newer philosophy in craniofacial surgery will be the technique of choice in many major craniofacial deficiencies.

References

1. Schendel SA, Wolford LM, Epker BN. Mandibular deficiency syndrome. III. Surgical advancement of the deficient mandible in growing children: treatment results in twelve patients. Oral Surg Oral Med Oral Pathol. 1978;45:364–77.
2. Guerrero C. Rapid mandibular expansion. Rev Venez Ortod. 1990;48:1–2.
3. Guerrero C, Contasti G. Transverse mandibular deficiency. In: Bell WH, editor. Modern practice in orthognathic and reconstructive surgery. Philadelphia: W.B. Saunders; 1992. p. 2383–97.
4. McCarthy JG, Schreiber J, Karp N, Thorne CH, Grayson BH. Lengthening the human mandible by gradual distraction. Plast Reconstr Surg. 1992;89:1–8.
5. Wangerin K, Gropp H. Die intraorale Distraktionsosteotomie des mikrogenen Unterkiefers zur Beseitigung der Atemwegsobstruktion. Dtsch Z Mund Kiefer Gesichtschir. 1994;18:236.
6. Guerrero C, Bell WH, Flores A, Modugno VL, Constasti G, Rodriguez AM, et al. Intraoral mandibular distraction osteogenesis. Odontol Dia. 1995;11:116–32.
7. Diner P, Kollar E, Martinez H, Vazquez M. Intraoral distraction for mandibular lengthening—a technical innovation. J Craniomaxillofac Surg. 1996;24:92–5.
8. Samchukov ML, Cope JB, Harper RP, Ross JD. Biomechanical considerations for mandibular lengthening and widening by gradual distraction. Am J Oral Maxillofac Surg. 1998;56:51–9.
9. Bell WH, Gonzalez M, Samchukov ML, Guerrero CA. Intraoral widening and lengthening of the mandible in baboons by distraction osteogenesis. J Oral Maxillofac Surg. 1999;57:548.

10. Guerrero CA, Bell WH. Intraoral distraction. In: McCarthy, editor. Distraction of the craniofacial skeleton. New York: Springer; 1999. p. 219–48.
11. Chin M, Toth B. Distraction osteogenesis in maxillofacial surgery using internal devices: review of five cases. J Oral Maxillofac Surg. 1996;54:45–4.
12. DeDeyne PG, Paley D, Herzenberg JE. Muscle and its connective tissue adaptation to distraction osteogenesis. Abstract #3 ASAMI North America, First International Meeting, New Orleans, Louisiana, March 1998.
13. Harper RP, Bell WH, Hinton RJ, Browne R, Cherkashin AM, Samchukov ML. Reactive changes in the temporomandibular joint after midline osteodistraction. Br J Oral Maxillofac Surg. 1997;35:20–5.
14. Bell WH, Gonzalez M, Samchukov ML, Guerrero CA. Intraoral widening and lengthening the mandible by distraction osteogenesis and histogenesis. J Oral Maxillofac Surg. 1999;57:548–62.
15. Guerrero CA, Bell WH, Contasti GI, Rodriguez AM. Intraoral mandibular distraction osteogenesis. Semin Orthod. 1999;5:35–40.
16. Ilizarov GA. The tension -stress effect on the genesis and growth of tissues: Part I. The influence of stability on fixation and soft tissue preservation. Clin Orthop. 1989;238:249.
17. Guerrero CA, Bell WH, Meza LS. Intraoral distraction osteogenesis. Maxillary and mandibular lengthening. In: Suzanne U. Stucki-McCormick, guest editor. Atlas of the oral and maxillofacial surgery clinics of North America (Distraction Osteogenesis); 1999. p. 7:1, 111–51.
18. Minoretti R, Triaca A, Antonini M, Merz B. Intraoral multiaxis mandibular distraction osteogenesis: clinical analysis of the first six years. In: Bell-Guerrero, editor. Distraction osteogenesis of the facial skeleton. Hamilton: BC Decker; 2007. p. 359–71.
19. Guerrero C, Bell W, Gonzalez M, Meza L. Intraoral distraction osteogenesis. In: Fonseca RJ, editor. Oral and maxillofacial surgery, vol. 2. Philadelphia: W.B. Saunders; 2000. p. 359–402.
20. Guerrero CA, Bell WH, Mujica EV, Gonzalez M, Dominguez E. Intraoral distraction osteogenesis. In: Fonseca: oral and maxillofacial surgery, 3rd ed. Elsevier Health Sciences. 2017. p. 3:196–221.
21. Gonzalez M, Bell WH, Guerrero CA, Buschang PH, Samchukov ML. Positional changes and stability of bone segments during simultaneous bilateral mandibular lengthening and widening by distraction osteogenesis. Br J Oral and Maxillofac Surg. 2001;39:169.
22. Guerrero CA, Bell HW, Gonzalez M. Mandibular remodeling: the fifth stage in distraction osteogenesis healing. In: Arnaud E, Diner PA, editors. 3rd International congress on cranial and facial bone distraction processes, Monduzzi Editore. Bologna; 2001. p. 267–73.
23. Guerrero CA, Figueroa F, Bell WH, Olmos-Malave Y, Rojas A, Gonzalez M. Surgical orthodontics in mandibular lengthening. In: Bell-Guerrero, editor. Distraction osteogenesis of the facial skeleton. Hamilton: BC Decker; 2007. p. 373–88.
24. Polley JW, Figueroa AA. Management of severe maxillary deficiency in childhood and adolescent through distraction osteogenesis with an external, adjustable, rigid distraction device. J Craniofac Surg. 1997;8:181.
25. Del Santo M, Guerrero CA, Buschang PH, et al. Long-term skeletal and dental effects of mandibular symphyseal distraction osteogenesis. Am J Orthod Dentofac Orthop. 1999;1–62.
26. Guerrero CA, Rivera H, Mujica E, Henriquez M, Gonzalez M. Principles of distraction osteogenesis. In: Bagheri S, Bell B, editors. Current therapy in oral and maxillofacial surgery, vol. 11. Elsevier Health Sciences; 2011. p. 101–11.
27. Gonzalez M, Guerrero C, Ding M. Distraction osteogenesis. In: Bagheri S, Bell B, Khan H, editors. Current therapy in oral and maxillofacial surgery, vol. 79. St Louis: Elsevier; 2011. p. 658–70.
28. Guerrero CA, Gonzalez M, Mujica EV: Mandibular intraoral distraction osteogenesis. In Kademani/Tiwana: Atlas of oral and maxillofacial surgery. Elsevier Health Sciences. 341–358. 2016.
29. Guerrero CA, Contasti G, Rodriguez A. Mandibular distraction osteogenesis. In: Naini FB, Gil DS, editors. Orthognathic surgery: principles, planning and practice, vol. 45. Wiley-Blackwell; 2017. p. 701.

30. Guerrero CA, Bell WH, Contasti G, Rodriguez A, Contasti R. In: McCarthy J, editor. Intraoral mandibular distraction, 2nd ed. Springer; 2017. p. 99–122.
31. Guerrero CA, Bell WH, Gonzalez M, Figueroa F. Maxillo-mandibular reconstruction by intraoral bone transport. In: Arnaud D, editor. 3rd international congress on facial distraction processes, vol. 1. Paris: Monduzzi; 2001. p. 569–74.
32. Fonseca RJ, Walker RV. Oral and maxillofacial trauma. Philadelphia: W.B. Saunders; 1991. p. 275.
33. Guerrero CA, Bell WH, Gonzalez M, Rojas A. Intraoral mandibular bone transport: a case report. In: Samchukov, Cope, Cherkashin, editors. Craniofacial distraction osteogenesis. St. Louis: Mosby; 2001. p. 372–5.
34. Guerrero CA, Bell WH, Gonzalez M, Figueroa F. Maxillo-mandibular reconstruction by intraoral bone transport. In: Arnaud D, editor. 3rd international congress on facial distraction processes. Bologna: Monduzzi editore; 2001. p. 569–74.
35. Guerrero CA, Rojas A, Figueroa F, Gonzalez M, Bell WH, Boyne P. Radiographic evaluation of traditional versus rhBMP-2 inducted intraoral bone transport in mandibular reconstruction. In: Arnaud D, editor. In: 4th international congress of maxillofacial and craniofacial distraction. Bologna: Monduzzi editore; 2003. p. 391–6.
36. Guerrero CA, Figueroa F, Gonzalez M. 3-D alveolar distraction osteogenesis. In: Diner PA, Arnaud E, editors. Proceedings of the 4th international congress of maxillofacial and craniofacial distraction; 2003 July 2–5; Paris. Bologna: Monduzzi Editore; 2003. p. 37–42.
37. Guerrero CA, Gonzalez M, Dominguez E. Bone transport by distraction osteogenesis for maxillomandibular reconstruction. In: Bell-Guerrero, editor. Distraction osteogenesis of the facial skeleton. Hamilton: BC Decker; 2007. p. 501–19.
38. Makarov MR, Kochutina LN, Birch JG, et al. Muscle histomorphology during distraction osteogenesis. In: Stein H, Suk SI, Leung PC, et al., editors. SIROT 99 international research society of orthopaedic surgery and traumatology, Sydney, Australia, April 16–19, 1999. Freund Publishing House LTD.: Tel Aviv, Israel; 1999. p. 647–52
39. Gonzalez M, Guerrero CA, Henriquez M, Figueroa F, Domínguez E. Docking site surgery in bone transport. In: Arnaud D, editor. In 5th international congress of maxillofacial and craniofacial distraction. Paris: Monduzzi editore; 2006. p. 99–104.
40. Hidding J, Lazar F, Zoeller JE. Vertical distraction of the alveolar process: a new technique for reconstructing the alveolar ridge. In: Samchucov ML, Cope JB, Cherkashin AM, editors. Craniofacial distraction osteogenesis. St. Louis (MO): Mosby; 2001. p. 393–400.
41. Oda T, Sawaki Y, Ueda M. Experimental alveolar ridge augmentation by distraction osteogenesis using a simple device that permits secondary implant placement. Int J Oral Maxillofac Implants. 2000;15:95–102.
42. Guerrero CA, Laplana R, Figueredo N, Rojas A. Surgical implant repositioning: a clinical report. Int J Oral Maxillofac Implants. 1999;14:48–54.
43. Guerrero CA, Gonzalez M, Laplana R, Rojas A. Reconstrução do rebordo alveolar mediante distração ostogênica para implantes osseointegrados. In: Dinato JC, Polido W, editors. Implantes osseointegrados: Cirugia e Prótese. Brazil: Artes Mèdicas; 2001. p. 423–39.
44. Razdolsky Y, Dessner S, El-Bialy. Correction of alveolar ridge deficiency using the ROD-5 distraction device: a case report. In: Samchucov ML, Cope JB, Cherkashin AM, editors. Craniofacial distraction osteogenesis. St. Louis (MO): Mosby; 2001. p. 454–8.
45. Ueda M. Maxillofacial bone distraction processes using osseointegrated implants and an intraoral device. In: Diner PA, Vasquez MP, editors. Proceeding of the international congress on cranial and facial bone distraction processes; 1997 June 19–21; Paris, France, vol. 26. Bologna: Monduzzi Editore; 1997. p. 75–84.

Facial Implants: Autogenous Bone Grafts and Alloplastic Implants

Jennifer E. Woerner and G. E. Ghali

Abstract

Facial asymmetry is a common condition impacted by a wide array of conditions. It often presents as a complex problem from the perspective of reconstruction. These conditions often require numerous surgeries throughout childhood and adolescence, and secondary procedures such as autogenous bone grafting and/or alloplastic implant placement may be necessary to normalize the facial skeleton. Fortunately, the ability to perform virtual surgical planning has improved the ability to compensate for bony and/or soft tissue loss and reduced operative time through the use of cutting guides, fixation templates, and/or fabrication of custom implants.

Keywords

Facial asymmetry · Custom implants · Alloplastic implants · Bone grafts

Introduction

Every human possesses some degree of facial asymmetry. For most people, this discrepancy between facial halves goes unnoticed. For the small percentage of people with obvious dysmorphology, it can affect function along with their psychosocial well-being. Minor nuances in facial symmetry can be present at birth or develop

J. E. Woerner
Shriners Hospital for Childrent, Shreveport, LA, USA

G. E. Ghali (✉)
Louisiana State University Health Sciences Center-Shreveport, Shreveport, LA, USA

Willis Knighton Health System, Shreveport, LA, USA
e-mail: gghali@wkhs.edu

P. Mehra, L. M. Wolford (eds.), *Management of Facial Asymmetry*,
https://doi.org/10.1007/978-3-030-44971-1_9

over time into adulthood. Over recent decades, the ability to diagnose and correct these deformities has dramatically improved. For many congenital deformities associated with asymmetry, autogenous bone grafting is the first line for normalizing the form, function, and aesthetics of the facial contours. Autogenous bone grafts can also be utilized during or following the time of orthognathic surgery as a secondary procedure. In contrast, the use of alloplastic implants is commonly employed as a secondary procedure to improve symmetry when osteotomies alone are not sufficient or to camouflage mild deformities without the utilization of osteotomies at all. Regardless of whether an autogenous source or alloplastic source is used, properties of a suitable maxillofacial implant include (1) ability to restore facial contours, (2) biocompatibility, and (3) mechanical stability [1, 2].

Common Causes of Facial Asymmetry

The etiologic causes of facial asymmetry are broad, but are commonly divided into congenital, developmental, and acquired deformities [3]. Kent [2] further breaks down congenital causes into those caused by over- or underdevelopment. Though determining the etiology of the facial asymmetry is essential, it is also important to determine whether this is due to the bony facial skeleton, the overlying soft tissue, impairment of animation, or a combination of these.

Osteotomies alone are often insufficient in correcting severe facial asymmetries. Therefore, the use of autogenous bone grafts, free tissue transfer, or alloplastic implants is often necessary to restore facial balance and harmony. A brief synopsis of the most common craniofacial conditions requiring maxillofacial implants will be outlined, as these are discussed in detail within other chapters in this text.

Craniosynostosis

Craniosynostosis is defined as the premature fusion of one or more cranial vault sutures. This can be a random, nonsyndromic, isolated incident or part of a spectrum of anomalies as evident in craniofacial dysostosis syndromes. The spectrum of findings and association with facial asymmetry is described in chapter "Facial Asymmetry: Management of the Oculo-auriculo-vertebral Spectrum (OAVS)". For the purposes of this chapter, we will discuss unilateral coronal synostosis as it is most commonly associated with facial asymmetry requiring secondary grafting procedures. Unilateral coronal synostosis has a prevalence of 1:10,000 live births and is the second most common form of craniosynostosis behind sagittal synostosis. Restricted growth across the affected coronal suture translates into recession of the frontal and parietal bones on the ipsilateral side. This then impacts the anterior skull base, along with the growth of the nose and orbit creating the characteristic twisted nasal architecture, displaced orbital location and shape, and hypoplasia of the zygoma on the affected side (Fig. 1) [4, 5]. This cranial base involvement can also affect the growth of the mandible resulting in asymmetry of the lower one third of

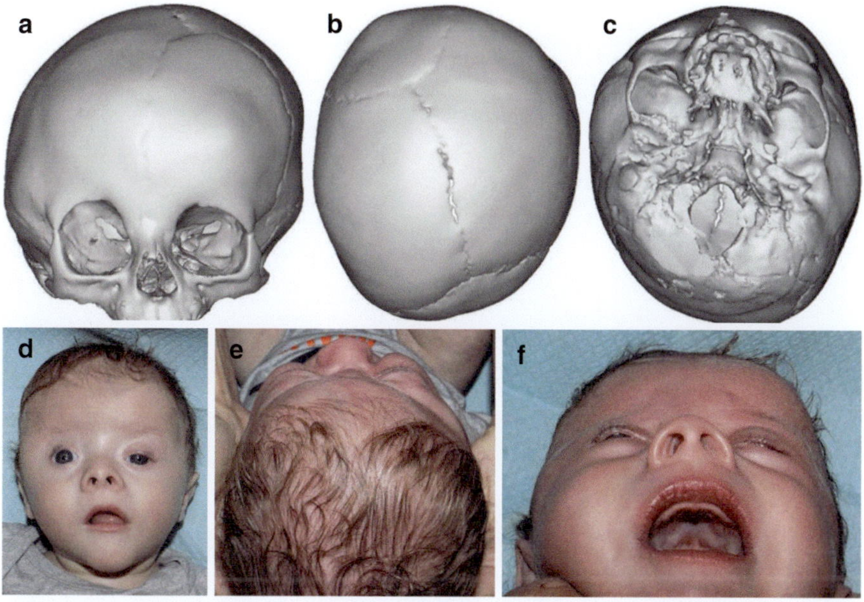

Fig. 1 3D reconstruction of infant born with right unilateral craniosynostosis with obvious anatomic deformity and asymmetry in (**a**) frontal, (**b**) birds eye, and (**c**) worms eye views. And another child with right unilateral craniosynostosis and resulting facial asymmetry in (**d**) frontal, (**e**) birds eye, and (**f**) worms eye views

the face. Secondary grafting of this area may be necessary to camouflage any remaining asymmetry following primary repair or to compensate for asymmetric growth as the child ages.

Oculo-Auriculo-Vertebral Spectrum

Oculo-auriculo-vertebral spectrum (OAVS) encompasses three disorders that were previously thought to be separate entities. In order of increasing severity, OAVS includes oculo-auriculo-vertebral disorder, hemifacial microsomia, and Goldenhar's syndrome. Facial deformities can affect any structures derived from the first and second branchial arches (Fig. 2). In 10–15% of cases, OAVS can occur bilaterally, though it is common for one side to be more severely affected than the other [6]. It is important to recognize that OAVS is not progressive in nature, and there is substantial evidence to support that growth rate on the affected side is no different from the non-affected side. This holds true regardless of the Kaban/Pruzansky grade or OMENS score [6–11]. Children with these conditions may require costochondral rib grafting, distraction osteogenesis, and/or formal orthognathic surgery. These procedures alone may not be adequate to address facial asymmetry, and grafting versus alloplastic implantation may be necessary to normalize facial appearance.

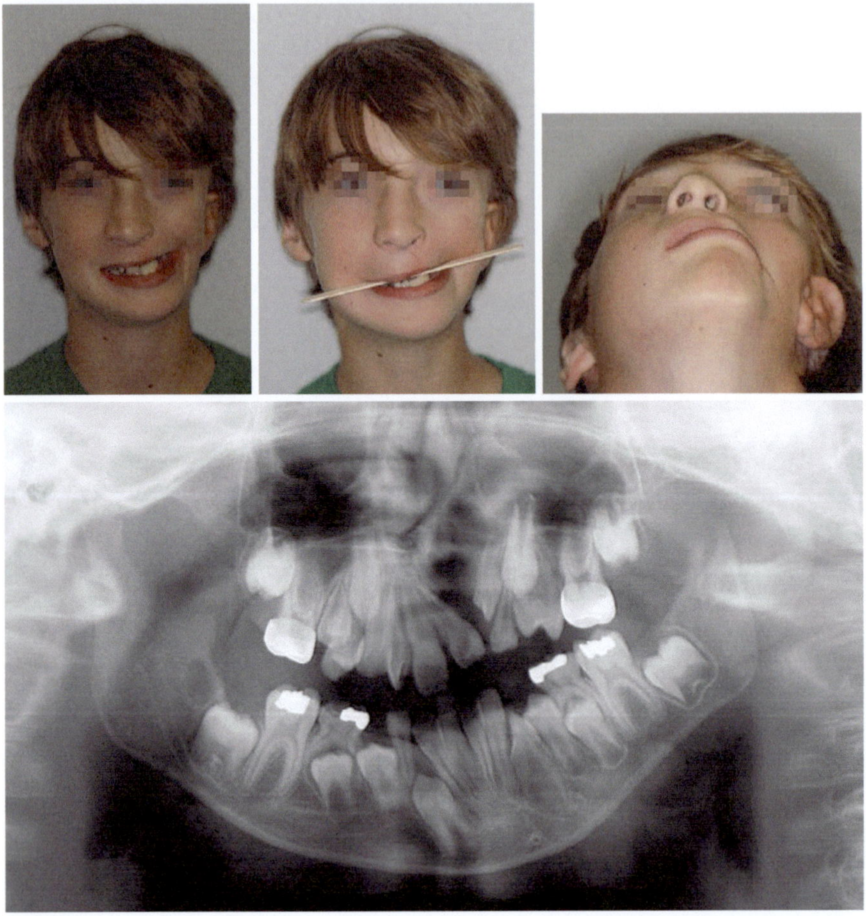

Fig. 2 A young boy on the OAV spectrum demonstrating many of the common facial features

Cleft Lip and Palate

According to a surveillance in 2006 by the Centers for Disease Control and Prevention (CDC), approximately 2650 babies are born with a cleft palate and 4440 babies are born with a cleft lip with or without a cleft palate annually in the United States [12]. Children born with CLP can present with unilateral or bilateral malformations with varying degrees of severity. This condition can affect the soft tissue and the underlying bone of the piriform rim, alveolus, and/or palate. Unilateral CLP patients have obvious facial asymmetry when compared to the non-cleft side (Fig. 3). In bilateral CLP, there can be asymmetry between the facial halves as well, depending on the severity of each independent cleft. Growth disturbance due to surgical repairs also contributes to facial asymmetry in this patient population. Numerous studies have shown impaired horizontal and vertical growth of the

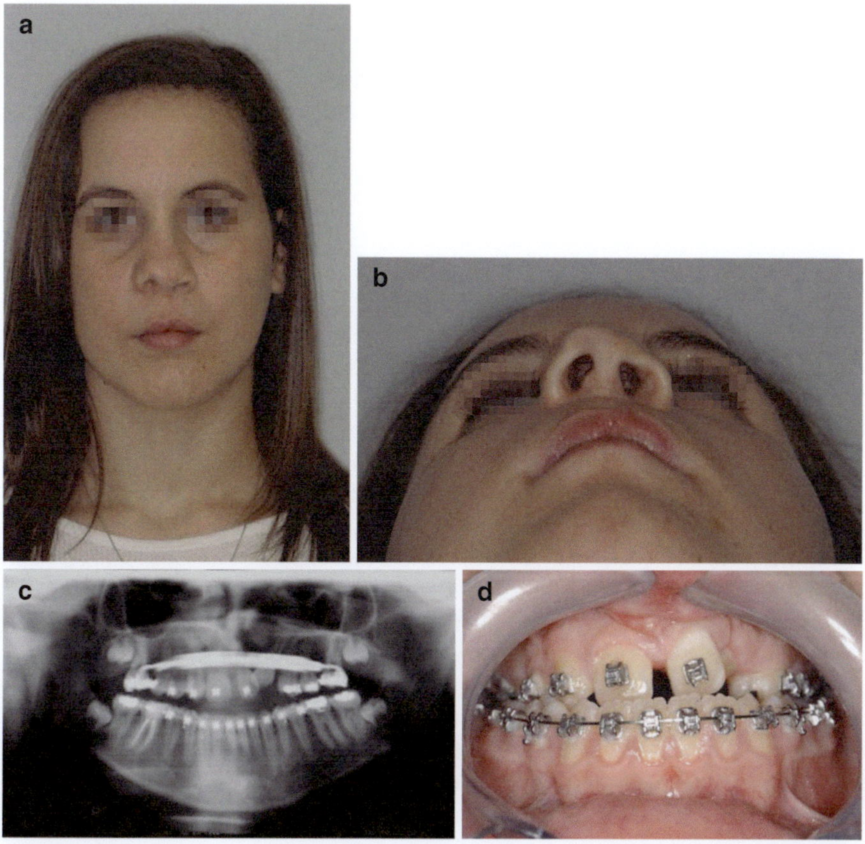

Fig. 3 Classic unilateral cleft lip and palate deformity in patient with unrepaired right oronasal fistula resulting in obvious facial asymmetry. (**a**, **b**) Mild asymmetry in frontal and worms eye view depicting poor support of upper lip and left alar cartilage due to bony cleft into maxilla and pyriform rim (**c**) Panoramic depicting alveolar cleft prior to repair (**d**) Intraoral photograph of fistula

maxilla resulting in a class III malocclusion requiring orthognathic surgery in approximately 25% of the patients [13–16]. Even following appropriately timed alveolar cleft bone grafting and orthognathic surgery, it is not uncommon for children with CLP to require additional grafting to address residual maxillary and nasal asymmetry.

Rare Craniofacial Clefts

In 1973, Tessier [17] presented his classification of craniofacial anomalies at the Second International Congress on Cleft Palate. The Tessier Classification System of Craniofacial Anomalies has since become the most widely utilized nomenclature for describing the soft tissue and corresponding bony deformities for rare facial clefts. With unilateral deformities, there is obvious asymmetry between the cleft and non-cleft side. Even Tessier 0–14 midline craniofacial clefts or bilateral Tessier 7 clefts associated with hemifacial microsomia can have varying amounts of asymmetry between the facial halves. Both autogenous and alloplastic maxillofacial implants may be necessary to attempt to normalize facial features in this group of patients by replacing missing or distorted bone, soft tissue, or entire facial subunits.

Condylar Hyperplasia/Hemimandibular Hyperplasia

Both condylar hyperplasia and hemimandibular hyperplasia are pathologic conditions that result in overgrowth of the mandible. These conditions can lead to significant facial asymmetry, poor esthetics, and functional deficits [18]. Significant controversy surrounds whether condylar hyperplasia and hemimandibular hypertrophy represent separate entities or a spectrum of the same disease [19]. For the purpose of this chapter, we will discuss them as a group in relation to addressing facial asymmetry. As nicely summarized by Posnick, the amount of facial asymmetry and facial phenotype produced is dependent on the timing between the condylar overgrowth and normal facial growth, along with the rate of overgrowth [20]. As discussed in chapter "Facial Asymmetry Caused by Condylar Hyperplasia", TMJ condylar hypertrophy, condylar overgrowth can result in significant mandibular asymmetry, along with secondary effects on the maxilla and chin. Depending on the phenotype and severity, grafting of the non-affected side may be necessary to enhance facial harmony. Refer to chapter "Facial Asymmetry Caused by Condylar Hyperplasia" for examples of facial asymmetry caused by condylar hyperplasia and hemimandibular hyperplasia.

Trauma/TMJ Ankylosis

Any form of facial trauma may result in facial asymmetry. Trauma occurring in infancy or childhood may impact growth, therefore resulting in asymmetry. The classical example is condylar head trauma in the growing child. This can create a hemarthrosis that can lead to pain and limited translational mobility. In severe cases, this can result in fibro-osseous ankylosis restricting facial growth. Early surgical intervention may reduce the adverse effects on facial growth and mandibular function. Ohno and colleagues [21] determined through serial growth studies that the two-year-old infants who underwent surgery for TMJ ankyloses had improved mandibular growth over those with delayed surgical intervention [21]. As discussed in chapter "Management of Facial Asymmetry in TMJ Ankylosis and Degenerative Joint Disease", there are numerous interventions for TMJ ankylosis in children, but the most current reconstruction includes costochondral bone grafting, fibula free flap reconstruction, or alloplastic total joint replacement when gross dysmorphology or displacement of the condylar head has

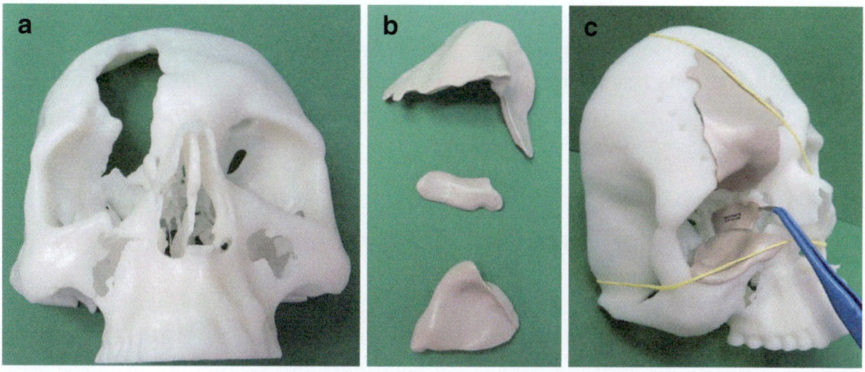

Fig. 4 Fronto-orbital defect following pedestrian versus automobile. (**a**) Stereolithic model depicting gross deformity of frontal bone, superior orbital rim, medial orbital wall, and floor of orbit (**b**) Three-piece custom implant of polyetheretherketone to reconstruct the defect (**c**) Positioning of alloplastic implant in model

occurred. Costochondral bone grafting remains the gold standard for TMJ reconstruction in the growing patient, but in recent years, Sinn [22, 23], along with Mercuri and Swift [24], has demonstrated the use of total joint prosthesis. For both authors, the use of total joint replacement in the pediatric population was limited to the reconstruction of severe cases or those that have re-ankylosed following a traditional surgical intervention [22–25]. In patients who have completed facial growth, Lee and colleagues found the literature supported TMJ reconstruction with a total joint prosthesis resulting in a significant reduction in complications and an improved quality of life [25, 26].

Trauma occurring before or after completion of facial growth may result in noticeable asymmetry if the patient is not appropriately reconstructed or proper anatomic contours are not achievable due to loss of soft tissue and/or bone. Residual deformities are not uncommon. Traumatic injuries commonly requiring secondary grafting to improve facial asymmetry include nasal bone fractures, ZMC/orbital floor blowouts, cranial vault deformities (Fig. 4), and ballistic injuries.

Degenerative Diseases

Rheumatologic conditions, steroid use, or other unknown factors may cause resorption of the mandibular condyle resulting in facial asymmetry. Of these, juvenile idiopathic arthritis (JIA) affecting the TMJ is the most common and can lead to varying degrees of growth disturbance and facial asymmetry. In regard to JIA, the TMJ is affected in 39–75% of cases and can be unilateral or bilateral [27, 28]. Patients with JIA commonly present with a class II malocclusion and an anterior open bite, and when the condition is unilateral in nature, a facial asymmetry occurs. It also carries the possibility of pain and limited range of motion [29]. When treating conditions such as JIA, the appropriate treatment and timing of intervention is highly debated. Regardless, there may be numerous indications to use autogenous bone grafts or alloplastic implants to correct facial asymmetry in this population. These interventions range from the primary correction of residual deformities following orthognathic surgery to reconstruction of the TMJ with CCG or alloplastic total joint replacement [29, 30].

Facial Hemiatrophy (Parry-Romberg Syndrome)

Facial hemiatrophy is a challenging facial asymmetry to treat and is characterized by progressive, unilateral, loss of bone, cartilage, and soft tissue bulk and thinning of skin (Fig. 5). Patients with facial hemiatrophy are commonly afflicted with hyperpigmentation, alopecia in the affected area, and Jacksonian epilepsy [3, 31]. The etiology of this condition is unknown with numerous theories which include infectious origins, neurologic sources, and autoimmune disease [3, 19, 32]. One of the most common thoughts is that this condition is a sub-type of scleroderma, much like morphea en coup de sabre [33]. Not only is this condition poorly understood, but it is also challenging to treat due the progressive nature of the disease and the severity of deformity that ensues. Once the condition stabilizes, the treatment is often reconstruction with a combination of numerous types of implants to include autogenous bone grafts, free tissue transfer, fat grafting, and alloplastic materials. Unfortunately, the results are often variable and only provide masking of the asymmetry.

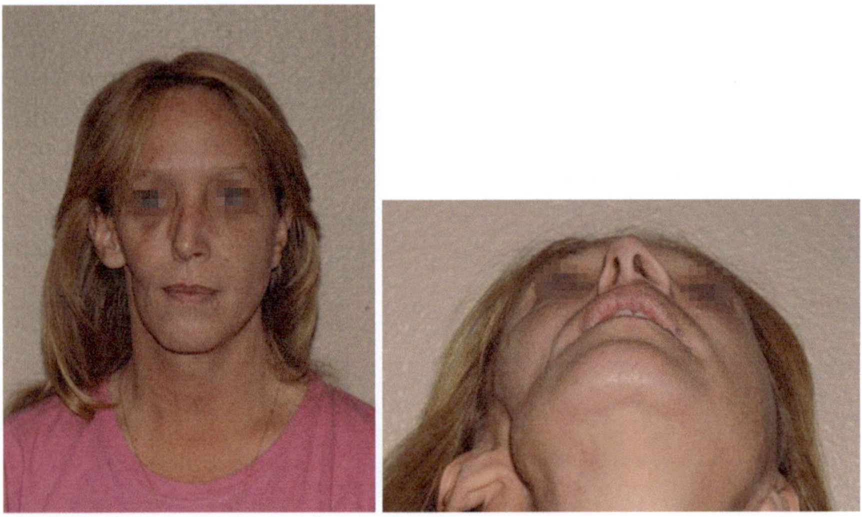

Fig. 5 45-year-old female with history of Parry-Romberg syndrome, demonstrating remarkable facial atrophy resulting in asymmetry

Sources for Autogenous Grafting

Autogenous bone grafts are still considered the gold standard and have been used for maxillofacial reconstruction dating back to the early 1900s [1]. There are a plethora of autogenous bone grafting sources that can be utilized to augment the facial skeleton. Regional bone stock will be briefly discussed, as it can be utilized during orthognathic surgery and for small areas requiring grafting. A majority of this section will focus on the most commonly utilized autogenous grafts from distant sites. Autogenous bone grafts to improve facial asymmetry are almost exclusively corticocancellous bone. Corticocancellous grafts provide cortical bone that can be easily fixated and will withstand pressure from the overlying soft tissue envelope and cancellous marrow that provides viable osteoblasts [1]. Autogenous grafts are well tolerated and revascularize over time.

Regional Sources of Bone

In correction of facial asymmetry, it is often necessary to remove bone from the hyperplastic side. It is useful to remove this bone in one piece that can then be grafted on the deficient side. With the advent of virtual surgical planning (VSP), the amount of reduction necessary can be planned preoperatively and cutting guides can be created. Other sources of regional bone that can be utilized include the mandibular ramus and symphysis. These locations provide small amounts of cortical bone that can be used for augmentation of the facial skeleton. Of the abovementioned conditions, this is most commonly utilized for asymmetry due to cleft lip and/or palate. A piece of ramus graft can be harvested to augment the pyriform rim and help correct the asymmetry of the nose and upper lip due to the inadequate bony support secondary to alveolar clefting (Fig. 6).

Costochondral Rib Graft

Costochondral bone grafts were the mainstay for grafting of the facial skeleton and are still the primary source of bone stock in children less than 9 years of age. When conditions with the OAVS or cases of severe ankylosis require mandibular and condylar reconstruction to improve function and facial esthetics, grafting from the contralateral fifth or sixth rib is most commonly employed (Fig. 7). It is important to leave the periosteum and perichondrium over the costochondral junction intact to help prevent the separation of the cartilage from the bone. Costochondral rib grafting prior to the age of 5 should be avoided if possible. The bone stock is small and difficult to fixate. It also shows a propensity for resorption when grafting is performed this early. One drawback of costochondral grafting is the unpredictable growth.

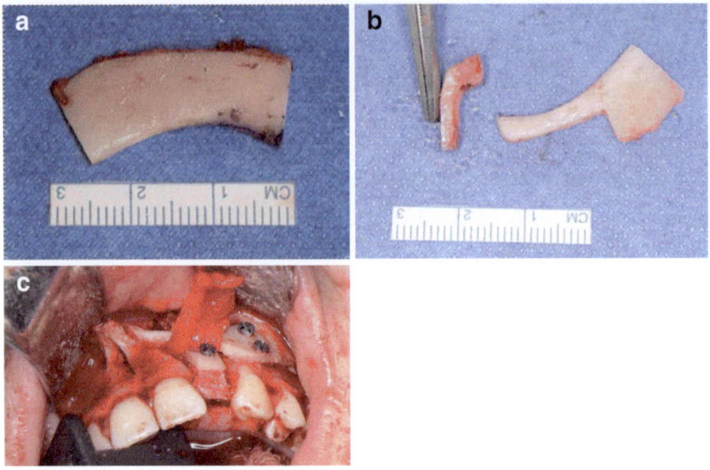

Fig. 6 (**a**) Ramus graft following harvest, (**b**) Shaping of ramus graft to augment the pyriform rim and (**c**) Ramus graft in place with additional augmentation of alveolar ridge with bone graft and BMP for later implant placement

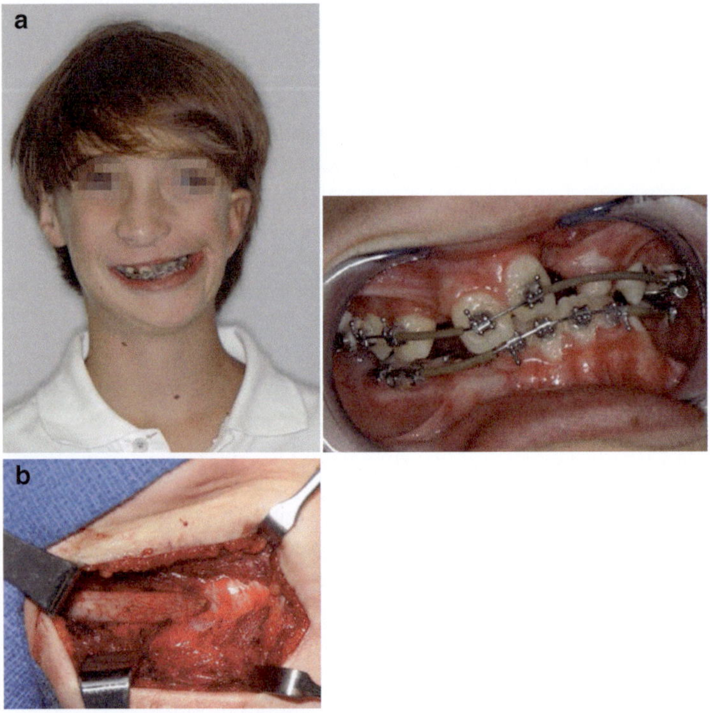

Fig. 7 The same child featured in Fig. 2 at age 8 before and after costochondral rib grafting. (**a**) Preoperative frontal and occlusal photographs, (**b**) Harvesting of fifth rib, (**c**) 6 weeks postoperative frontal and occlusal photographs following placement of costochondral rib graft to reconstruct the left mandibular ramus and Le Fort 1 osteotomy, and (**d**) Preoperative and postoperative Panorex following reconstruction

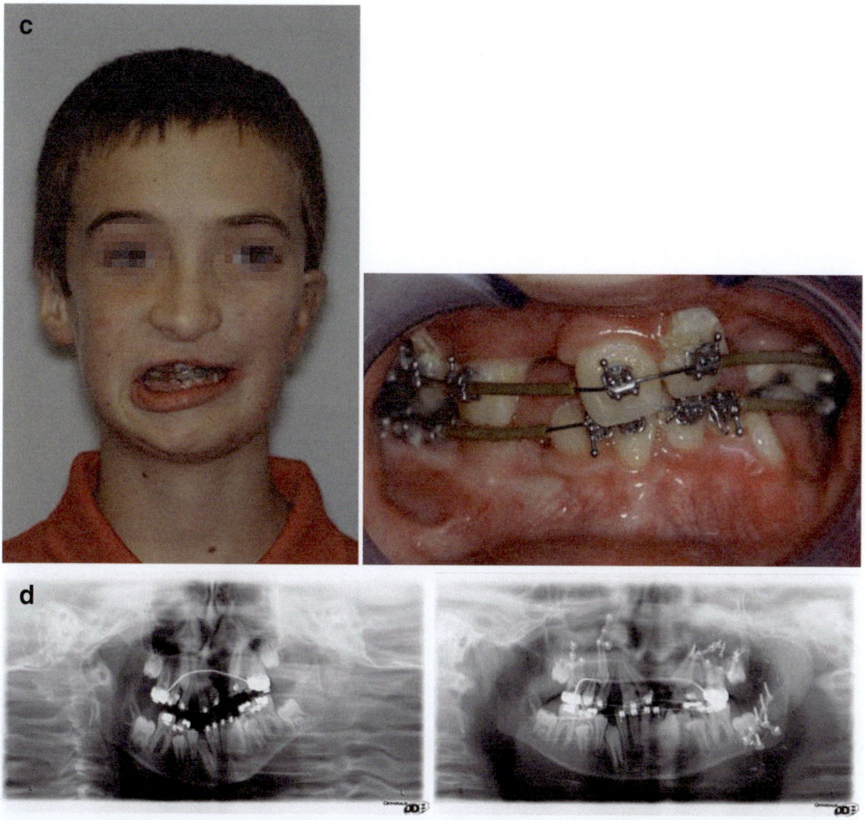

Fig. 7 (continued)

Iliac Crest

Iliac crest can be harvested from the anterior or posterior ilium, depending on the volume of bone required for reconstruction (Figs. 8 and 9). The anterior ilium can supply up to 50 cc of corticocancellous bone and bicortical or tricortical harvest can be performed if necessary. The posterior ilium can supply more than twice as much cancellous bone as the anterior iliac crest, but cortical bone harvest is limited to the lateral cortex due to the sacroiliac joint present on the medial aspect. Some advantages of iliac crest include ease of operation, low morbidity rate, and a large volume of bone available. Disadvantages of the anterior approach include the possibility of a transient gait disturbance and damage to surrounding sensory nerves. When considering a posterior approach, disadvantages include requirement of prone positioning of patient and inability to perform a two-team approach, both adding to operative time. Harvesting of cortical blocks is not recommended in children below the age of 9 due to the potential for growth disturbance.

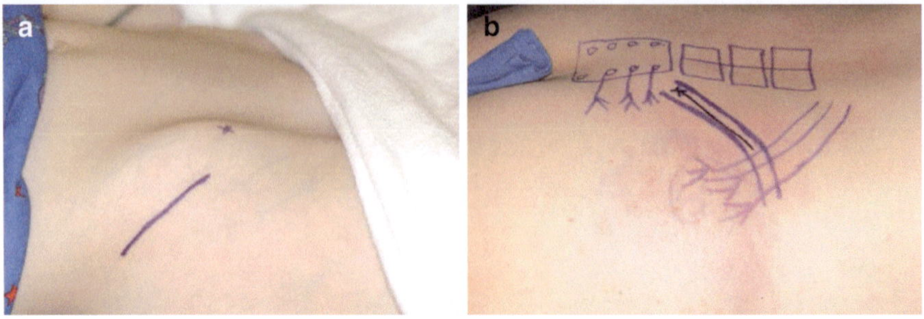

Fig. 8 (**a**) Preoperative marking for anterior iliac crest harvest and (**b**) Preoperative markings for posterior iliac crest harvest

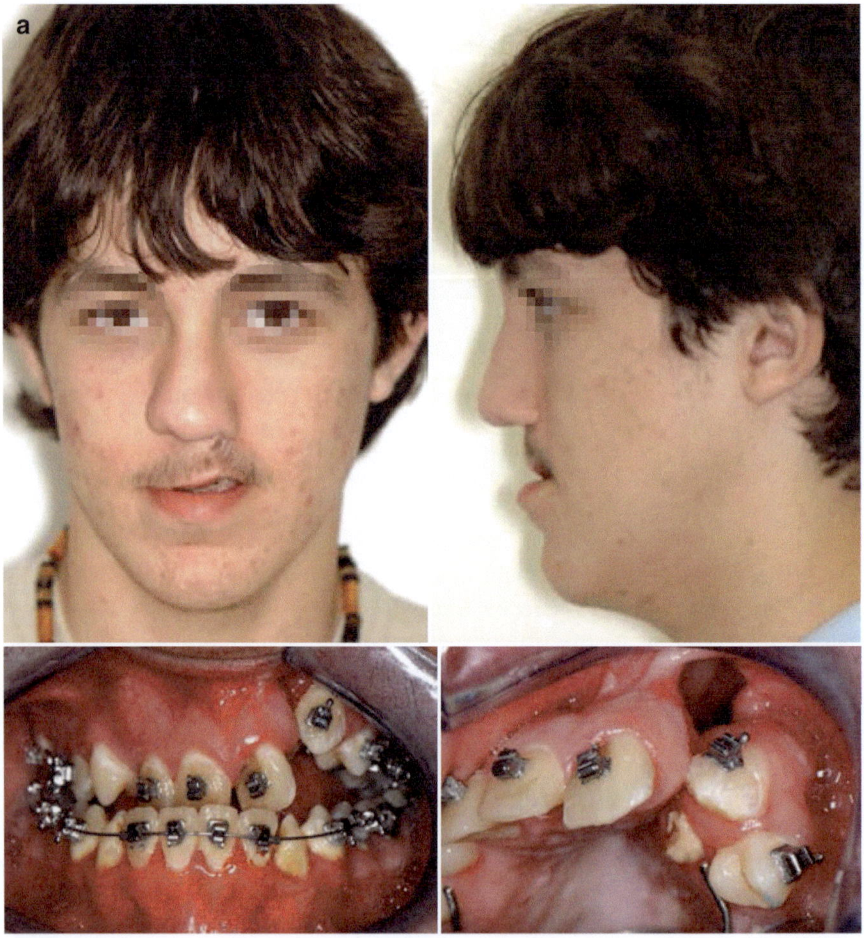

Fig. 9 15-year-old male with (**a**) ungrafted alveolar cleft, poor upper lip, and left alar support due to large oronasal fistula and (**b**) 6 months status post iliac crest bone graft to left pyriform and alveolus, along with oronasal fistula closure

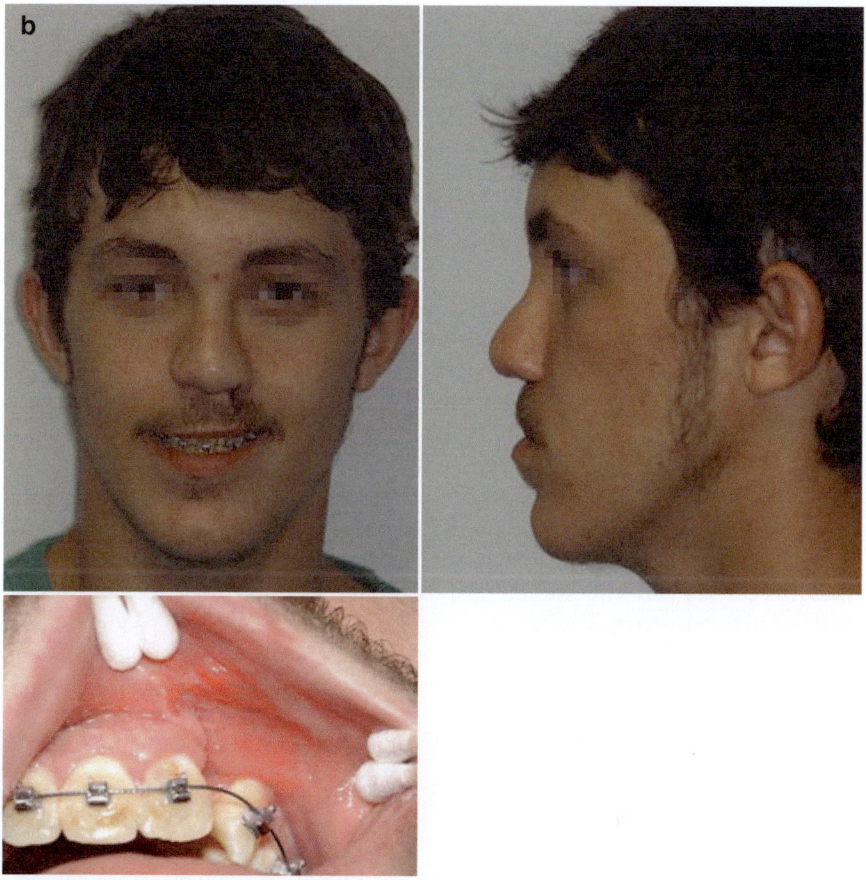

Fig. 9 (continued)

Cranial Bone Graft

Since Tessier's article in 1982, calvarium has been a common bone grafting source in craniofacial reconstruction due to the ease of access, decreased surgical time, and low morbidity [17]. It is commonly utilized during procedures already requiring a coronal incision, such as high-level Le Fort advancements, hypertelorism correction, cranial vault remodeling, and orbital, zygomatic, and/or nasal reconstructions. Cranial bone grafts can also be harvested utilizing linear incisions in the parietal-occipital region of the skull. The dense nature of the cortical bone makes it ideal for onlay grafting and reduces resorption while still allowing for rapid revascularization. The incidence of major complications is small, but some disadvantages include possibility of dural tear, contour deformities, scarring and alopecia, and minimal availability of cancellous bone [34, 35]. Cranial bone is commonly harvested as a split-thickness graft, but can be taken as a full-thickness piece through the use of a craniotomy. Full-thickness harvesting is more commonly employed during procedures already requiring a transcranial approach such as cranial vault reconstruction, monobloc advancements, and high-level Le Fort osteotomies. When acquiring split-thickness grafts, the parietal bone is the most commonly harvested location as it averages about 6 mm in thickness and can be easily harvested as a split thickness leaving the inner cortical table intact [36, 37].

Free Tissue Transfer

Free tissue transfer can be utilized for restoration of facial contours in patients with facial asymmetry. Free tissue transfer allows incorporation of skin, subcutaneous fat, fascia, muscle, and/or bone and can be tailored to the individual deformity. Advantages of vascularized flaps include maintenance of viability, decreased resorption and remodeling, and the ability to reconstruct large areas. Disadvantages include donor site morbidity, possible need for flap debulking, and technical demands. The most common free flap employed for autogenous bone grafting is the fibula free flap. It has excellent bone stock with the ability to harvest 20–26 cm of bone if necessary, allowing for multiple osteotomies to give proper contours to the graft. It can be harvested as bone only, or with a thin and pliable skin paddle to assist in soft tissue bulking. The vascular pedicle for the fibular free flap is derived from the peroneal artery and provides adequate length for midface and mandibular reconstruction [38].

Alloplastic Augmentation

Though autogenous grafting is still considered the gold standard for facial augmentation in the correction of asymmetry, numerous alloplastic materials have become popular in recent years. According to Kent and Craig [2], the two important considerations when choosing an alloplastic implant include (1) physical properties allowing adaptation to the facial skeleton and (2) biocompatibility. One advantage of alloplastic materials is that they can be created preoperatively and customized to fit a patient-specific defect, therefore reducing operative time [39]. Alloplastic implants are often an excellent choice for large deformities or complex contours where autogenous bone stock would be inefficient or unable to create a proper contour [39–42]. Through the use of computer-assisted surgery, alloplastic materials can be created to mask a lack of bone and/or soft tissue. There is also the capability to fashion these prostheses with predrilled holes for fixation, helping to reduce stress on the implant and possible fracture, along with planning for ideal screw placement accounting for the anatomy of the facial skeleton and the quality of bone stock available. Depending on the material, alloplastic implants are available in smooth and porous forms. In general, porous implants allow for some soft tissue ingrowth and prevent migration of the implant upon healing.

Silicone

Silicone has the longest and most accepted history of all alloplastic implants to date and has been placed since the 1950s [2, 43]. They are available in a wide range of preformed sizes and shapes to match areas of the facial skeleton and come in porous and nonporous varieties for augmentation. Silicone has some significant advantages to include its resistance to degradation and high biocompatibility. Silicone implants also maintain their shape during sterilization and the vulcanized form can be trimmed intraoperatively. Due to the inertness of silicone, a soft tissue capsule typically forms around the implant and soft tissue ingrowth does not occur. Unfortunately, this does allow for some mobility of the implant. It has also been reported that silicone implants cause a variable amount of bone resorption. This is more common in areas of muscle attachment and function, such as the chin. For this reason, much controversy surrounds the use of silicone implants in this region [44]. Silicone implants also have the ability to migrate and extrude without proper fixation and soft tissue coverage.

Polymethylmethacrylate

Polymethylmethacrylate is most commonly employed as a hard tissue replacement (HTR) (Biomet Microfixation, Jacksonville, FL, USA). It is a porous, polymeric composite that is non-resorbable. It is sintered with a coating consisting of polyhydroxyethylmethacrylate and calcium hydroxide. It is a rigid material with high compressive strength and a porosity that ranges from 150 to 350 μm. If necessary, the material can be trimmed by utilizing a handpiece and bur [43]. Considering the porosity resulting in soft tissue ingrowth, it has little mobility once placed and secured with screw fixation (Fig. 10).

Porous Polyethylene

Porous polyethylene is an ultrahigh-density, non-resorbable material that has characteristically good biocompatibility and tensile strength. Commercial varieties include MedPor and SynPor (Stryker Corporation, Newman, GA, USA). Pore size ranges from 125 to 250 μm [45]. This creates a thin, fibrous pocket around the implant, therefore preventing migration of the material [46]. This material is available in multiple sizes and shapes. Using prefabricated, three-dimensional stereolithic models, this material can be carved preoperatively to fit the patient-specific defect. Due to its porous nature, there is rapid soft tissue and vascular ingrowth. Some studies have shown bony ingrowth into porous polyethylene as well [45, 47]. Due to the limited potential for migration of porous polyethylene, fixation of the implant is not always necessary though recommended when possible. Porous polyethylene is commonly employed in the repair of enophthalmos, along with infraorbital rim defects [48].

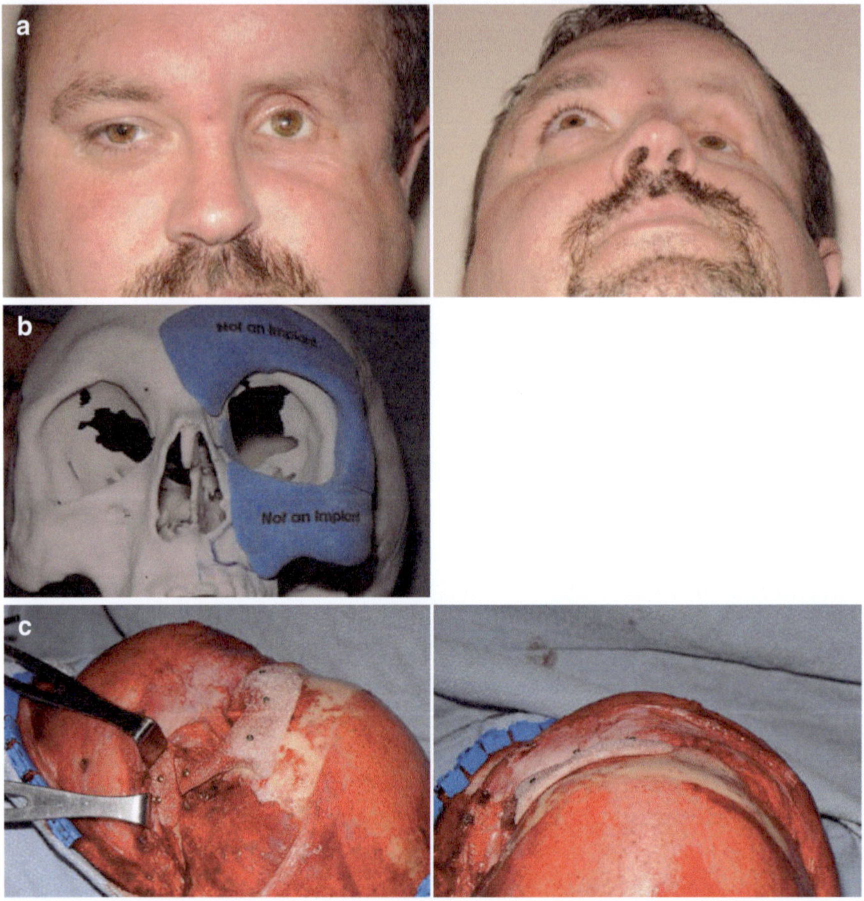

Fig. 10 Middle-aged male with significant orbital deformity due to late effects of radiation treatment. (**a**) Preoperative photographs, (**b**) model planning of two-piece custom polymethylmethacrylate implant, and (**c**) intraoperative screw fixation of the custom implant

Polyetheretherketone

Polyetheretherketone (PEEK) is a semicrystalline, polyaromatic linear polymer. It is chemically inert and resistant to chemicals and radiation and has high strength, excellent thermoplastic properties, and biocompatibility. PEEK has a longer history of success within the orthopedic and spinal surgery literature but has recently gained popularity in craniomaxillofacial reconstruction [49]. If needed, it can be trimmed intraoperatively with the use of a handpiece and bur. PEEK implants can be created with predrilled holes for fixation or titanium plates and screws can be utilized to secure the prosthesis (Fig. 11). Unfortunately, the rigidity of PEEK can make surgical placement difficult requiring either larger surgical access or reconstruction of a defect using a multipiece implant.

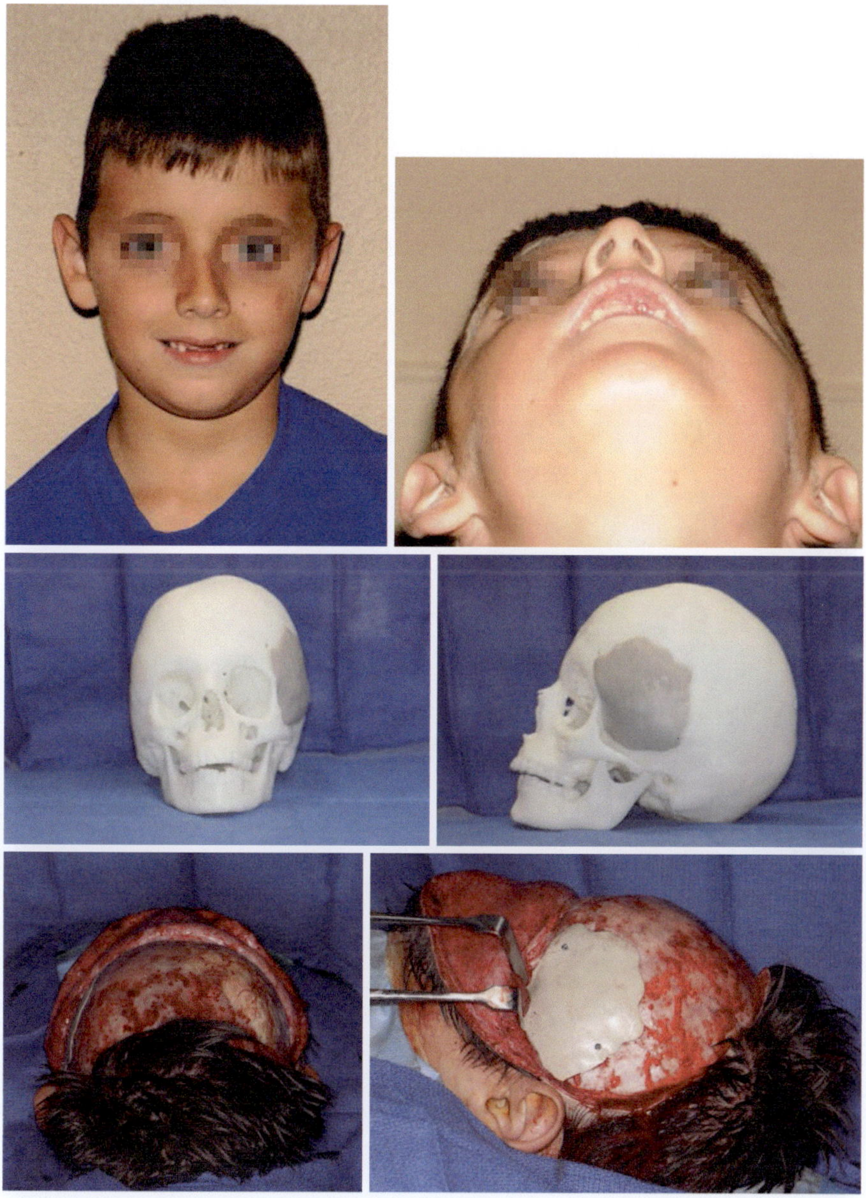

Fig. 11 This young male patient had significant cranial asymmetry involving the left temporal area. A PEEK implant was custom formed to reconstruct the defect. After insertion, the implant was stabilized in position with bone screws

Calcium Phosphate Cement

Most calcium phosphate cements, pastes, or puddies are classified as "polycrystalline" ceramics and have excellent biocompatibility. They have compressive strength similar to bone, but have lower tensile strength making them brittle [50]. The cements are often mixed intraoperatively and have a set time for application, molding, and carving prior to hardening of the material. These materials do, however, directly bond to bone and over time are incorporated into the living bone tissue, as they trigger osteoconduction (Fig. 12) [2].

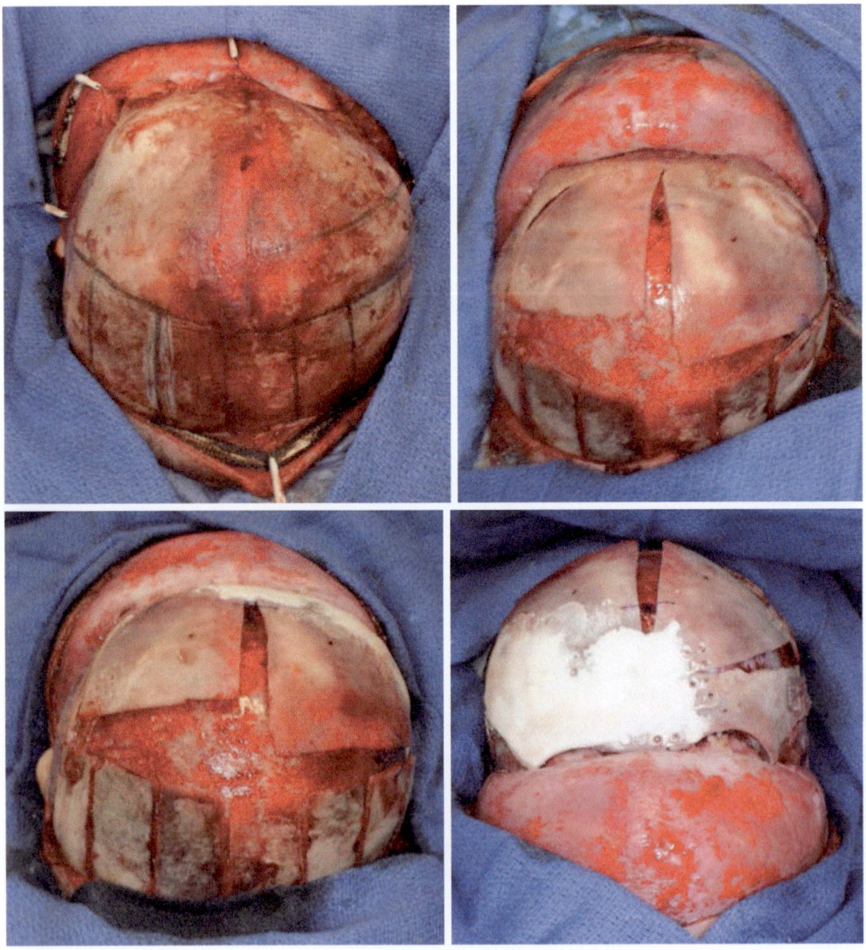

Fig. 12 Cranial vault deformity reconstructed with osteotomies, repositioning of the cranial bone segments, and large osseous defect rebuilt with calcium phosphate cement

Hydroxylapatite

Hydroxyapatite is a calcium phosphate salt and is the most prevalent mineral found in bone. The synthetic formulation (C_{10} $(PO_4)_6(OH)_2$) has been available for over three decades for maxillofacial reconstruction. It is available as a ceramic in a block form or a nonceramic paste form. The block form is difficult to carve and is not replaced with bone over time [50, 51]. It is highly biocompatible, but also possesses low tensile strength making it very brittle. This can make fixation of block grafts very difficult [51]. The nonceramic paste has been used in craniomaxillofacial defect reconstruction and is osteoconductive in nature [52]. An injectable variety, Radiesse (Radiesse, Bioform, San Mateo, CA), has been approved by the FDA and is commonly used for hard tissue augmentation of the angles, cheeks, and contour defects following osteotomies [53].

References

1. Bloomquist DS. Bone grafting in dentofacial defects. In: Bell WHP, White RP, editors. Surgical correction of dentofacial deformities, vol. II. Philadelphia, PA: W.B. Saunders Company; 1980. p. 1502–23.
2. Kent JN, Craig MA. Secondary autogenous and alloplastic reshaping procedures for facial asymmetry. (1061-3315 (Print)).
3. Sándor GKB, McGuire TP, Ylikontiola LP, Serlo WS, Pirttiniemi PM. Management of facial asymmetry. Oral Maxillofac Surg Clin. 2007;19(3):395–422. https://doi.org/10.1016/j.coms.2007.05.001.
4. Ghali GE, B. A. Nonsyndromic craniosynostosis. In: Miloro MGGELPWP, editor. Peterson's principles of oral and maxillofacial surgery, vol. 2. 3rd ed. Shelton: People's Medical Publishing House; 2012. p. 979–94.
5. Posnick JC. Anterior plagiocephaly: unilateral coronal synostosis and skull molding. In: Posnick JC, editor. Craniofacial and maxillofacial surgery in children and young adults, vol. 1. 1st ed. Philadelphia: W.B. Saunders Company; 2000a. p. 128.
6. Posnick JC. Hemifacial microsomia: evaluation and treatment. In: Posnick JC, editor. Craniofacial and maxillofacial surgery in children and young adults, vol. 1. 1st ed. Philadelphia: W.B. Saunders Company; 2000c. p. 419–45.
7. Ongkosuwito EM, van Neck Jw Fau-Wattel E, Wattel E Fau-van Adrichem LN, van Adrichem Ln Fau-Kuijpers-Jagtman AM, Kuijpers-Jagtman AM. Craniofacial morphology in unilateral hemifacial microsomia. (1532-1940 (Electronic)).
8. Ongkosuwito EM, van Vooren J, Fau-van Neck JW, van Neck Jw Fau-Wattel E, Wattel E Fau-Wolvius EB, Wolvius Eb Fau-van Adrichem LN, van Adrichem Ln Fau-Kuijpers-Jagtman AM, Kuijpers-Jagtman AM. Changes of mandibular ramal height, during growth in unilateral hemifacial microsomia patients and unaffected controls. (1878-4119 (Electronic)).
9. Rune B Fau-Selvik G, Selvik G Fau-Sarnas KV, Sarnas Kv Fau-Jacobsson S, Jacobsson S. Growth in hemifacial microsomia studied with the aid of roentgen stereophotogrammetry and metallic implants. (0009-8701 (Print)).
10. Rune B, Sarnas KV, Selvik G, et al. Roentgen stereometry with the aid of metallic implants in hemifacial microsomia. Am J Orthod. 1983;84:231.
11. Rune BSG, Sarnas KV, et al. Growth in the hemifacial microsomia studied with the aid of roentgen stereophotogrammetry and metallic implants. Cleft Palate J. 1981;18:128.
12. Parker, S. E., Mai Ct Fau-Canfield MA, Canfield Ma Fau-Rickard R, Rickard R Fau-Wang Y, Wang Y Fau-Meyer RE, Meyer Re Fau-Anderson P, Correa A, et al. Updated National Birth

Prevalence estimates for selected birth defects in the United States, 2004–2006. (1542-0760 (Electronic)).
13. Bardach J. The influence of cleft lip repair on facial growth. Cleft Palate J. 1990;27(1):76–8. https://doi.org/10.1597/1545-1569_1990_027_0076_tioclr_2.3.co_2.
14. Ross RB. Treatment variables affecting facial growth in complete unilateral cleft lip and palate. Part 3. Alveolus Repair Bone Grafting. 1987;24(1):33–44.
15. Semb G. A study of facial growth in patients with unilateral cleft lip and palate treated by the Oslo CLP team. Cleft Palate Craniofac J. 1991;28(1):1–21. https://doi.org/10.1597/1545-1569_1991_028_0001_asofgi_2.3.co_2.
16. Shaw, W. C., Dahl E, Fau-Asher-McDade C, Asher-McDade C, Fau-Brattstrom V, Brattstrom V, Fau-Mars M, Mars M, Fau-McWilliam J, McWilliam J, Fau-Molsted K, et al. A six-center international study of treatment outcome in patients with clefts of the lip and palate: Part 5. General discussion and conclusions. (1055-6656 (Print)).
17. Tessier P. Autogenous bone grafts taken from the calvarium for facial and cranial applications. Clin Plast Surg. 1982;9:531–8.
18. Wolford LM. Facial asymmetry: diagnosis and treatment considerations. In: Turvey TA, editor. Oral and maxillofacial surgery, vol. III. St. Louis: Saunders Elsevier; 2009. p. 272–315.
19. Waite PDU, S.D. Facial asymmetry. In: Miloro MGGELPWP, editor. Peterson's principles of oral and maxillofacial surgery, vol. 2. 3rd ed. Shelton: People's Medical Publishing Hous; 2012. p. 1396–410.
20. Posnick JC. Asymmetrical mandibular prognathism with and without maxillary deformity. In: Posnick JC, editor. Craniofacial and maxillofacial surgery in children and young adults, vol. 2. Philadelphia: W.B. Saunders Company; 2000b. p. 1057–80.
21. Ohno K, Fau-Michi K, Michi K, Fau-Ueno T, Ueno T. Mandibular growth following ankylosis operation in childhood. (0300-9785 (Print)).
22. Sinn DP. Total joint replacement in the pediatric patient. Paper presented at the AAOMS Annual Meeting, Las Vegas, NV; 2016.
23. Sinn DP. Pediatric TMJ total joint replacement. Paper presented at the AAOMS Annual Meeting, San Francisco, CA; 2017.
24. Mercuri LG, Swift JQ. Considerations for the use of alloplastic temporomandibular joint replacement in the growing patient. (1531-5053 (Electronic)).
25. Mercuri LG. Costochondral graft versus total alloplastic joint for temporomandibular joint reconstruction. Oral Maxillofac Surg Clin North Am. 2018;30(3):335–42. https://doi.org/10.1016/j.coms.2018.05.003.
26. Lee WY, Park YW, Kim SG. Comparison of costochondral graft and customized total joint reconstruction for treatments of temporomandibular joint replacement. (2288-8101 (Print)).
27. Cannizzaro E, Schroeder S, MuLler LM, Kellenberger CJ, Saurenmann RK. Temporomandibular joint involvement in children with juvenile idiopathic arthritis. J Rheumatol. 2011;38(3):510.
28. Ringold S, Cron RQ. The temporomandibular joint in juvenile idiopathic arthritis: frequently used and frequently arthritic. (1546-0096 (Electronic)).
29. Abramowicz, S., Kim, S., Prahalad, S., Chouinard, A. F., & Kaban, L. B. Juvenile arthritis: current concepts in terminology, etiopathogenesis, diagnosis, and management. (1399-0020 (Electronic)).
30. Granquist EJ. Treatment of the temporomandibular joint in a child with juvenile idiopathic arthritis. Oral and Maxillofac Surg Clin. 2018;30(1):97–107. https://doi.org/10.1016/j.coms.2017.08.002.
31. Cohen MM Jr. Perspectives on craniofacial asymmetry. IV. Hemi-asymmetries. (0901-5027 (Print)).
32. Moss M, Fau-Crikelair GF, Crikelair GF. Progressive facial hemiatrophy following cervical sympathectomy in the rat. (0003-9969 (Print)).
33. Tolkachjov, S. N., Patel, N. G., & Tollefson, M. M. Progressive hemifacial atrophy: a review. (1750-1172 (Electronic)).

34. Zouhary KJ. Bone graft harvesting from distant sites: concepts and techniques. Oral Maxillofac Surg Clin North Am. 2010;22(3):301–16. https://doi.org/10.1016/j.coms.2010.04.007.
35. Ruiz RL, Turvey TA, Costello BJ, Tejera TJ. Cranial bone grafts: craniomaxillofacial applications and harvesting techniques. Atlas Oral Maxillofac Surg Clin North Am. 2005;13(2):127–37. https://doi.org/10.1016/j.cxom.2005.07.002.
36. Choi HJ, De Silva RK, Tong DC, De Silva HL, Love RM, Athens J. The thickness of parietal bones in a New Zealand sample of cadaveric skulls in relation to calvarial bone graft. (1943–3875 (Print)).
37. Moreira-Gonzalez A, Papay Fe Fau-Zins JE, Zins JE. Calvarial thickness and its relation to cranial bone harvest. (1529-4242 (Electronic)).
38. Likhterov I, Roche AM, Urken ML. Contemporary osseous reconstruction of the mandible and the maxilla. Oral Maxillofac Surg Clin North Am. 2019;31(1):101–16. https://doi.org/10.1016/j.coms.2018.08.005.
39. Guevara-Rojas G, Figl M, Schicho K, Seemann R, Traxler H, Vacariu A, Watzinger F, et al. Patient-specific polyetheretherketone facial implants in a computer-aided planning workflow. J Oral Maxillofac Surg. 2014;72(9):1801–12. https://doi.org/10.1016/j.joms.2014.02.013.
40. Eufinger H, Wehmöller M, Machtens E, Heuser L, Harders A, Kruse D. Reconstruction of craniofacial bone defects with individual alloplastic implants based on CAD/CAM-manipulated CT-data. J Cranio-Maxillofac Surg. 1995;23(3):175–81. https://doi.org/10.1016/S1010-5182(05)80007-1.
41. Gerbino G, Zavattero E, Zenga F, Bianchi FA, Garzino-Demo P, Berrone S. Primary and secondary reconstruction of complex craniofacial defects using polyetheretherketone custom-made implants. J Cranio-Maxillofac Surg. 2015;43(8):1356–63. https://doi.org/10.1016/j.jcms.2015.06.043.
42. Lethaus B, Poort ter Laak M, Laeven P, Beerens M, Koper D, Poukens J, Kessler P. A treatment algorithm for patients with large skull bone defects and first results. J Cranio-Maxillofac Surg. 2011;39(6):435–40. https://doi.org/10.1016/j.jcms.2010.10.003.
43. Goldsmith D, Horowitz A, Orentlicher G. Facial skeletal augmentation using custom facial implants. Atlas Oral Maxillofac Surg Clin. 2012;20(1):119–34. https://doi.org/10.1016/j.cxom.2011.12.002.
44. Karras SC, Wolford LM. Augmentation genioplasty with hard tissue replacement implants. (0278-2391 (Print)).
45. Maas CS, Merwin Ge Fau-Wilson J, Wilson J, Fau-Frey MD, Frey Md Fau-Maves MD, Maves MD. Comparison of biomaterials for facial bone augmentation. (0886-4470 (Print)).
46. Gui L, Huang L, Zhang Z. Genioplasty and chin augmentation with medpore implants: a report of 650 cases. Aesthet Plast Surg. 2008;32(2):220–6. https://doi.org/10.1007/s00266-007-9106-6.
47. Berghaus A. Porous polyethylene in reconstructive head and neck surgery. (0003-9977 (Print)).
48. Hwang SM, Park SH, Lee JS, Kim HD, Hwang MK, Kim MW. Improvement of Infraorbital Rim contour Using Medpor. (2287–1152 (Print)).
49. Staal F, Pluijmers B, Wolvius E, Koudstaal M. Patient-specific implant for residual facial asymmetry following orthognathic surgery in unilateral craniofacial microsomia. (1943–3875 (Print)).
50. Kao ST, Scott DD. A review of bone substitutes. Oral Maxillofac Surg Clin North Am. 2007;19(4):513–21. https://doi.org/10.1016/j.coms.2007.06.002.
51. Potter JK, Malmquist M, Ellis E. Biomaterials for reconstruction of the internal orbit. Oral Maxillofac Surg Clin North Am. 2012;24(4):609–27. https://doi.org/10.1016/j.coms.2012.07.002.
52. Costantino PD, Friedman CD. Synthetic bone graft substitutes. (0030-6665 (Print)).
53. Mohamed WV, Perenack JD. Aesthetic adjuncts with orthognathic surgery. Oral Maxillofac Surg Clin. 2014;26(4):573–85. https://doi.org/10.1016/j.coms.2014.08.010.

Structured Fat Grafting for Correction of Facial Asymmetry

Eduardo Arias and Pravin K. Patel

Abstract

There are a multitude of conditions that can result in facial asymmetry. For many of these patients, the asymmetry affects multiple tissue planes from the underlying skeletal framework to the overlying soft tissue and the skin envelope. This may include patients with conditions such as hemifacial microsomia, Parry-Romberg disease, traumatic injury, and tumor resection with resultant contour deficiency and facial asymmetry. To address each of the components of facial asymmetry involves skeletal, soft tissue, and functional facial elements. The ability to restore volume and contours using soft tissue can camouflage skeletal components that may not be amenable to osseous reconstruction. This chapter will focus on fat grafting augmentation techniques to improve facial symmetry.

Keywords

Soft tissue volume deficiency · Three-dimensional surface imaging · Cone-beam computed tomography · CBCT · Virtual surgical planning · VSP · Fat graft

E. Arias · P. K. Patel (✉)
Division of Plastic, Reconstructive and Cosmetic Surgery, The University of Illinois at Chicago, The Craniofacial Center, Chicago, IL, USA
e-mail: ariase@uic.edu; pkpatel@uic.edu

P. Mehra, L. M. Wolford (eds.), *Management of Facial Asymmetry*,
https://doi.org/10.1007/978-3-030-44971-1_10

Introduction

There are a multitude of conditions that can result in facial asymmetry. For many of these patients, the asymmetry affects multiple tissue planes from the underlying skeletal framework to the overlying soft tissue and the skin envelope. In patients with congenital condition such as hemifacial microsomia and its variants, the asymmetry extends to ear microtia, mircoophthamia, and perioral lip elements. Patients with Parry-Romberg disease will present with hemifacial progressive soft tissue atrophy. Patients from traumatic injury and tumor resection will present with acquired contour deficiency and resulting facial asymmetry. Thus, the surgeon must have within his or her armamentarium a large number of procedures to be able to address each of the components of facial asymmetry involved—skeletal, soft tissue, and functional facial elements. Restoring the symmetry of skeletal framework is addressed in Chap. 11. The ability to restore volume and contours using soft tissue can camouflage skeletal components that may not be readily amenable. This chapter will focus on our approach to address the soft tissue component to improve the facial symmetry.

Objective Studies

As with all patients, careful clinical exam remains the foundation to document the regional extent of the asymmetry and the tissue planes that are involved. Only by tactile feel can the surgeon determine the depth and quality of the soft tissue involvement. The surgeon's eye can more readily determine the topography and contours of the face that are missed in the conventional two-dimensional photographic documentation because of the lack of depth perception. Today, three-dimensional surface imaging and 3D cone-beam computed tomography (CBCT) scan can objectively quantify the degree of asymmetry. Moreover, the various digital modalities (CBCT, optical dental scan, facial imaging) can be combined or fused to create a "digital" head of the patient that can be manipulated with various available software (Fig. 1).

In determining the measure of asymmetry, a critical initial step is determining the midsagittal plane. This may pose a significant challenge in patients with severe skeletal and soft tissue asymmetry. One approach is to use the basion, sella, and nasion as skeletal landmarks to establish the midsagittal plane as it is then projected onto the soft tissue, with the caveat that the cranial base is unaffected and relatively symmetric. This establishes the sagittal plane about which each half of the patient's face (the hemiface) can then be mirrored against each other. Differences in the facial topography occur when the right hemiface is mirrored on the left hemiface and similarly when the left hemiface is mirrored on the right. These regional asymmetries can then be corrected by skeletal osteotomies and repositioning, by skeletal contouring procedures, and by soft tissue procedures (Fig. 2). Currently, available

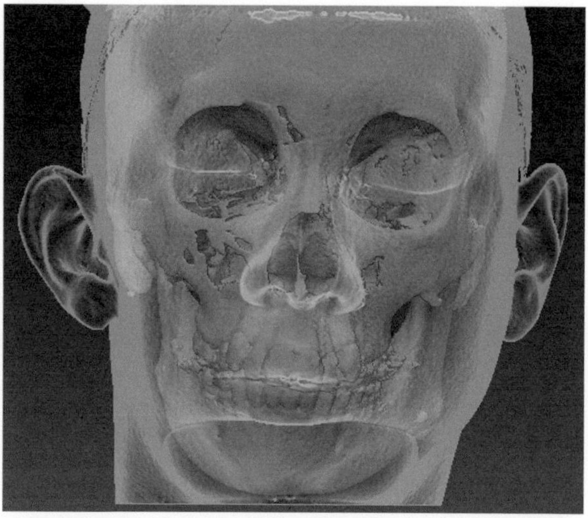

Fig. 1 Digital model of a patient with facial asymmetry with skeletal framework and overlying soft tissue envelope

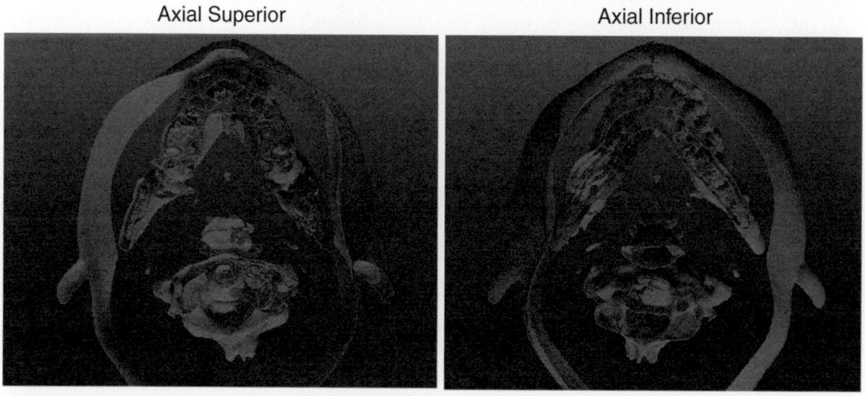

Fig. 2 Mirror image of the unaffected left hemiface onto the right hemiface. This illustrates the difference at the mandibular level. Note the difference in the bone and in the soft tissue

digital surgical planning software have greatly enhanced our ability to quantify the anatomy and optimize the operative treatment planning [1, 2].

Volumetric Soft Tissue Reconstruction

Once the regions of soft tissue volume deficiency are determined, there are two practical questions that arise: what "filler" material and how to distribute that volume to "match" the desired contour.

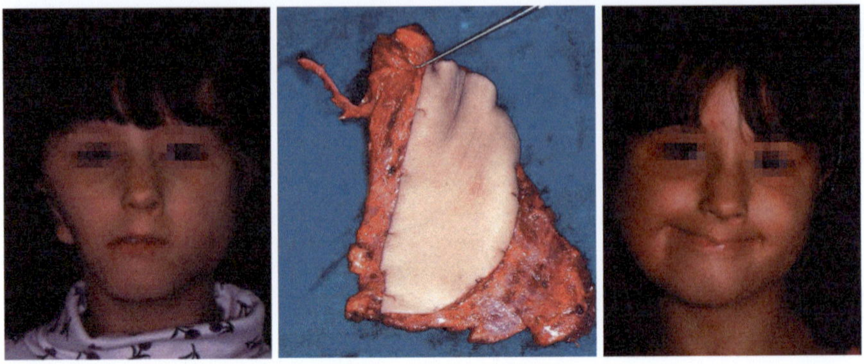

Fig. 3 Patient born with right hemifacial microsomia who previously underwent left mandibular distraction. While soft tissue reconstruction is ideally performed after skeletal maturity and orthognathic surgery, we performed a scapular free flap rather early in childhood for psychological-social reasons at school age

There is a wide variety of biologic (autologous and allograft) materials and synthetically manufactured materials that the surgeon can have access to. While the various available "fillers" and "injectables" can be used for minor asymmetry, the well-established procedures for autogenous vascularized (Fig. 3) and non-vascularized tissue transfer and fat grafting remain the cornerstone for patients with significant asymmetry.

Since the series of publications by Sydney Coleman [3] on structural fat grafting, there is increasing clinical evidence that significant asymmetry can be lessened by autogenous fat without the need for lengthy procedures that involve vascularized tissue transfer. While the clinical outcomes of autologous fat grafting generally yield good results, it varies from case to case and the assessment is qualitative. Such variations have been attributed to unpredictable graft resorption [4, 5] and the variety of techniques for fat grafting [6]. While surgeon dependent, there is a need to approach the volumetric restoration quantitatively to be able to more accurately assess the outcome against a prediction [6]. Our approach [7] is detailed as follows.

Data Acquisition

We obtain 2D photographs, 3D facial photographs (3dMD, Atlanta, GA, USA), and cone-beam computed tomography (CBCT) scans. CBCT scan data of each patient is captured for virtual surgical planning (VSP) using an iCAT scanner (Next Generation 17–19, Imaging Sciences International, Hatfield, PA, USA). The scans are captured in 17.9 s with extended field of view (23 cm diameter and 17 cm height). The voxel size measured 0.3 × 0.3 × 0.3 mm. DICOM (Digital Imaging and

Communications in Medicine) image files are imported and segmented to create STL files of patient-specific virtual models in Mimics (Mimics, Materialise, Leuven, Belgium).

Facial Landmark Selection

The STL files are imported into ZBrush (Pixologic, LA, CA, USA). In ZBrush, each virtual model of the patient's head is repositioned to the Frankfurt horizontal plane (FH) as the standard reference plane.

The soft tissue cephalometric landmarks are marked, where 11 regions are used as standard sites to define the area of interest for each patient (Fig. 4a). These cephalometric landmarks included six midline points (nasion, nasal tip, subnasale, A point of upper lip, B point of lower lip, and mentalis) and five bilateral points (zygomatic, ala, lateral commissure, mental nerve, and tragus).

Surgical Guide Design

We use the MaskPen function in ZBrush (Pixologic, LA, CA, USA). The unaffected side is highlighted and "masked" (area defined) based on the 11 cephalometric anatomical landmarks on the preoperative soft tissue surface to determine the area to be copied (Fig. 4b). The selected unaffected side of the patient's face is copied at 1.5 mm thickness (Fig. 4c) forming a shape that fits flush with the skin surface of the unaffected side. This shape was mirrored and positioned on the affected side to simulate the best aesthetics for optimal facial symmetry (Fig. 3). An image of each patient's face is constructed with the mirrored unaffected side to serve as a reference for the postoperative evaluation of facial symmetry, representing the targeted clinical outcome. The simulated postoperative mask, named "post-op," is exported as STL files for printing and 3D printed in a clear photopolymerizing resin (Formlabs, Somerville, MA, USA) (Fig. 5).

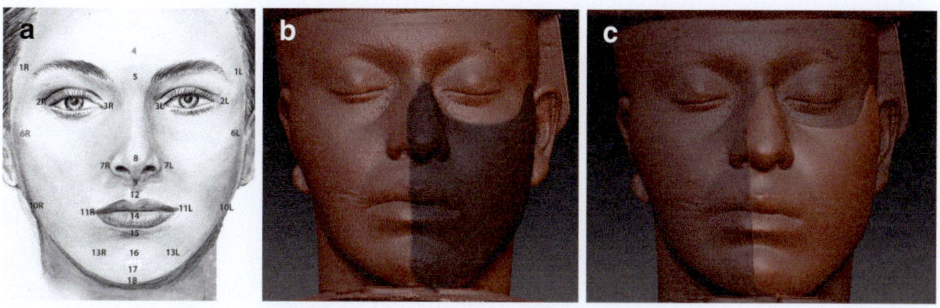

Fig. 4 (**a**) Soft tissue landmarks are defined. (**b**) The unaffected region (mask) is copied as a reference for symmetrization. (**c**) This shape is mirrored and positioned on the affected side to simulate the optimal facial symmetry

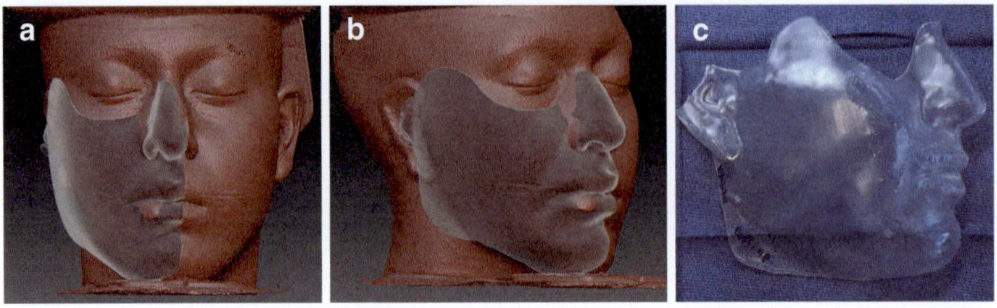

Fig. 5 (**a**) Shape mirrored and positioned on the affected side to simulate the desired facial symmetry, (**b**) Right oblique view of the desired correction. (**c**) 3D printed mask used by surgeon at the end of the procedure and during follow-up clinic visit to verify and evaluate accuracy of the fat grafting placement

Pre-op Mask Design and Volumetric Measurements

The affected side topography is analyzed for areas of interest and facial compartments that are lacking volume and symmetry. Selected areas are defined and "masked" following our described facial landmark protocol. A 1.5-mm-thick mask incorporating areas of anatomical detail that would assist with positive registration on the soft tissue surface of the affected side, i.e., the nose and lip contours, is fashioned . This affected surface mask and the mirrored simulated soft tissue are superimposed and fused together digitally. This new surgical guide with volumetric containers defining volume differences is virtually designed (ZBrush, Pixologic, LA, CA, USA) based on the specific facial compartments and locations of volume deficit to produce the virtual volumetric surgical mask (Fig. 6a).

Both the volumetric surgical guide mask and the "post-op" facial mask of the targeted surgical outcome are extended to incorporate the nose, tragus, and chin of each patient for accurate placement. The surgical guides are printed on a Form 2 (Formlabs, Somerville, MA, USA) stereolithography 3D printer with a layer thickness of 1.5 mm in clear biocompatible photopolymerizing resin (Fig. 6b). The volume deficit is marked and calculated in cubic centimeters (cc). The precise volume of the volumetric containers are verified by filling the container with water via a syringe with measurement in cc. The volumetric containers of the surgical guides allowed for precise measurement of autologous fat needed and defined the location for fat injection to restore facial symmetry.

Operative Technique

The areas and amounts of fat to be injected are based on the surgical guide with volumetric containers fabricated for each patient. The areas of fat injections are marked in the surgical field through guide perforations (Fig. 7). The patient-specific "post-op" facial mask is registered on the patient's face intraoperatively to verify appropriate fat injection volumes.

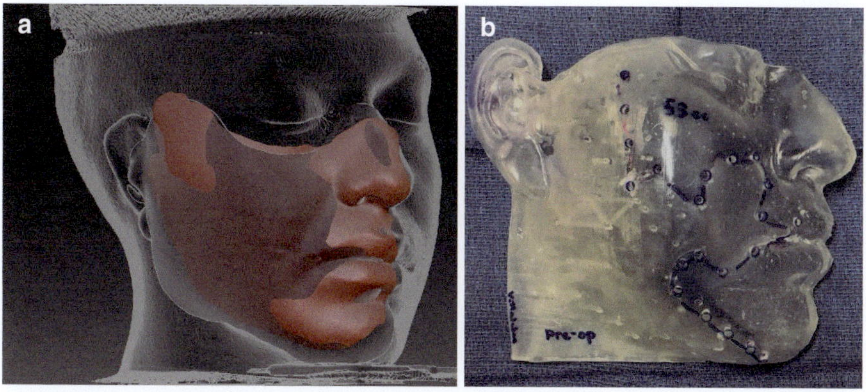

Fig. 6 (**a**) Technique used to determine the volumetric difference between the two surfaces: the initial facial deformity and the desired correction. Affected and unaffected side superimposed together to design volumetric container. (**b**) 3D printed mask that is two layers with the internal layer flush with the facial deformity and the outer layer as the planned correction. The volume between the two layers can be measured and the depth regionally measured to more accurately place the fat

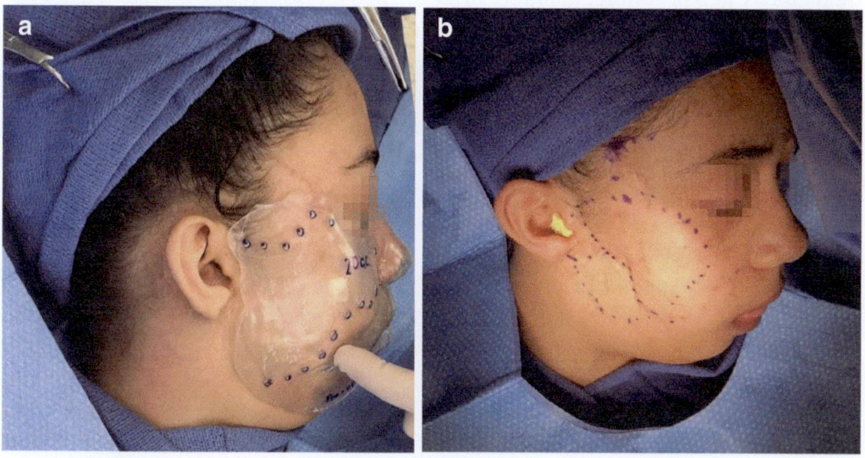

Fig. 7 Intraoperative use of the three-dimensional printed surgical guide with volumetric container. (**a**) Surgical guide seated on the affected side of the patient (**b**) Margins proposed fat grafting marked with skin marker

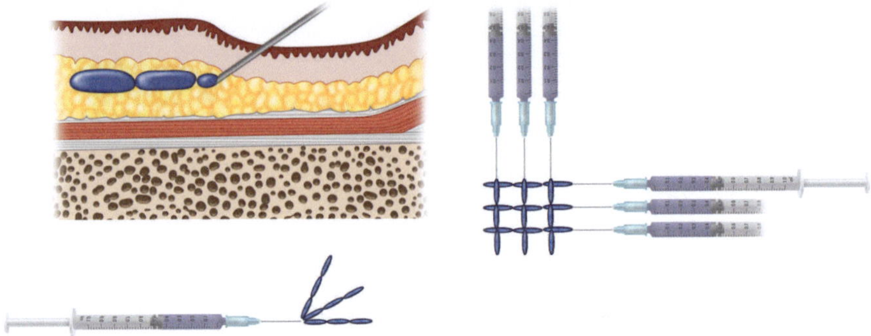

Fig. 8 This illustrates the technique of linear placement of fat droplets through various vectors to control the grafting and to optimize graft take as described by Coleman [3]

The donor site is prepared and infiltrated with a tumescent fluid. The fat is harvested using blunt tip harvesting cannula attached to 10 ml Luer-Lock syringes. With gentle negative pressure, the fat with tumescent fluid is aspirated. Once the syringes are filled, they are positioned vertically to allow gravity to separate the fat from the fluid. This is then distilled onto a telfa pad that allows absorption of the fluid and by gentle rolling, the fat is isolated. The fat is then transferred to a combination of 3 ml and 1 ml syringes for placement. The placement cannula sizes vary in the range 18–20 gauge and are blunt tip with a single hole. The fat is instilled in small aliquots as the cannula is withdrawn to allow the soft tissue to collapse around the deposit. This is done in multiple planes from multiple vectors (Fig. 8). The endpoint of placement of the fat is based on the guides.

Clinical Applications

We illustrate the soft tissue augmentation approach in the following series of patients with facial asymmetry. Figure 9 shows a patient who presented with traumatic loss of soft tissue without a skeletal component. Figure 10 illustrates a patient with right hemifacial microsomia who underwent right maxillary-mandibular distraction and required autogenous fat augmentation. Figure 11 illustrates a patient who underwent conventional skeletal surgery followed by fat augmentation because of the soft tissue deficit.

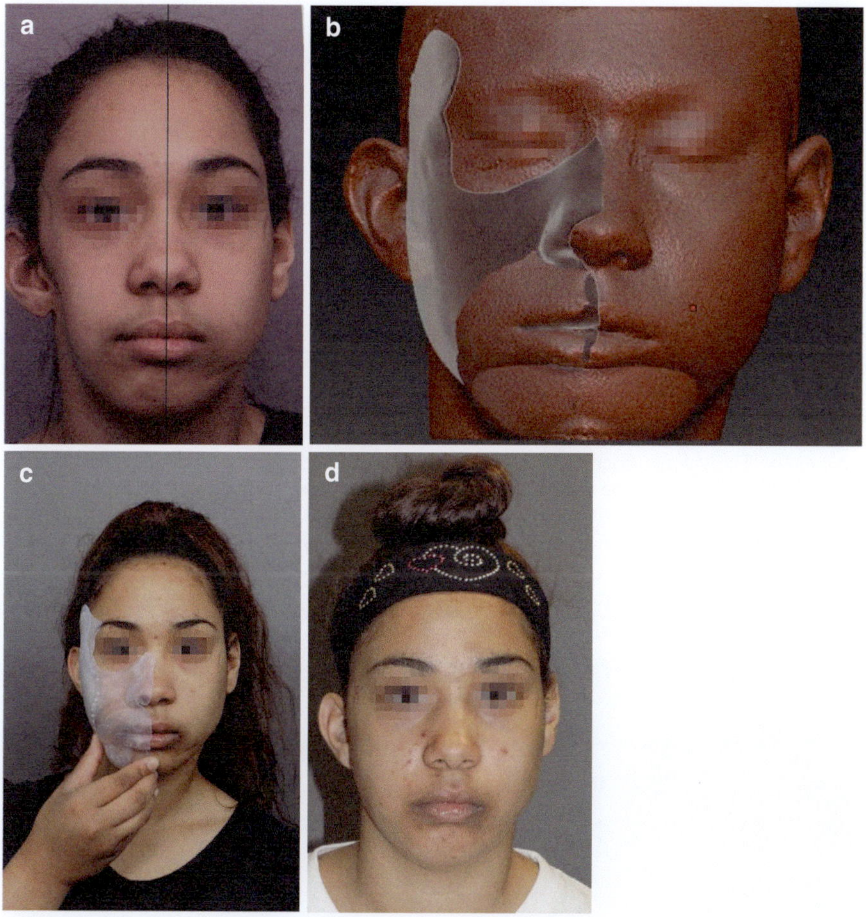

Fig. 9 (**a**) 13 years old, right post-traumatic tissue loss. (**b**) Digital design of the mask for intraoperative guidance. (**c**) Patient in clinic fitted with mask prior to the procedure. (**d**) Postoperative outcome after injection with 27 ml of autogenous fat guided by the mask

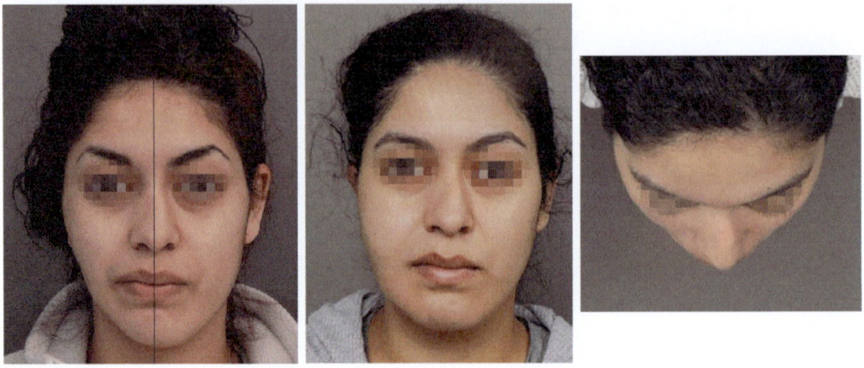

Fig. 10 Patient was born with right microtia and hemifacial microsomia, status-post right ear reconstruction and right maxillary-mandibular distraction, presented with residual right facial asymmetry. The volume discrepancy between the left and right face was 23 mL with the most pronounced asymmetry at the right latero-posterior zygoma. She was treated with surgical autologous fat grafting with the assistance of the 3D printed surgical guide with volumetric containers. The patient-specific "post-op" facial mask was successfully registered on the patient's face intraoperatively to verify target fat injection volumes

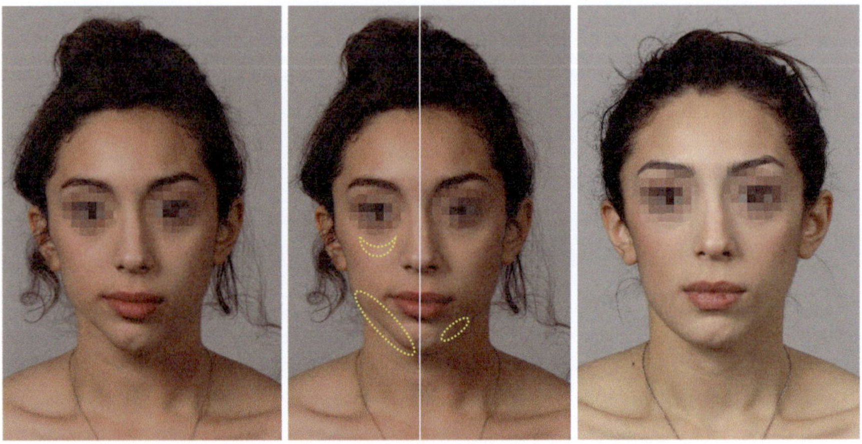

Fig. 11 This case illustrates a patient who underwent conventional skeletal surgery (skeletally based implants) with residual soft tissue asymmetry and benefited from further refinement with autogenous fat grafting

Summary

The surgeon must have ~~a~~ within his or her armamentarium a wide range of procedures to be able to address each of the components of facial asymmetry involved—skeletal, soft tissue and functional facial elements. Once the skeletal framework is corrected with conventional osteotomies and repositioning, there is often a residual asymmetry because of the "shape" of the bone itself. The skeletal shape can be addressed with custom prosthetic implants using mirror-imaging technique. However, in many circumstances, correction of the bone does not necessarily translate to facial symmetry when there is volumetric asymmetry of the soft tissue envelope. Today, the addition of soft tissue contouring with regional liposuction and fat augmentation gives the ability to the surgeon to refine the outcome at multiple tissue levels [6, 8, 9].

References

1. Zhao L, Patel PK, Cohen M. Application of virtual surgical planning with computer assisted design and manufacturing technology to cranio-maxillofacial surgery. Arch Plast Surg. 2012;39:309–16.
2. Khambay B, Ullah R. Current methods of assessing the accuracy of three-dimensional soft tissue facial predictions: technical and clinical considerations. Int J Oral Maxillofac Surg. 2015;44:132–8.
3. Coleman SR. Structural fat grafting: more than a permanent filler. Plast Reconstr Surg. 2006;118(Suppl):108S–20S.
4. Xie Y, Zheng DN, Li QF, et al. An integrated fat grafting technique for cosmetic facial contouring. J Plast Reconstr Aesthet Surg. 2010;63:270–6.
5. Gir P, Brown SA, Oni G, et al. Fat grafting: evidence-based review on autologous fat harvesting, processing, reinjection, and storage. Plast Reconstr Surg. 2012;130:249–58.
6. Guibert M, Franchi G, Ansari E, et al. Fat graft transfer in children's facial malformations: a prospective three-dimensional evaluation. J Plast Reconstr Aesthet Surg. 2013;66:799–804.
7. Arias E, Huang Y-H, Zhao L et al. Virtual surgical planning and three dimensional printed guide for soft tissue correction in facial asymmetry. J Craniofac Surg. [in press] 2019.
8. Clauser LC, Tieghi R, Galie M, et al. Structural fat grafting: facial volumetric restoration in complex reconstructive surgery. J Craniofac Surg. 2011;22:1695–701.
9. Denadai R, Raposo-Amaral CA, Buzzo CL, et al. Isolated autologous free fat grafting for management of facial contour asymmetry in a subset of growing patients with craniofacial microsomia. Ann Plast Surg. 2016;76:288–94.

Skeletal Corrections of Facial Asymmetry

Timothy A. Turvey and Caitlin B. L. McGraw

Abstract

Facial asymmetries can manifest in all thirds of the face and in all planes (sagittal, transverse, and vertical). Significant asymmetry in adolescence and adults can result in esthetic as well as functional consequences such as malocclusion, nasal airway impairment, and temporomandibular joint dysfunction (TMD). In infants and children, asymmetry may also involve the cranial base, forehead, orbits, and neurological consequences. Etiologies may include congenital or developmental deformities, trauma, overgrowth, resorption of condyles, tumors, dysplasia, etc. Comprehensive diagnoses include etiology, age of onset, involved structures (hard and soft tissues), and degree of deformity, progressive or static, etc. Using appropriate diagnostic methods including clinical, imaging, lab tests, etc. will provide a detailed diagnosis and treatment approach to provide optimal treatment outcomes. This chapter focuses on the diagnostics as well as the planning and surgical techniques to correct asymmetries of the facial skeletal structures.

Keywords

Facial asymmetry · Hyperplasia · Hypoplasia · Osteotomies · Bone grafts · Alloplastic implants

T. A. Turvey (✉)
Department of Craniofacial and Surgical Services, University of North Carolina at Chapel Hill, Chapel Hill, NC, USA
e-mail: tim_turvey@unc.edu

C. B. L. McGraw
Portland, OR, USA

P. Mehra, L. M. Wolford (eds.), *Management of Facial Asymmetry*,
https://doi.org/10.1007/978-3-030-44971-1_11

Introduction

Subtle facial asymmetry is consistent with the human phenotype. Asymmetries can manifest in all thirds of the face and in all planes (sagittal, transverse, and vertical). It is subtle asymmetry that makes the face interesting to observe and adds to attractiveness. When asymmetry is beyond subtle and it is more eye-catching, it can result in functional as well as esthetic consequences. In adolescents and adults, the most common consequences in addition to esthetics are malocclusion, nasal airway impairment, and temporomandibular joint dysfunction (TMD). In infants and children when asymmetry involves the cranial base and forehead, neurological consequences are of concern. Ophthalmological consequences are rare except in posttraumatic situations (diplopia being the most common) or congenital conditions which may lead to amblyopia or optic atrophy.

When facial asymmetry exceeds normal, patients may develop awareness of it and seek treatment. Straight face views or three-quarter views rather than profile are much more important to this population since these are the views where the expression is most obvious. Patients who experience facial asymmetry as a result of trauma, overgrowth, resorption of condyles, etc. are more likely to complain and will compare the pre-onset appearance to their current situation. Patients with congenital conditions may seek treatment but are more accepting of their situation since it is a birth defect and they lack the awareness of "the way it used to be."

Thorough recognition of every asymmetry in every third of the face is of paramount importance. Including the orthodontist and other pertinent care providers is a critically important part of diagnosing and comprehensive treatment planning. Not recognizing or underemphasizing a lesser facial asymmetry may lead to dissatisfaction when a major facial asymmetry is addressed and postsurgically the lesser asymmetry becomes more apparent.

Incidence and Etiology

According to Proffit, facial asymmetry is clinically apparent in approximately one-third of the dentofacial deformity population with the lower third of the face being most commonly involved (75% have chin asymmetry, 36% have middle face asymmetry, and 5% have upper face asymmetry) [1, 2]. For many people, the right face is larger, and when overgrowth conditions occur, the right side is usually affected. The reason for this is unknown and has nothing to do with dexterity dominance. What we know about facial asymmetry is that when it occurs in association with other growth issues of the face (sagittal or vertical problems), it is usually the other growth issues that are the chief complaint and the asymmetry is a secondary concern [1, 2]. For most patients, transverse asymmetries are more noticeable than vertical asymmetries. The malocclusion associated with facial asymmetry varies. Class I and Class III malocclusions have equal distributions of skeletal asymmetry, but class II malocclusion is less frequently associated with skeletal asymmetry for reasons unknown. It is the authors' impression that the asymmetry is present but it goes unnoticed because the chin is retropositioned. There are multiple causes of facial asymmetry and in general they are associated with either bone, soft tissue, or neural tissue innervating the area (Table 1).

Birth defects, development defects (including intrauterine and postnatal issues), trauma, pathology (including tumors both benign and malignant), cysts, dysplasias, postural issues, functional issues, etc. are all factors that may cause or at least contribute to facial asymmetry. Determining the cause of asymmetry is more than an academic exercise since identifying the cause may have therapeutic implications For instance, recognizing that torticollis may have a profound effect on head and facial development may lead to physical therapy being recommended to improve facial asymmetry when it is recognized early in life.

There is overlap with the categories of facial asymmetry as presented, and commonly the condition falls into more than one category.

Table 1 Conditions causing facial asymmetry

Developmental conditions	Congenital conditions
Tumors or cyst of the maxilla or mandible	Facial clefts
Unilateral condyle hyperplasia	Craniosynostosis
• Elongation	Multiple other syndromes and overgrowth conditions
• Hyperplasia	
Trauma	
Resorptive conditions	
• Arthritis	
• Non-arthritic (idiopathic condylar)	
Degenerative processes	
• Osteoarthritis	
• Autoimmune arthritis (rheumatoid, psoriatic)	
• Autoimmune diseases (Perry-Romberg disease)	
Pathological conditions	
• Tumors	
• Cyst	
• Neurofibromatosis	
• AV malformations	
• Dysplasias	
– Fibrous dysplasia	
– Cherubism	
• Endocrine related hypertrophy	

Recognition and Diagnosis

Careful examination of the face in natural head position is critical. To achieve natural head position, the patient should look into a mirror that is positioned 6 feet away. Orbital dystopia is much more common than realized, and positioning the head so that the interpupillary line is parallel to the floor introduces artifact and does not reflect the reality of how the patient postures themselves. Ear canals can also be on different levels and using a cephalostat head positioner with both ear rods in place may also introduce faulty recordings. Scoliosis and torticollis are other conditions that can present with facial asymmetry and can influence head posture. If scoliosis correction, torticollis correction, or orbital dystopia correction is planned, it is best to address these conditions prior to improving the facial asymmetry since their correction may affect head posture.

Each third of the face should be evaluated independently and collectively in relation to the other two-thirds. Focusing on just the area of major asymmetry and underrecognition of what may be minor degrees of asymmetry should be discouraged. Once the major asymmetry is corrected, minor asymmetries may become more apparent and become a concern.

Examining and comparing photographs (especially grade school photos) in addition the patient's or family's observation is sometimes helpful in determining the onset of resorptive or overgrowth condition. It is common to discover that a recently recognized asymmetry was present earlier in life but was less noticeable prior to the adolescent growth spurt.

Nuclear Medicine Imaging (Radionuclide Scan, SPECT Scan)

Nuclear medicine imaging including SPECT (single-proton emission computerized tomography) scans is a helpful tool in determining the metabolic activity of areas of the facial skeleton that are changing. It is important to use this technology and to interpret the results in consideration of the clinical findings. The nuclear tracers are not capable of discriminating growth from resorption; their uptake is dependent on blood flow. Technetium is the usual nuclide employed for identifying growth or lytic skeletal changes. SPECT scanning is a newer technology that allows for quantitative measuring of the uptake marker and the ability to compare one side to the other. It is not an exacting science and a 5% difference in the sides being compared is the threshold used for indicating differential uptake [3]. The author finds these scans to be much more useful for overgrowth conditions rather than for resorptive conditions.

Treatment Considerations

There are four critical elements to consider when treating facial asymmetry including:

1. Determining if the process is due to overgrowth (hyperplasia), underdevelopment (hypoplasia), or resorptive processes (arthritis, Parry–Romberg syndrome, etc.)
2. Assessing the degree of growth or resorptive activity
3. Determining if the asymmetry is secondary to an active or a quiescent process
4. Considering the age of the patient

The most common type of asymmetry treated by this author is developmental in origin. Obwegeser's contribution has improved the understanding of the condyle hyperplasias and other developmental conditions [4, 5]. Of the developmental conditions, condyle hyperplasia of the elongation variety has the greatest frequency followed by trauma. Condyle resorption can arise idiopathically or from arthritic conditions. It can also be secondary to previous surgery of the jaw. Unilateral condyle hyperplasia of the hypertrophy variety is much less frequent and true neoplasia of the condyle (osteochondroma) is even rarer. Asymmetries can arise from tumors or cysts anywhere in the maxilla, mandible, or frontal bone.

Once facial asymmetry has been thoroughly analyzed, a treatment plan must be developed. The treatment plan should be patient driven, not parent or referral source driven. Treatment plans can range from no treatment to relatively simple contouring procedures with implant placement, osteoplasty, or contour bone grafting. Complex plans involving orthodontics, orthognathic surgery, and occasionally transcranial surgery are sometimes necessary. Treating both developmental and congenital facial asymmetries can be challenging diagnostically and therapeutically. The author's experience suggests that thorough recognition of every asymmetry of every third of the face is of paramount importance from the onset.

Treatment Options

Reduction Osteoplasty

Reduction osteoplasty yields the least predictable changes in soft tissues since the procedure relies on bone removal and the soft tissue adaptation to the recontoured skeleton. Edema, hematoma, formation, and soft tissue variables such as thickness, fat content, elasticity, collagen makeup of the skin, etc. all contribute to less than predictable changes. In general, younger patients with thin soft tissues and good skin quality respond more predictably than older patients with thicker soft tissues and less elasticity. Meticulous attention to hemostasis is critically important when using this option to improve asymmetry. Hematoma formation may result in more scarring and thicker tissue. Preoperative, intraoperative, and postoperative administration of corticosteroids may help reduce the edema and improve the predictability of the procedure. Pressure dressings may also be of help.

Contouring with Bone Grafts and Alloplast

The results of contour bone grafts and alloplastic materials are more predictable than reduction osteoplasty since these add support to the overlying soft tissues and do not rely on shrinkage of soft tissue. In general, adding to the skeleton provides a more predictable change in soft tissue than removing support. The materials used for osseous contouring also matter. The decision to use alloplastic versus autogenous material must be left up to the comfort level of the surgeon. It is author's preference to use autogenous bone grafts for contour rather than alloplastic material, in most instances. Contemporary implant materials are well tolerated by the body, but bone resorption on the cortical surface where the implant is placed will occur and is most dependent on the pressure and activity of the overlying soft tissues. Bone grafts have the potential to resorb since they must re-vascularize and remodel. Cranial bone, because of its cortical density, rich Haversian system (designed for survival in a hypoxic environment), and rapid revascularization is favored for facial contouring. Furthermore, its convex contour makes it well suited for most areas of the face. Observations after thirty years of placement of these grafts indicate that they seem to maintain their integrity and support of the soft tissues. Alloplastic materials are foreign bodies and may become infected even years after placement and may require removal.

Certain areas of the face are prone to bone graft resorption and therefore the site of placement is a consideration when using implants. An example is the angle of the mandible where the masseter muscle is responsible for the contour. The symphysis of the mandible is another region where muscular activity influences the contour more than other areas of the face. In general, the muscles of mastication seem to have more influence on bone morphology than the mimic muscles. When trying to contour the angle of the mandible, alloplastic materials may have an advantage. However, for most regions of the face, autogenous bone grafts appear ideal. Free bone grafts in the chin area predictably resorb. Vascularized bone grafts will remodel but overall do well. Alloplastic implants always cause some cortical bone resorption, and for this reason and the fact that autogenous material has no foreign body reaction, the authors favor the use of autogenous material whenever possible. Consideration of the area to be augmented sometimes tempers this generalization.

Osteotomies

Osteotomies with vascular pedicles yield the most predictable results when reducing or enhancing contour. When the soft tissues remain attached and the bone segment is moved, there is closer soft tissue to hard tissue response.

When orthognathic surgery is utilized to improve facial asymmetry, the results are relatively predictable. When planning asymmetrical osteotomies, the effect of movement of the segments in all dimensions must be considered. In 1993, Bell and Erickson published on the planning of facial osteotomies describing the aeronautical terms of pitch, roll, and yaw [5]. Many surgeons were aware of the complexity of the skeletal movements but were unaware of how interdependent the movements were on different facial landmarks. For example, the effects of pitch, roll, and yaw have direct influence on chin position and these movements are major considerations when planning facial osteotomies in the presence of asymmetry. The application of computer simulated virtual surgical planning is extremely helpful in planning complex asymmetry cases because it assists in visualizing the effects of these movements on different landmarks [6, 7]. Stereolithic models of the facial skeleton are also very helpful in the planning of complex asymmetry corrections [8].

The most predictable results of altering facial asymmetry occur when osteotomies are designed to preserve as much soft tissue attachment to the segments as possible. Osteotomies with robust vascular pedicles yield the most predictable results when reducing or enhancing contour. When the soft tissues remain attached and the bone segment is moved, there is a more direct soft tissue to hard tissue response.

Age of Treatment

Another important consideration when treating facial asymmetry is the patient's age. In general, when asymmetry is treated early, there is less secondary deformity. For example, when mandibular ankylosis is untreated from early childhood, not only does the mandible lack the forward and downward growth stimulus from function, but the mandible becomes secondarily deformed because of the abnormal muscle tensions (flatness on the affected side and bowing on the unaffected side). The secondary deformities are very difficult to eliminate once they develop. Another example is anterior plagiocephaly secondary to unilateral coronal craniosynostosis. The lack of forward development of the supraorbital rim and forehead and the anterior cranial base from coronal synostosis on the affected side results in profound changes in the middle and lower facial development and shape. Orbital dystopia, nasal bridge and tip asymmetry, and cheek and mandibular asymmetry can occur in addition to the occipital deformities and contralateral overgrowth on the non-affected side in this condition. Correction of this condition early in life can reverse some of the abnormalities by creating a more favorable symmetrical growth environment. The effect of early surgery on growth must be considered and the benefits of early surgery must outweigh the potential growth alteration resulting from surgery.

When dealing with lower facial asymmetry, the decision to operate early must be weighed against the effects of early surgery on subsequent facial growth. With cranial base and vault abnormalities, surgery within the first year is usually indicated since it allows the brain (which has explosive growth the first year of life and is the primary driver of upper and middle face development) to continue to guide head and facial growth. Similarly, temporomandibular joint ankylosis release early allows function to resume and its influence on mandibular growth can favorably improve the outcome. However, the decision to operate must be tempered by the child's and parents' ability to comply with the necessary postsurgical physical therapy. Surgery introduces scarring and unless a rigorous physical therapy regimen is employed with ankylosis release, postsurgical relapse is predictable. Sometimes delaying surgery is the most prudent course of action in light of certain social or behavioral circumstances that reduce the patient's and parent's compliance. In general, a decision to proceed with surgery is prudent when the effects of surgery on growth are neutral or if it will provide a better environment for growth to occur.

Craniofacial microsomia is an example of a condition where the hypoplasia of the affected side may be interfering with the vertical maxillary development in a growing child. Early mandibular surgery to elongate the ramus provides an improved environment for the vertical development of the maxilla and midface to the extent that it may eliminate the need for maxillary surgery later in life. If orthodontic appliance therapy is felt to offer the same potential, a decision to proceed with surgery must be tempered by the orthodontic possibilities. A child who has experienced a mandibular condyle fracture early in life is yet another example. Maintaining function, projection, and symmetry of the mandible are the post-injury goals. Occasionally, these goals can be accomplished with orthodontic therapy alone, whereas sometimes early surgical intervention is indicated to prevent secondary deformities from developing.

Facial asymmetry requires careful consideration when determining the timing of surgery. One school of thought is to delay surgery until the process becomes quiescent. This makes logical sense but ignores the psychosocial aspects of the patients' life and it assumes that there is an end point to the pathology. Orthodontic appliances, school vacations, work schedules, and the patient's thoughts on the urgency/non-urgency must be weighed into the decision of when to proceed with surgery. However, if there are no pressing psychosocial issues, then the most predictable result can be obtained by delaying surgery until growth maturation.

With overgrowth conditions, such as condyle hyperplasia, removing the condyle head seems to abort the overgrowth condition and can lead to long-term stability, when done in conjunction with definitive orthodontic care and orthognathic surgery. These overgrowth conditions however can continue into the third, fourth. and even fifth decades of life. The process is not well understood and the condition is characterized by episodic, not constant, growth. What triggers the overgrowth is unknown. Similarly, what causes the condition to become quiescent is unknown. What is known is that the condition may become active again after a period of quiescence. Removing the condyle head appears to be protective and seems to lead to long-term stability [5, 9–11].

Case Reports

Case 1

A 20-year-old man complained of anterior open bite, facial asymmetry, masticatory problems, speech issues, and TMD symptoms consisting of popping, clicking, and pain. The patient felt that his mandibular asymmetry was worsening with time.

The original facial evaluation revealed elongation of the face, lip incompetency, vertical maxillary excess, maxillary deficiency, and retrogenia. Class III asymmetrical malocclusion with open bite and anterior and lateral cross bites was also noted. The pre-surgical orthodontic plan included the removal of four premolars with complete leveling of the mandibular arch and segmental mechanics in the maxilla to facilitate leveling and transverse correction by surgery. The interdental osteotomies in the maxilla were planned between the cuspids and premolars bilaterally.

When the patient returned for pre-surgical evaluation, the open bite worsened as did the anterior and lateral cross bites consistent with removal of dental compensations. (Fig. 1a–f). The face height increased slightly and consistent with bite opening. The patient's and surgeon's impression was that the lower facial asymmetry worsened over this 1-year pre-surgical orthodontic phase. Tracking maxillary mandibular midline discrepancies is not accurate for monitoring skeletal change since teeth are moving with orthodontic preparation.

A SPECT scan revealed increased uptake (beyond the 5% threshold) in the right condylar head consistent with overgrowth (Fig. 1g). The panoramic radiograph demonstrated a normal appearing condyle with elongation of the condylar neck on the right. The mandibular midline was shifted to the left of the maxillary midline which was centered with the facial midline. A cross bite on the left was also noted. The range of mandibular movements was normal.

When the surgery was performed, a three-piece segmental maxillary osteotomy with superior repositioning of the posterior segments independent of the anterior segment and maintenance of the maxillary midline was achieved. Maxillary advancement and leveling of the cant were also corrected by elevation of the right posterior maxilla more than the left. Bilateral sagittal osteotomies of the mandibular ramus, a condylectomy, and an asymmetrical genioplasty were simultaneously performed. The planning was done virtually and an interim and final splint were printed (Fig. 1h).

The surgery was conducted transorally except for the condylectomy. This was performed with a temporally extended tragal incision along the crest of the tragus. A nerve stimulator is always used to avoid injury to the facial nerve. This approach exposes the posterior lateral condyle and facilitates the condylectomy. The condylar head (approx. 8 mm) was excised and the proximal segment of the sagittal osteotomy was rotated posteriorly and superiorly into the glenoid fossa. The surgery was performed with preservation of the meniscus, and when the stump was positioned into the fossa, it was not secured with force. Positional screws were used to fixate the proximal and distal segments placed transorally (Fig. 1i). When performing the condylectomy, subperiosteal dissection around the entire condyle and neck is critically important to avoid injury to the internal maxillary artery.

Plates and screws were used to secure all maxillary and mandibular segments. No wire inter-maxillary fixation was employed post-surgery but a splint wired to the maxilla and guiding elastics were used. The patient was encouraged to move the jaw immediately following surgery. Physical therapy was begun after 2 weeks and consisted of opening and closing, lateral excursive and protrusive exercises. Chewing was discouraged as was forceful stretching for the first 6 weeks.

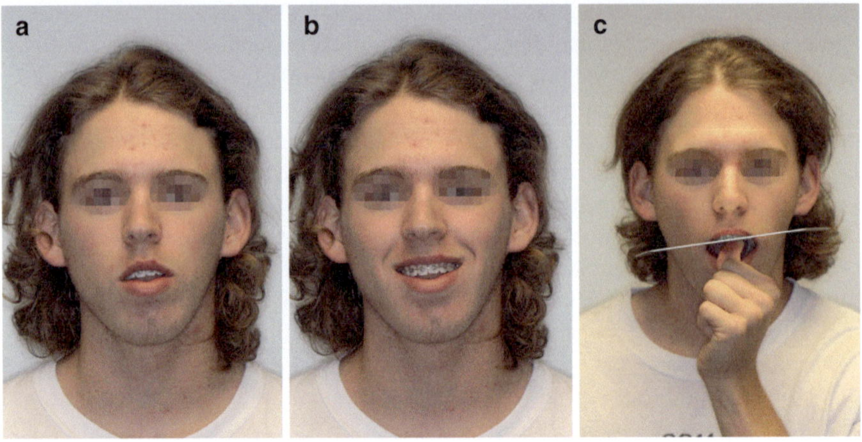

Fig. 1 Case 1. Unilateral condylar hyperplasia hemi-elongation variety. (**a** and **b**) Preoperative full-face view demonstrating lip incompetency, elongation of the lower face, and mandibular asymmetry with deviation of the chin to the left. During animation, the cant of the maxilla becomes more apparent with the right side down. Note that the maxillary incisor midlines is coincident with the facial midline. (**c**) With the Fox plane in place, the cant of the maxilla is obvious with the right lower. (**d** and **e**) The profile views confirm elongation of the lower facial third, adequate nasolabial support, and retrogenia. (**f**) The occlusion is class III with an anterior open bite. Segmental orthodontic mechanics in the maxilla has leveled and aligned the three maxillary segments independently. Four premolars have been removed (one in each quadrant) to facilitate arch alignment and to leave adequate space between the maxillary cuspid and premolar to facilitate the interdental osteotomies in the maxilla. The extraction spaces in the mandible have been closed and the arch has been aligned and leveled. (**g**) The preoperative radiographs. Notice that the maxillary extraction spaces have been closed but the maxillary cuspid-premolar interspace has the roots divergent to facilitate the interdental osteotomies for the three-piece LeFort I. In the mandibular arch, the extraction spaces have been closed entirely and the arch has been leveled and aligned entirely. (**h**) The surgery was planned virtually. Notice the leveling of the maxilla has been done in three pieces, and the bite has been closed by superior repositioning of the entire maxilla with posterior segments moving higher than the anterior and with the left posterior maxilla raising more than the right. The mandible was mobilized via sagittal osteotomies bilaterally with the left side advancing and shifting to center the midline. Notice the interference between the proximal and distal segments of the left sagittal osteotomy (gray overlapping the blue). This requires reduction of the proximal portion of the distal segment to permit the segments to meet flush. A condylectomy was also performed on the right with immediate reconstruction by moving the condyle stump into the fossa. The chin has also been advanced to achieve a 1:1 Holdaway ratio. (**i**) Postoperative radiographs demonstrating plates and screws used to secure the maxillary segments. Screws alone have been used to stabilize the mandible. A high condylectomy was performed on the right and the condyle stump was positioned superiorly and secured in the fossa with screw fixation. (**j** and **k**) One-year postoperative full-face photos demonstrating the improved facial harmony and symmetry. Notice lip competency and the shorter face with better lip and chin relationships. (**l** and **m**) One-year postoperative profile views demonstrating improved balance and projection of the chin, lips, and nose. Slight elevation of the nasal tip has been complimentary. (**n**) One-year postoperative occlusion with bite closure, coincident midlines, class I cuspid and molar relationship, and absence of cross bite. (**o**) Composite CT scans demonstrating the preoperative condition (left) and the right condylectomy with immediate construction (middle). The right image documents the reformation of a cortical cap on the right condyle and good remodeling. This occurs by functional adaption (restoring normal range of mandibular movement)

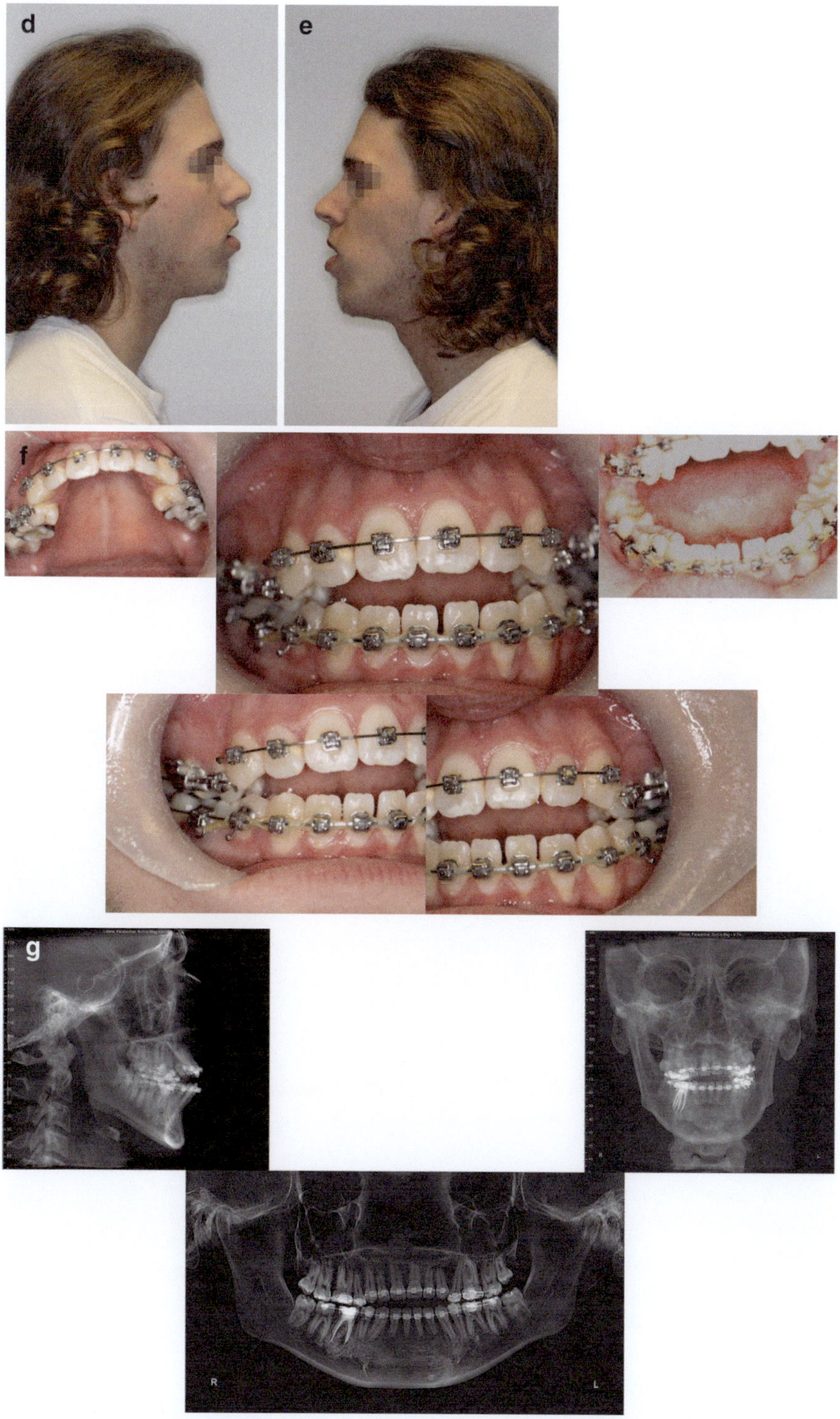

Fig. 1 (continued)

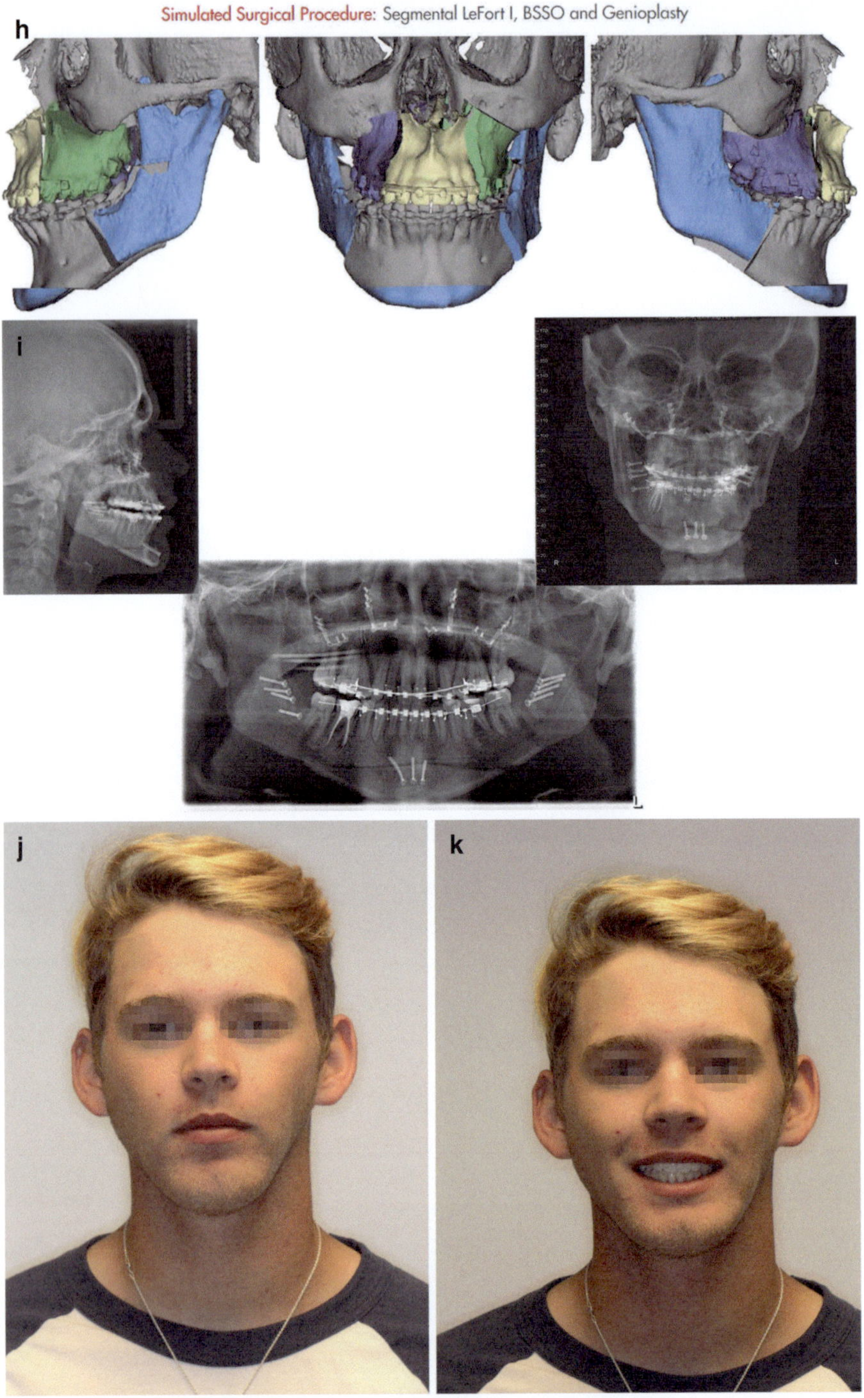

Fig. 1 (continued)

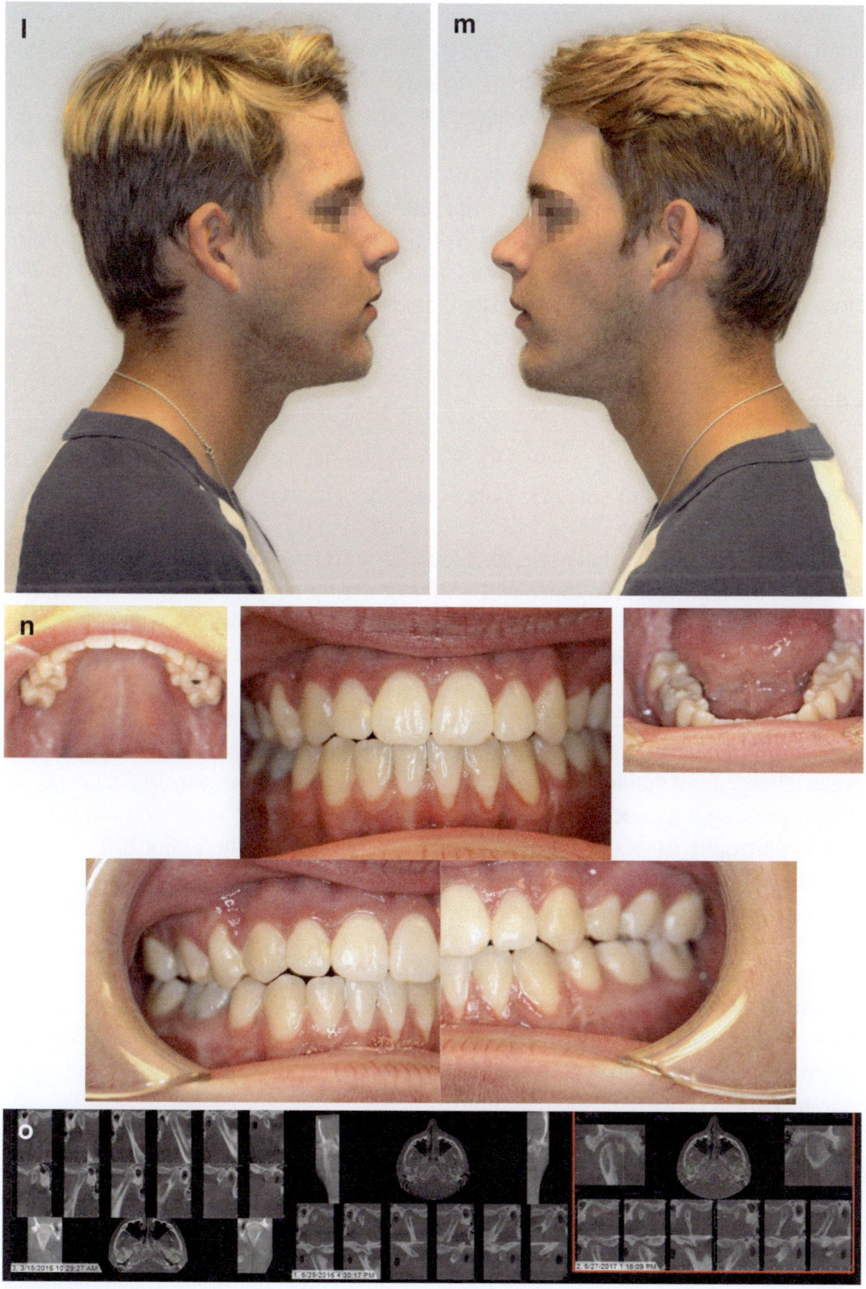

Fig. 1 (continued)

When a high condylectomy is performed, the lateral pterygoid muscle attachment must be removed from the condylar head that is removed. Occasionally, this results in restricted lateral movement to the side opposite the condylectomy, and the jaw may also deviate on protrusion to the side of the condylectomy. Patients are instructed to practice in front of a mirror to regain symmetrical movements. With time and practice, this is often achievable.

One year following surgery, the improvement of the symmetry, projection, and balance of the face can be observed (Fig. 1j, k). The bite is closed and the maxilla has been leveled (Fig. 1l). A remodeled condylar head can be observed with regeneration of a cortical cap (Fig. 1m). There are no TMD symptoms or pain.

Case 2

A 26-year-old woman was referred by her orthodontist because of concerns of facial asymmetry. The patient was also concerned about dental esthetics and increasing TMD symptoms.

The facial exam revealed noticeable facial asymmetry with the left exceeding the length of the right. At rest, there was a cant of the lip commissures; during animation, a cant of the occlusal plane with the left more inferior was noted. The maxillary and mandibular midlines were off slightly and the cuspid and molar relationships were Class I. Cross bite was not present (Fig. 2a–e).

The radiographs confirmed unilateral condyle hyperplasia of the hypertrophy variety. The author prefers the term hypertrophy since this is more consistent with organ enlargement and hyperplasia is more consistent with the histological description of increased numbers of cells. This condition is not the same etiologically as hemihypertrophy associated with endocrine disturbances. The major difference is the lack of endocrinopathy in this condition. This condition's etiology, as are all unilateral condyle hyperplasias, is unknown. The hypertrophy variety is distinct from the elongation variety in a number of ways. The overgrowth is always vertical and hardly ever does it result in a cross bite. In this condition, the dental midlines are almost always coincident but sometimes, the mandibular dental midline can be to the affected side as seen in this patient. Occasionally, there is a posterior open bite which suggests rapid growth to the extent that the maxilla could not keep up with the vertical overgrowth of the mandible.

Radiographically, the mandible is always larger on the affected side. The condyle head, neck, ramus, body, and a portion of the symphysis are always three dimensionally enlarged. Unlike endocrinopathy-related hypertrophy, the teeth are of normal size. The inferior alveolar neurovascular bundle is always displaced inferiorly in this condition and the antigonial notch is flattened (Fig. 2f).

Palpation of the inferior border of the mandible in the symphyseal region usually reveals a distinct step where the condition joins the opposite, non-affected side.

The author's experience suggests that the non-affected side is always vertically shorter than expected. This has been confirmed with anthropometric and cephalometric measurements in a series of affected individuals. The author routinely

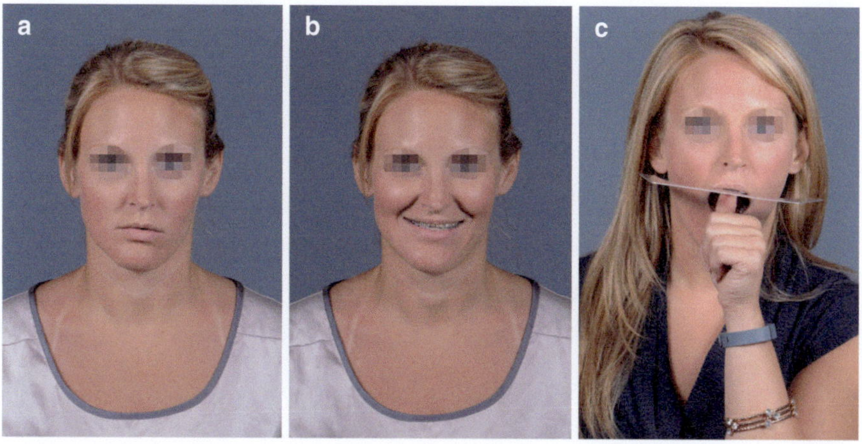

Fig. 2 Case 2. Unilateral condylar hyperplasia-hypertrophy variety. (**a** and **b**) Full-face view demonstrating elongation of the left face and shortness of the right. The midline of the chin is coincident with the facial midline. The lip and commissures are canted with the left inferior (2). With the Fox plane in place, the cant is confirmed. (**d** and **e**) The profile views are different with shortness and more prominence of the right ramus and body of the mandible. (**f**) The occlusion is class I with near coincident maxillary and mandibular dental midlines (The mandibular midline is slightly to the left which is not unusual with this condition). Notice the left posterior open bite suggesting vertical growth of the mandible beyond the compensatory growth of the maxilla. Four premolars were removed for orthodontic purposes and the spaces have been closed and the arches aligned and leveled. (**g**) The radiographs are highly consistent with unilateral condyle hyperplasia of the hypertrophy variety. Notice the enlargement of the entire left mandible and vertical displacement of the angle with absence of an antigonial notch. The lateral cephalometric radiograph demonstrated the left and right inferior mandibular border differences. Notice also the inferior displacement of the neurovascular canal. (**h**) Mirror imaging of the left and right face. The middle photo is the patients presenting deformity. The left photo is a mirror image of the right face (too short). The right photo is a mirror image of the left face (too long). The authors find mirror imaging helpful in determining whether to shorten or lengthen the face. In this situation, a decision was made to lengthen the right face and shorten the left. (**i**) The virtual image planning demonstrating the LeFort I downgrafting on the right maxilla and shortening of the left maxilla as well as the inverted L osteotomy defect in the right mandibular ramus and right symphysis and body area of the mandible. Notice the interim splint constructed to reflect maxillary surgery completed before mandibular surgery. (**j**) Eighteen-month postsurgical radiographs demonstrating elongation of the right face and shortening of the left face via LeFort I osteotomy, an inverted L osteotomy of the mandible on the right, sagittal osteotomy on the left, a condylectomy on the left, and asymmetrical genioplasty with elongation on the right and shortening on the left. Split-thickness cranial bone grafts were inserted into all osteotomy defects. Notice that the left condyle stump was positioned superiorly into the glenoid fossa. (**k**) Eighteen-month postsurgical CT scan demonstrating regeneration of the left condyle head with a cortical cap. (**k** and **l**) Eighteen-month postsurgical photos demonstrating the improvement of facial symmetry, the absence of a canted maxilla, and leveled lip commissures. (**m** and **n**) One-year postsurgical profile views. Notice the minimal evidence of the right neck scar and left temporotragal scar. (**o**) Postsurgical occlusion with closure of the left posterior bite. Notice the fixed gingival graft placed pre-surgically to protect the crestal gingival height of the mandibular anterior teeth

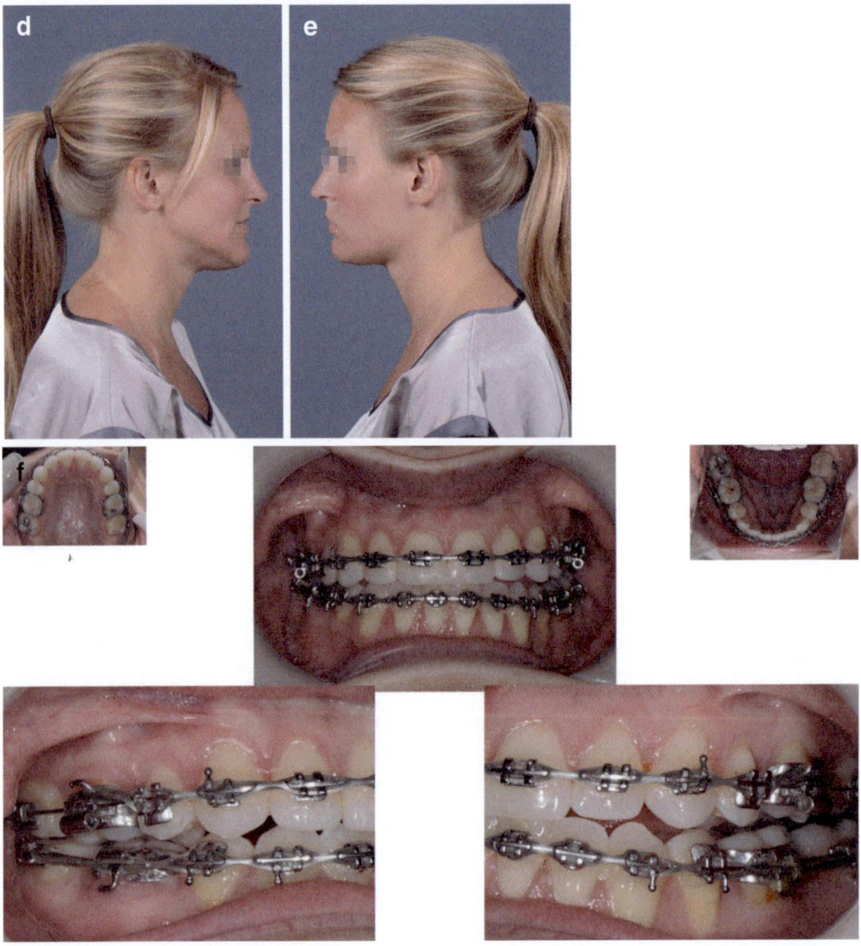

Fig. 2 (continued)

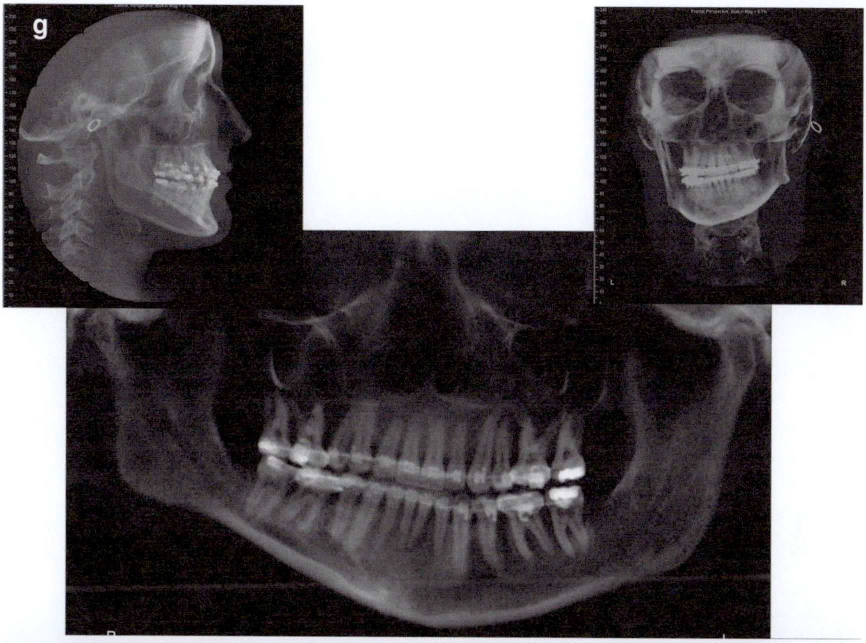

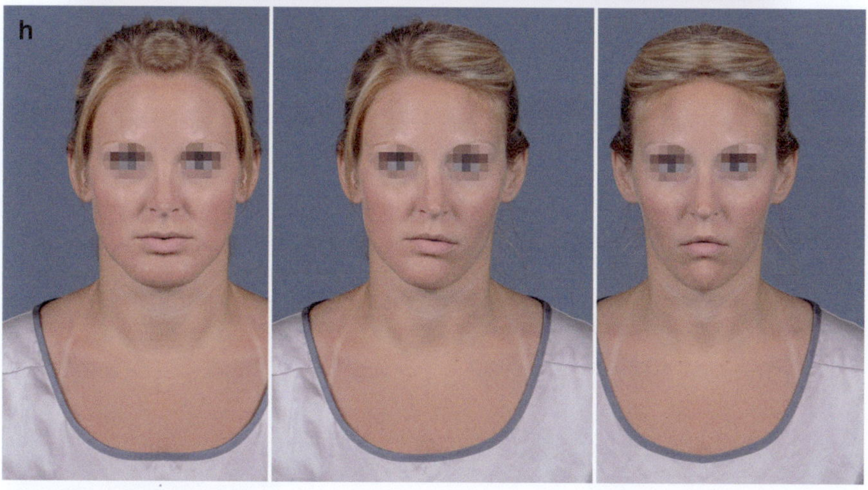

Fig. 2 (continued)

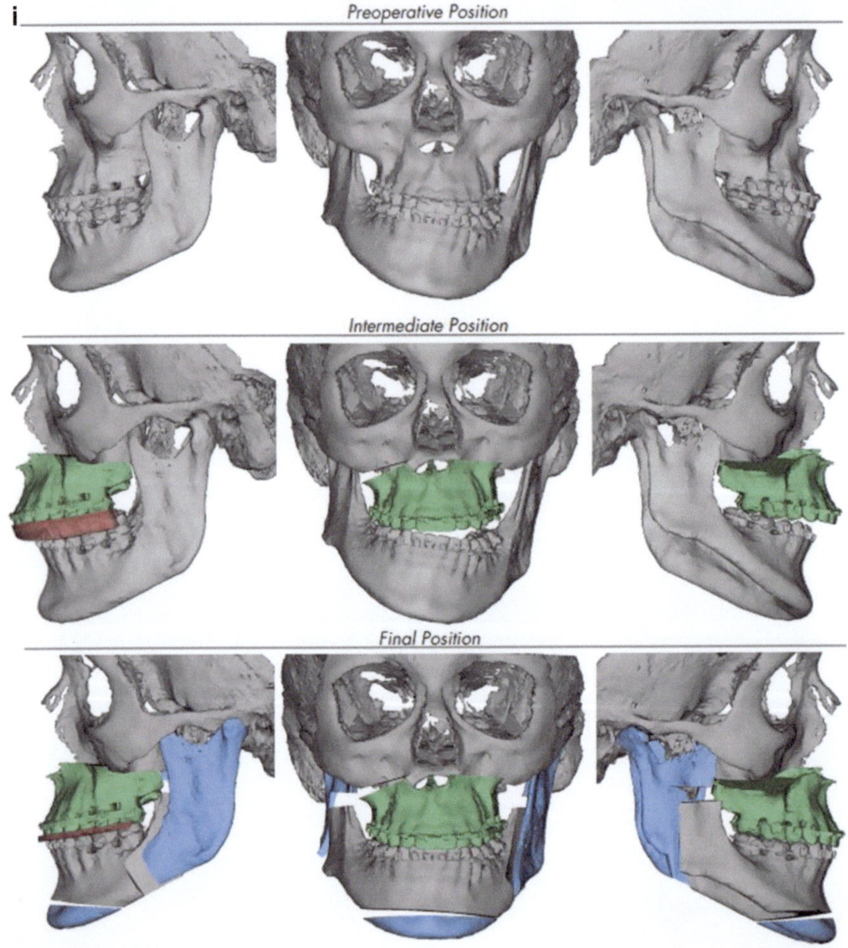

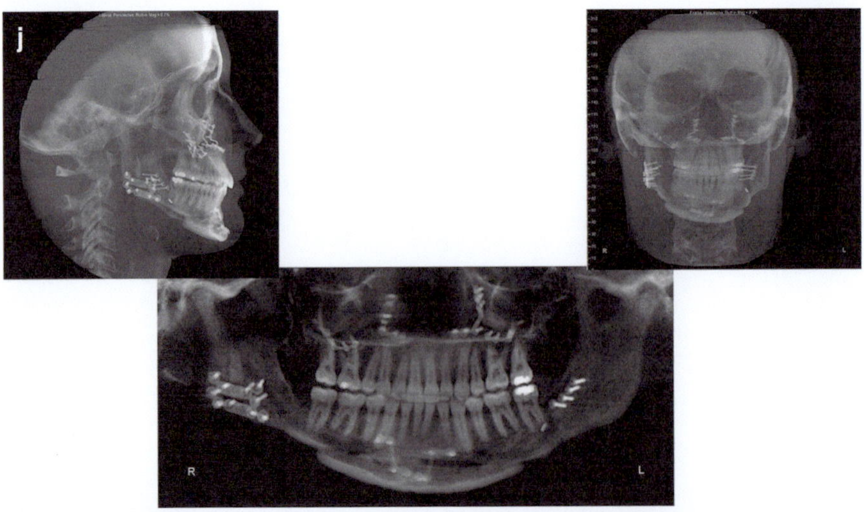

Fig. 2 (continued)

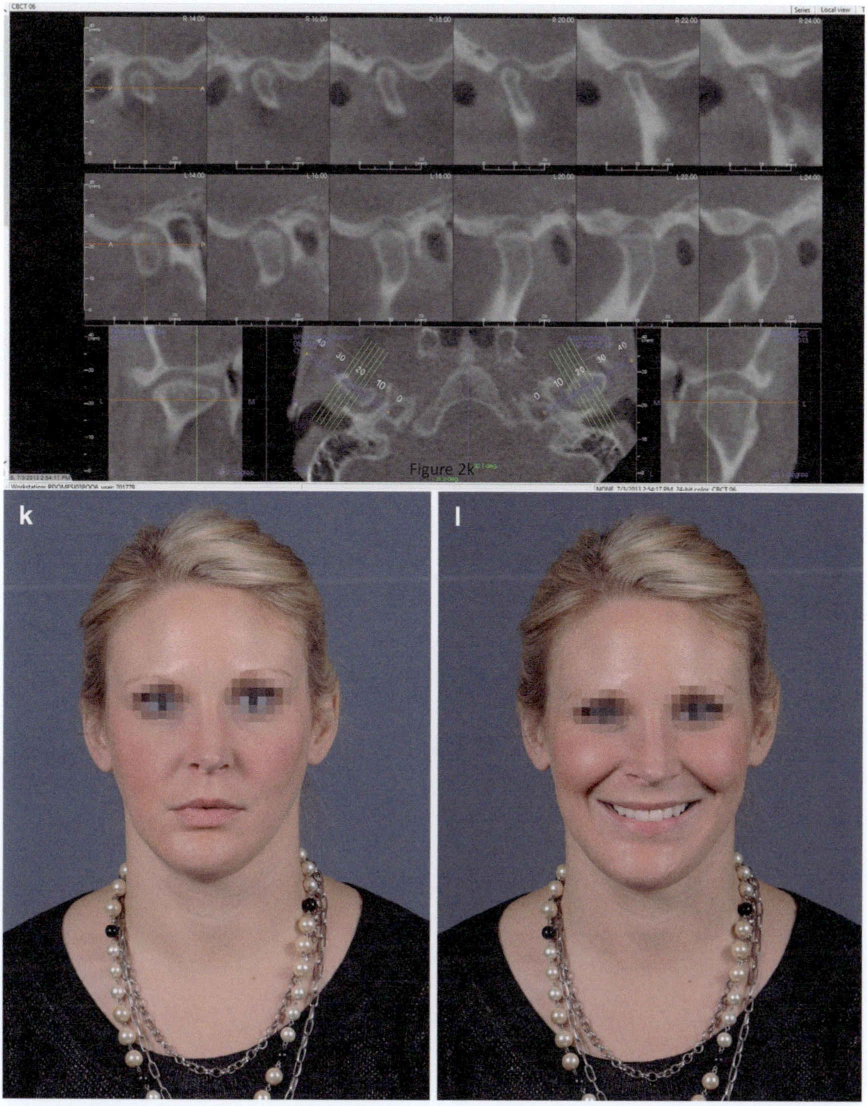

Fig. 2 (continued)

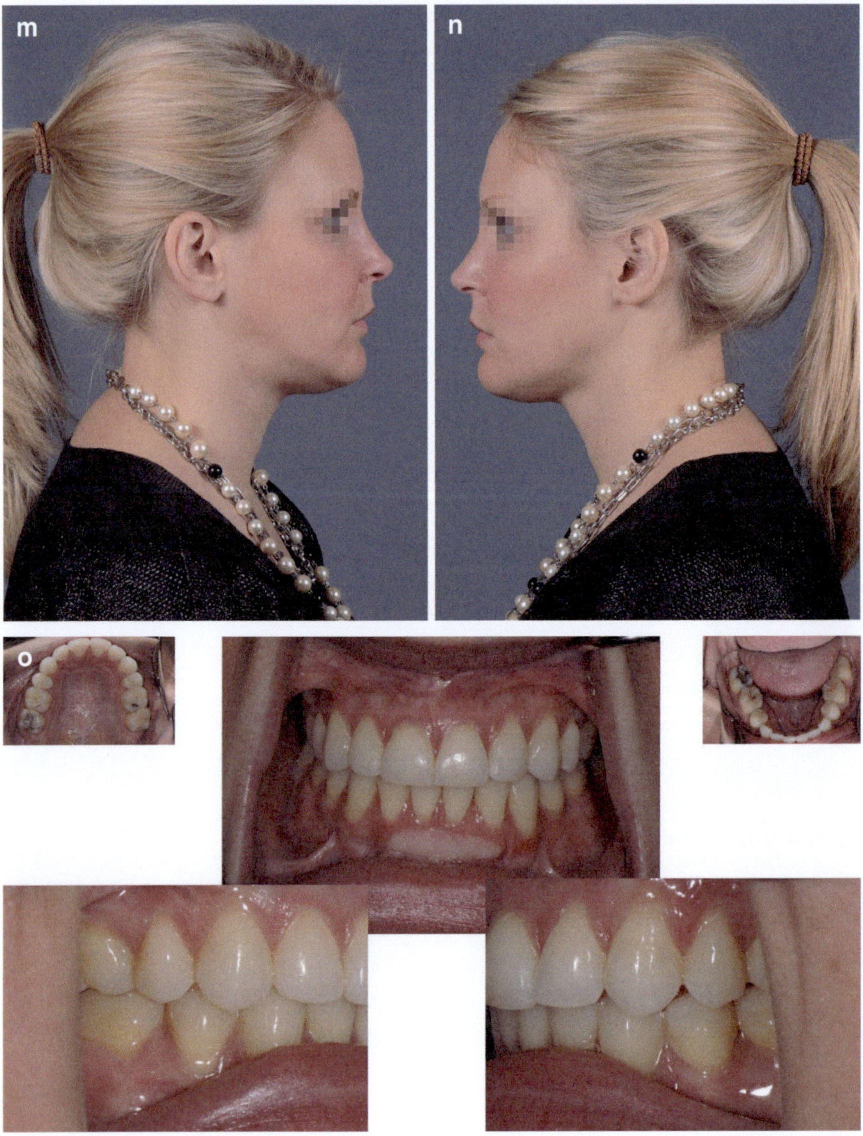

Fig. 2 (continued)

employs photographic mirror imaging to help determine if the long side requires shortening or if the short side requires lengthening (Fig. 2g). Invariably, almost always lengthening of the short side and shortening of the long side is required and a genioplasty is almost always employed as well to lengthen the short side, shorten the long side, and maintain the chin in the midline.

The surgery to address this condition is very complex and requires three-dimensional conceptualization and a clear understanding of the effect of altering pitch, roll, and yaw. The maxilla, mandible, and chin must be mobilized; and if the condyle remains actively growing, a condylectomy is also performed with simultaneous reconstruction. The SPECT scan confirmed active condylar head growth on the left.

This patient's treatment plan was conducted virtually (Fig. 2h). The alternative requires carefully executed model surgery on a semi-adjustable articulator with a face bow transfer. Stereolithic model surgery is an excellent way of helping understand the complexities of the skeletal movements and their effect on the midline.

Elongation of the short side is much more difficult than shortening. The maxilla is usually mobilized and repositioned first in the sequence of surgery. The maxilla must be stabilized with plates and screws and bone grafts should be used to encourage healing. The author prefers the use of an inverted L osteotomy conducted via a neck incision for the mandibular elongation. Using a neck incision allows for complete release of the pterygomasseteric sling, displacement of the body of the mandible inferiorly, and the use of bone plates, screws, and bone grafts to stabilize the complex. Although there will always be remodeling of the angle (pterygomasseteric activity), the increase in mandibular body height anterior to the angle remains long term. The neck scar is designed to blend with the natural skin lines.

When the condylectomy is performed, the segment removed is approximately 8 mm of the head. This is approached through a temporal tragal erect skin incision which provides clear access to the lateral pole of the condylar head. The stump of the remaining neck of the condyle is positioned superiorly against the meniscus which remains in the glenoid fossa. Repositioning this segment is done through the intraoral sagittal osteotomy incision with a periosteal elevator rotating the segment superiorly. Once the sagittal osteotomy is completed and the tooth bearing segment is wired in the correct maxillomandibular relationship, the proximal segment is guided posteriorly and superiorly through the transoral sagittal osteotomy incision. A finger is inserted through the temporal tragal incision to palpate the condylar stump and to guide it into the fossa. The condylar stump should not be forced against the skull base but it must be seated in the fossa and secured with screws and/or plates as would be done with any sagittal osteotomy.

Adding to the complexity of the surgery is the concern of sterility of the surgical fields. It is impossible to perform this surgery without cross contamination of the intraoral and extraoral wounds. All patients are administered antibiotics (cephalosporin or clindamycin if penicillin allergic) and very generous irrigation before wound closure. Steroids are also administered to help control the swelling.

In general, the unilateral sagittal osteotomy is performed first, (but not split) followed by the completion of the maxillary surgery and stabilization with bone plates, screws, and interpositional bone grafts. The condylectomy and inverted L osteotomies are next completed after glove change and this is done using skin incisions. Once the inverted L osteotomy of the mandible is completed, the wound is packed and the intraoral sagittal osteotomy is completed. Intermaxillary fixation is established with wires. The proximal segment is positioned as described above. The inverted L osteotomy is next stabilized through the neck wound using plates and screws and bone grafts inserted into the defects. The intraoral wounds are then closed entirely, gloves are changed, and the skin wounds are then closed after through irrigation. To date, the author has had minimal problems with infection and no long-term infection morbidity using this sequence and approach.

Postsurgical radiographs demonstrate that all osteotomies are well secured with plate and screw fixation and osseous defects are bone grafted (Fig. 2i). Condylar head remodeling takes place as the patient functions (Fig. 2j).

Eighteen months following surgery, the facial symmetry is improved (Fig. 2k, l) and the occlusion is also improved (Fig. 2m).

Case 3

A 16-year-old man with grade III craniofacial microsomia presented for improvement of the condition. Complicating his situation was the previous placement of a costochondral graft on the affected side of the mandible and maxillary and mandibular osteotomies. These were performed at age 7 at another institution. Ear reconstruction was done in three stages at yet another institution.

The facial exam revealed severe lower facial asymmetry with the mandible displaced to the right (opposite the affected side). This occurred as the overgrowth of the rib became more disproportionate over the course of puberty. (Rib grafts grow like ribs not like the mandible). Hypoplasia of all of the soft tissues of the affected side was noted as was scarring from the previous surgery. The mandibular displacement to the non-affected side intensified the soft tissue deficiencies of the affected side. A cant of the maxilla as well as maxillary deficiency was noted. The zygoma on the affected side was also hypoplastic (Fig. 3a–d). Orthodontic appliances were placed and the arches were decompensated (Fig. 3e). The radiographs confirmed severe skeletal asymmetry including overgrowth of the rib graft (Fig. 3f).

LeFort I osteotomy with advancement and leveling was performed as well as bilateral sagittal osteotomies of the mandible. On the non-affected side, this was conducted routinely; on the affected side, the split was accomplished along the overlap junction of the rib graft with the native mandible. Furthermore, a genioplasty was performed to center the chin with the face. Biodegradable bone plates and screws secured the segments of the maxilla and mandible. Split-thickness cranial bone was inserted into the osteotomy defects in the maxilla. Additional bone grafts were onlayed onto the deficient zygoma and body and angle of the mandible (Fig. 3g).

The patient healed well and was able to be debanded within 6 months of surgery with coincident dental midlines and class I cuspid relationship. Although the

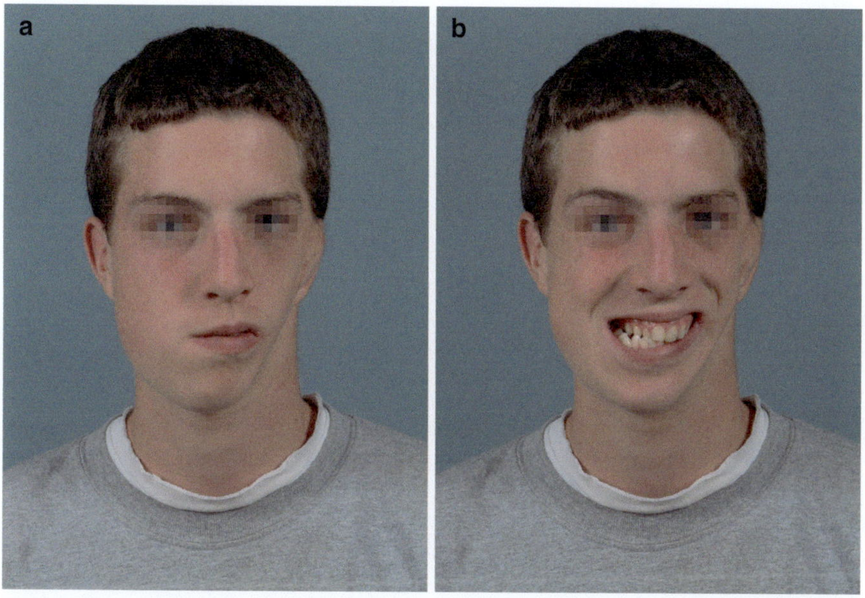

Fig. 3 (**a**, **b**) Case 3. Left craniofacial microsomia. Facial view in repose and during animation. The remarkable degree of tissue hypoplasia on the left is exaggerated because of the overgrowth of the previously placed costochondral graft. There is a cant to the lips and maxilla and midline discrepancies between the maxilla and mandible. (**c**, **d**) The left and right profiles demonstrate elongation of the face and little definition of the left mandibular angle and body as well as retrogenia. There is also scarring in the left preauricular area. The left ear has been reconstructed and is well positioned and of equal size and projection. (**e**) Occlusion views demonstrating severe midline discrepancy between the arches, complete cross bite on the right and asymmetrical class III malocclusion bilaterally. (**f**) The radiographs demonstrate the severe skeletal asymmetry and overgrowth of the costochondral graft on the left. The bone plates and screws are from previous skeletal surgery done elsewhere at age 7. (**g**) Postsurgical radiographs demonstrating LeFort I osteotomy, bilateral sagittal osteotomies, and asymmetrical genioplasty with interpositional bone grafts on the left and onlay bone grafts to the mandible, maxilla, and zygoma. The fixation was completed with biodegradable plates and screws. (**h**, **i**) One-year postsurgical photos demonstrate that the skeletal changes resulted in improvement of the condition but inadequate restoration of the soft tissues. (**j**) One-year postsurgical occlusion. Notice class I relationships, coincident midlines, and absence of cross bite. (**k** and **l**) Final result after placement of a polyethylene mandibular angle implant and two sessions of fat injections (30 cc each) spaced 6 months apart. Photos taken 2 years after last surgery. (**m** and **n**) Final profile views. Notice the well-defined mandibular angles and inferior mandibular body

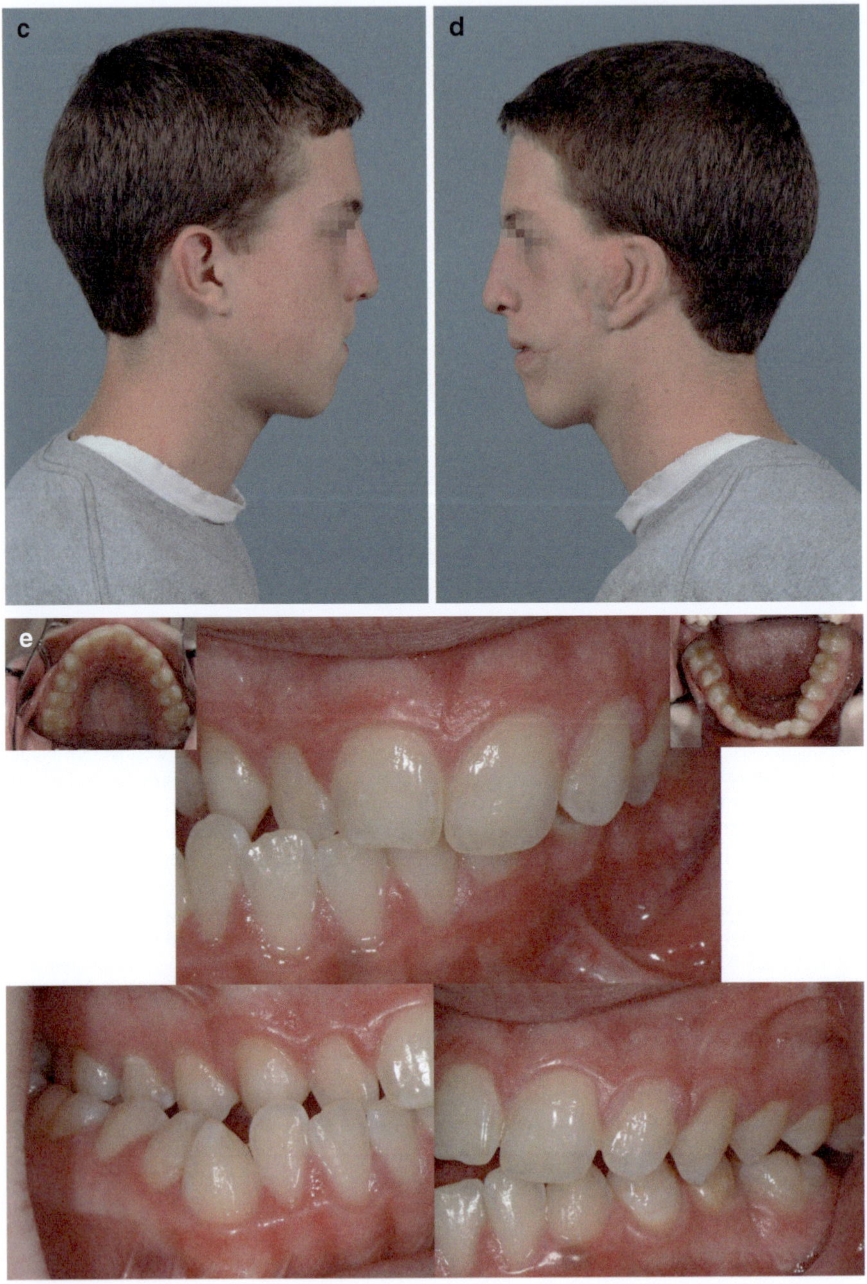

Fig. 3 (continued)

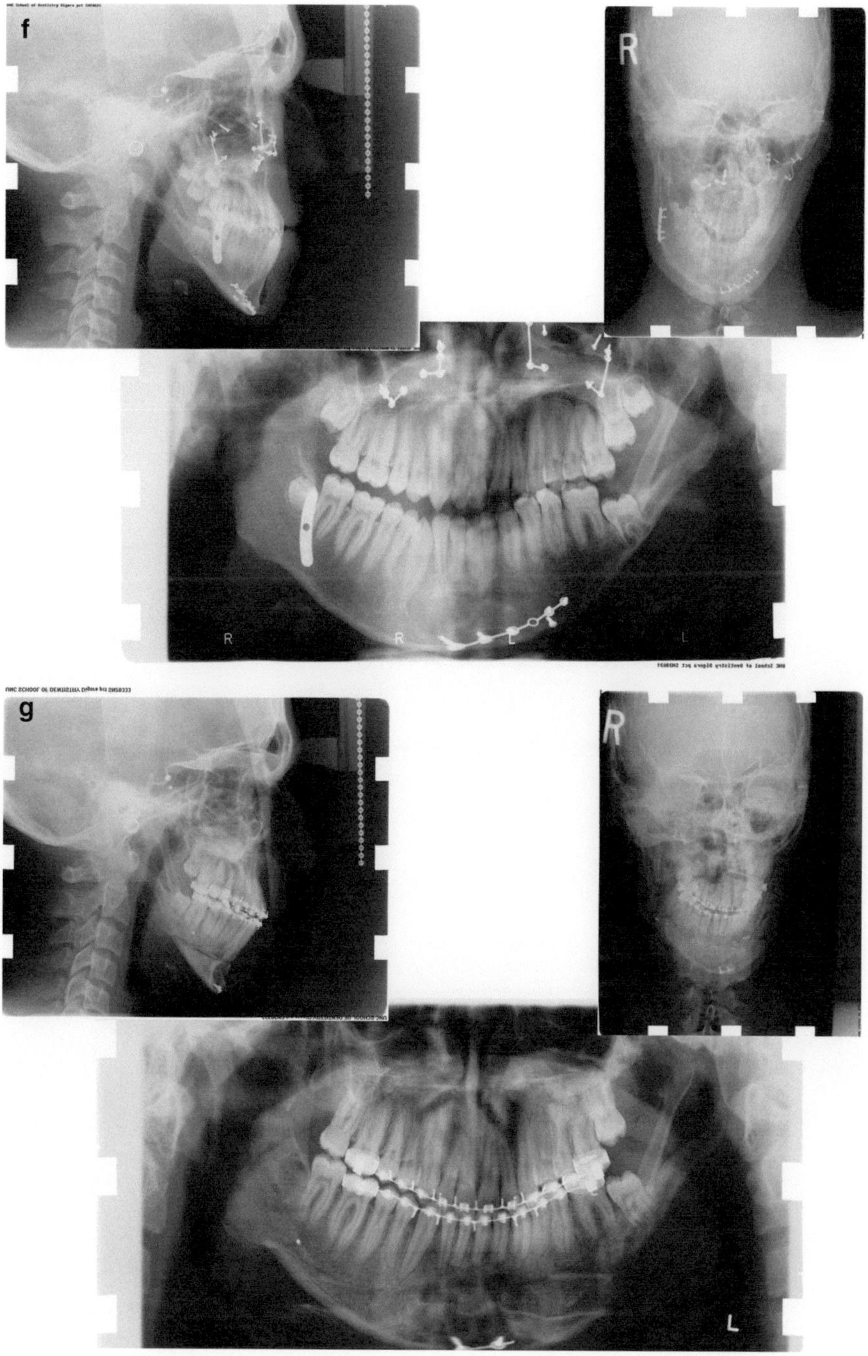

Fig. 11.3 (continued)

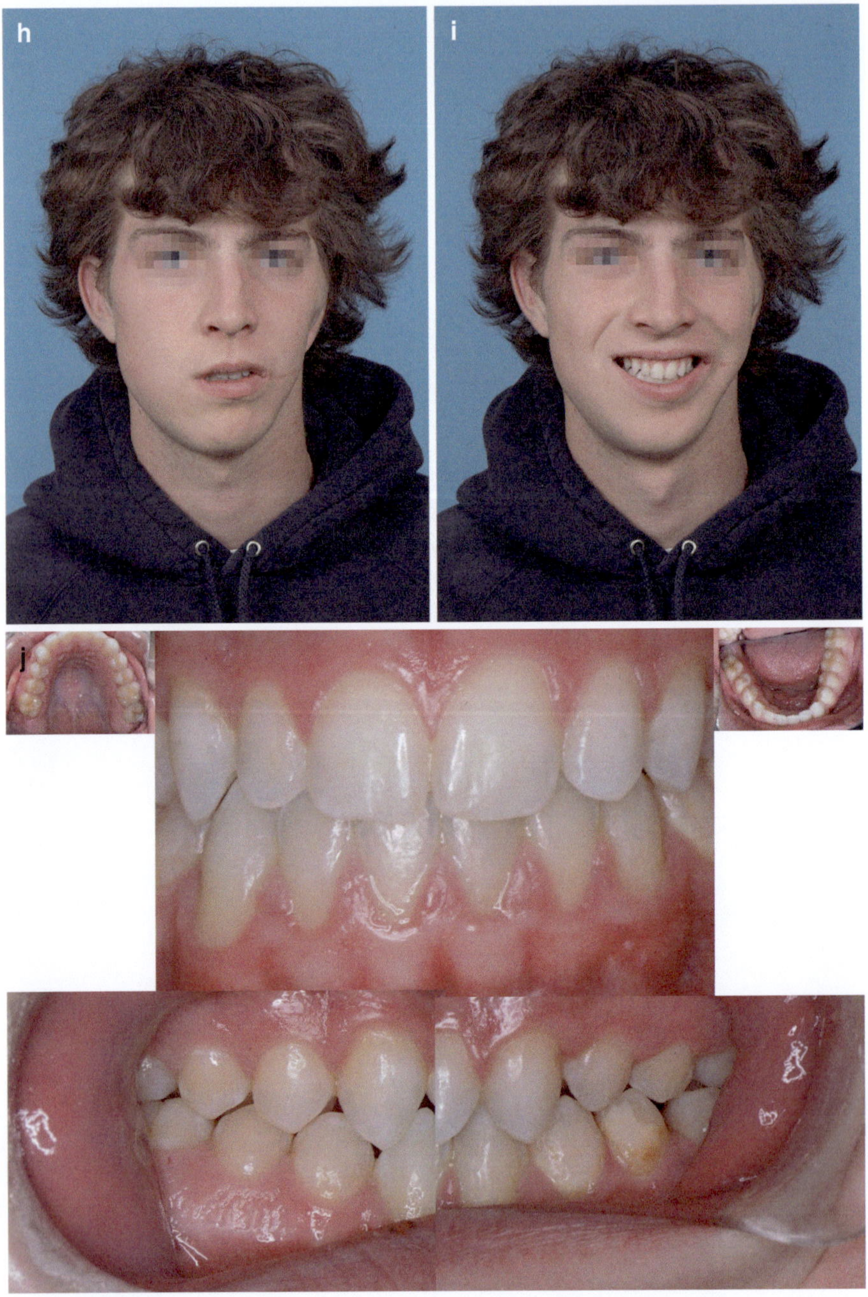

Fig. 3 (continued)

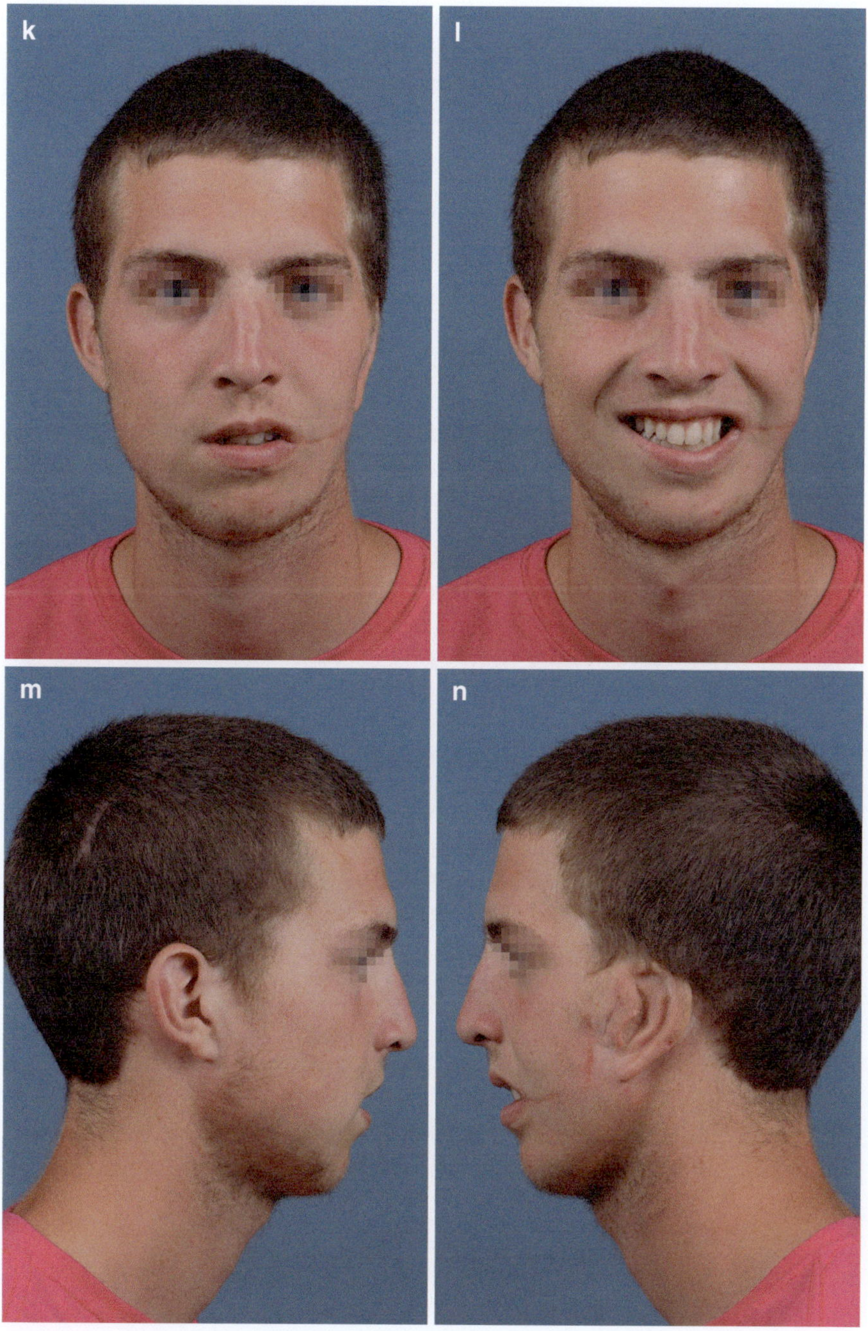

Fig. 3 (continued)

skeletal correction was adequate, the soft tissue discrepancy remained (Fig. 3h–j). At that point, the patient elected to have a polyethylene mandibular angle implant placed on the affected side as well as autogenous fat grafting to the left face. The fat grafting was repeated 6 months later and the patient was satisfied with the result (Fig. 3k–n).

When dealing with severe asymmetry, often alloplastic implants and fat grafting can complement the changes that occur with osteotomies and contour bone grafting.

Case 4

A 15-year-old woman with grade II craniofacial microsomia affecting the right side sought improvement of the facial appearance and the occlusal discrepancy. Soft tissue and skeletal hypoplasia of the right face from the right lateral canthus to the mandibular inferior border was observed. The mandible was more deficient on the right and the chin was deviated to the right as well as being hypoplastic. The right lateral canthus was elevated and there was a cant of the maxilla with the right side up. The cheek on the right was also deficient (Fig. 4a and c).

Once she was orthodontically prepared, osteotomies were designed to improve the condition. These consisted of LeFort I on the left and modified orbital maxillary osteotomy on the right extending to the right zygomatico-frontal suture. This asymmetrical osteotomy design allowed the maxilla and orbit to be advanced and leveled by bringing the right side inferiorly and centering the maxillary midline which was deviated to the right. An inverted L osteotomy of the mandible on the right and sagittal osteotomy on the left allowed the mandible to be advanced and leveled by inferior positioning of the right ramus. These movements facilitated centering the chin, and a genioplasty enhanced the chin projection (Fig. 4e and f).

Split-thickness cranial bone was used to fill the osteotomy defects in the maxilla and mandible. Additionally, onlay bone grafts were used to contour the cheek and the mandibular body on the right.

A hemi-coronal incision was used to access the right midface and a neck incision was used to conduct the inverted L osteotomy on the mandible. The remaining surgery was conducted transorally. Bone plates and screws were used to fixate all segments (Fig. 4f–i). Eighteen-month postsurgical facial changes are apparent (Fig. 4b, d) with minimal evidence of scarring.

This case illustrates the versatility of creative osteotomy design and the use of split-thickness cranial bone grafts to contour areas of deficiency. Careful planning is of paramount importance.

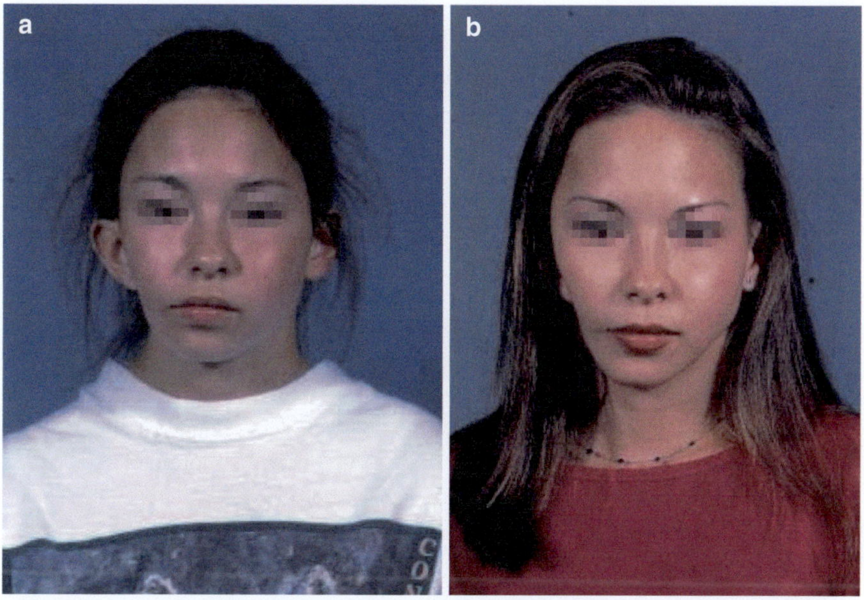

Fig. 4 Case 4. Right craniofacial microsomia (**a** and **b**) Preoperative (**a**) and 18-month postoperative (**b**) views of a patient who underwent asymmetrically designed midface and mandibular osteotomies to improve the symmetry of the face. (**c** and **d**) Preoperative (left) and 18-month postoperative profiles of the same patient. Notice the elongation of the right posterior face and definition of the mandibular angle. There is also improvement of the chin position. (**e** and **f**) The illustrations on the left demonstrate the preoperative condition. The right illustration demonstrated LeFort I on the left, a modified zygomatico-orbital osteotomy on the right, onlay bone graft to the right infraorbital rim and zygoma, a sagittal osteotomy of the left mandible, an inverted L osteotomy of the right mandible, and an asymmetrical genioplasty. These hybrid osteotomies addressed the patient's malformations. (**f**) Coronal incision to gain access to the right orbit and zygoma with bone plate and bone grafts to stabilize the right middle face. (**g**) The intraoperative occlusion demonstrating leveling of the maxilla by inferior movement on the right. (**h**) Intraoral view demonstrating plate fixation of the right maxilla with bone grafts in place. (**i**) Intraoral view demonstrating plate fixation of the left maxilla

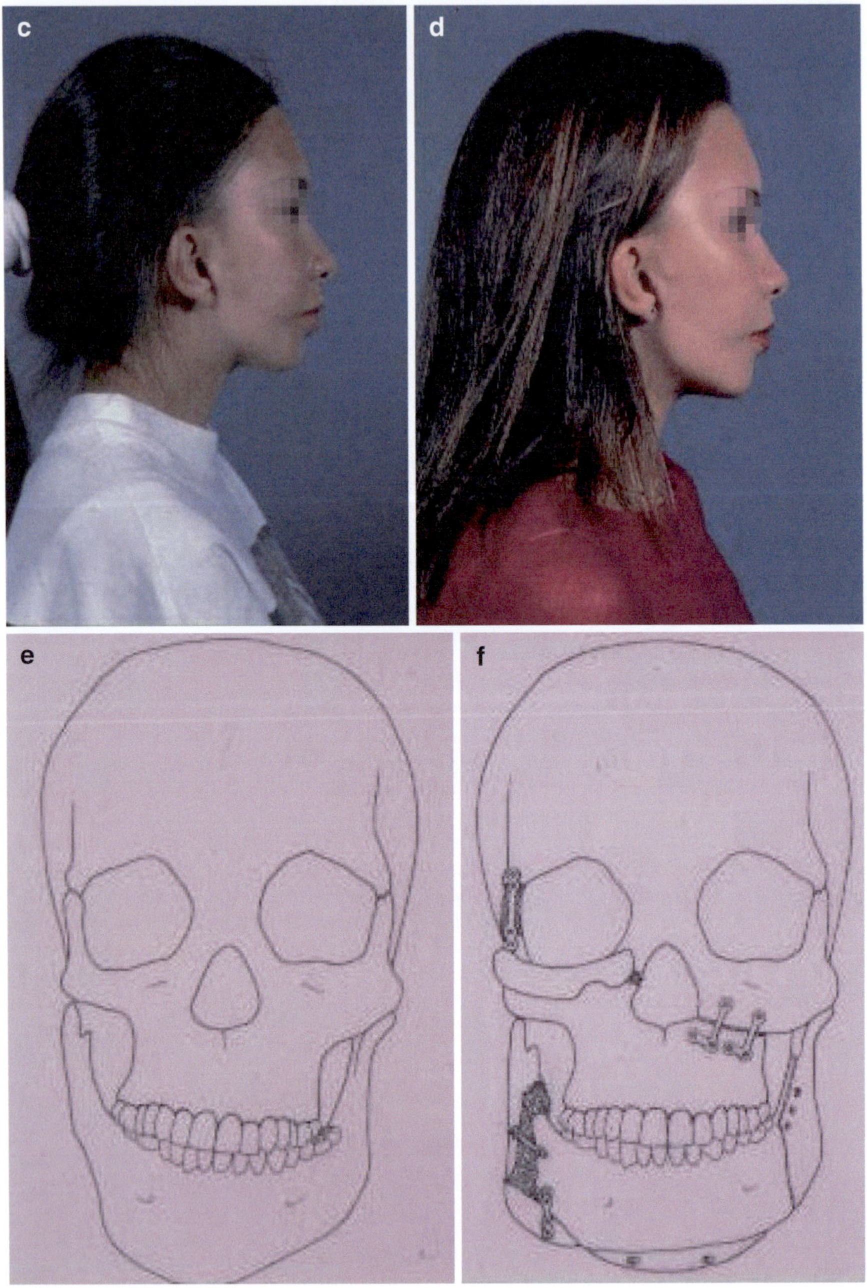

Fig. 4 (continued)

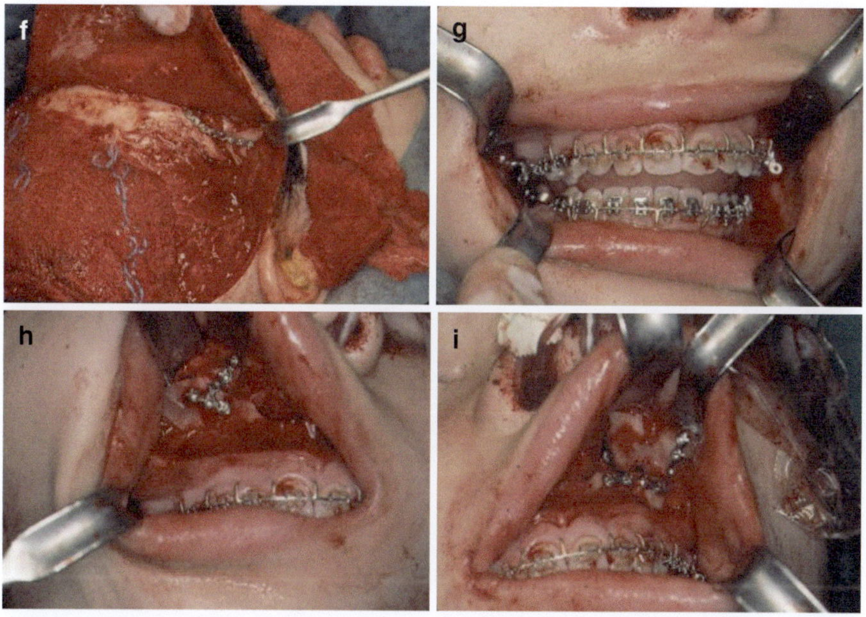

Fig. 4 (continued)

Case 5

This 28-year-old active duty military officer was referred because of facial asymmetry. According to the patient, the asymmetry was noted earlier in life, worsened about the time of puberty, and then stabilized. The patient was treated with orthodontic appliances as a youth with removal of multiple teeth from the right posterior maxilla. He was debanded at about 16 years of age and he reports that his posterior teeth were never able to be erupted into occlusion.

The facial exam revealed severe hypoplasia of the right check and buccal regions extending from the orbit to the inferior border of the mandible. The ophthalmological exam was normal with no fundoscopic abnormalities noted, reactive pupils of the same size, and a full range of extraocular movements. The facial nerves were completely functional in all branches. The nose was midline and the nasal airways were equally patent on both sides. The oral exam revealed no occlusion on the right with a cant on the maxilla (right side up). The cant began at the midline and there was multiple missing teeth in the right maxilla. The mandible appeared normal as were the teeth on the same side.

The incisal opening and range of mandibular movements were normal. The skin of the right face was tight, lacked fat, and had a reddish hue compared to the unaffected skin. The right infraorbital rim and zygoma were hypoplastic. There was no neurosensory disturbance (Fig. 5a and b).

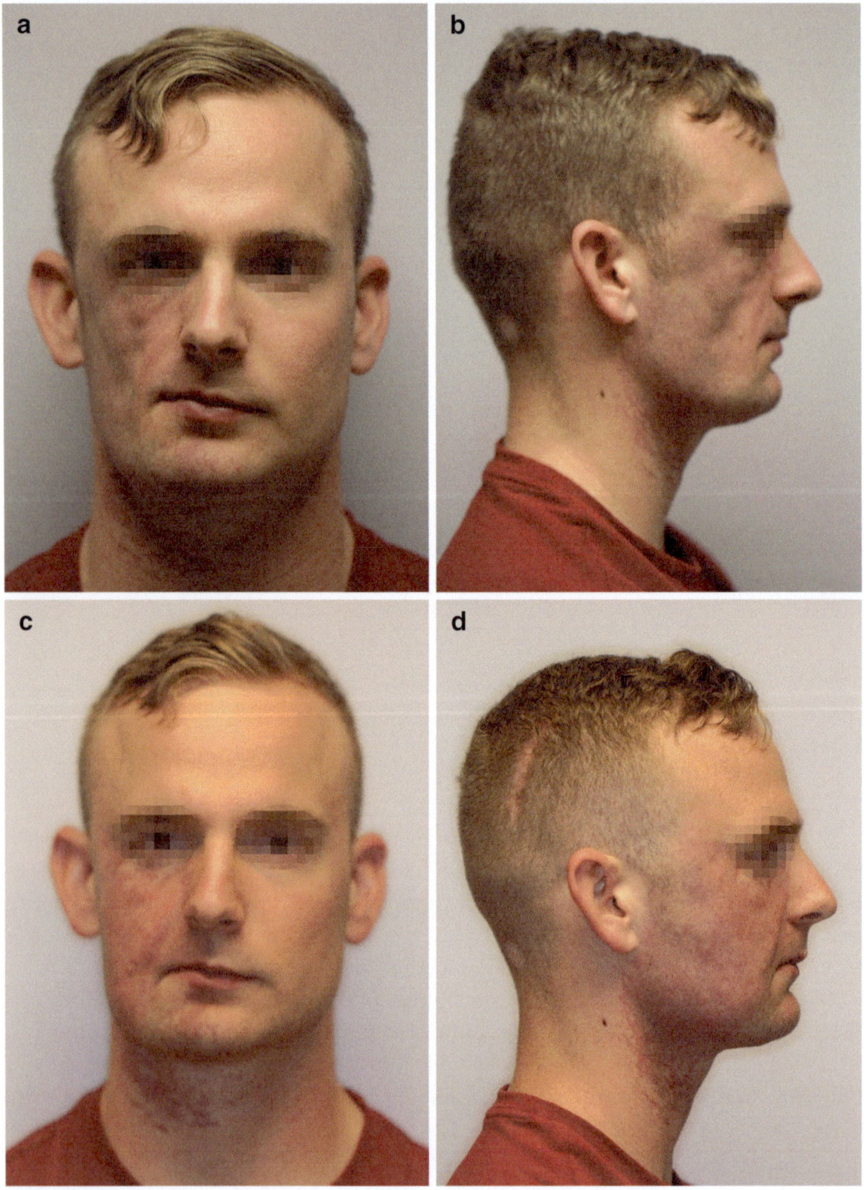

Fig. 5 Case 5. Parry-Romberg syndrome (hemifacial atrophy) (**a** and **b**) Preoperative facial and profile views demonstrating both skeletal and soft tissue atrophies secondary to the autoimmune-induced change association with the condition. Notice the skin color change and the contracture of the soft tissues of the right face. (**c** and **d**) The improved symmetry resulted from split-thickness cranial bone grafts to enhance the skeletal support of the cheeks and infraorbital area. The subcutaneous injection of fat harvested from the buttocks improved the skin thickness and quality taking it from a dried leather appearance and texture to more normal, soft, and supple consistency. (**e** and **f**) Preoperative and postoperative views demonstrating improved symmetry secondary to skeletal support from split-thickness cranial bone grafts and subcutaneous fat injection

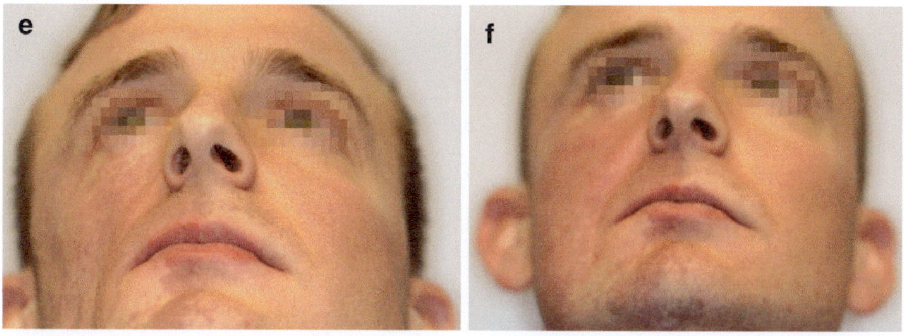

Fig. 5 (continued)

A genetics evaluation confirmed Perry-Romberg Syndrome (Hemifacial Atrophy)

Several treatment plans were presented including a surgical and orthodontic option. The patient's concern was primarily esthetic, and he opted for split-thickness calvarial bone grafts and fat injection into the subdermal layers on the affected side. These procedures were conducted simultaneously using an intraoral approach to the infraorbital rim and zygoma. Multiple stacked layers of split-thickness cranial bone were used to highlight the cheek and infraorbital region. The area to be injected with fat on the right face was outlined and fine cannulas were used to undermine the skin layer. Three stab incisions (one above the zygoma, one over the posterior mandible, and one anteriorly near the lip commissure) were used as the entry of the cannulas and multiple tunnels were dissected. The fat was harvested from the right buttocks and was washed and injected. A total of 60 cc was injected.

This case illustrates that often, in addition to skeletal surgery, the soft tissue problem can also be addressed for a good outcome. In this situation, autogenous fat was used with success (Fig. 5c–e).

Case 6

This girl presented at age 8 being referred by a pediatric dentist who noticed facial and occlusal asymmetry. The family was aware of facial asymmetry and decided to investigate this further. The only thing of significance in her history was a difficult vaginal delivery requiring suction and forceps. There were no other reports of trauma nor did the patient have any complaints of TMJ dysfunction.

The examination revealed asymmetry of the maxilla and mandible (Fig. 6a). The maxilla was canted with the left side up (Fig. 6b). The profile was convex, consistent with mandibular deficiency (Fig. 6c and d). The oral exam indicated a class II asymmetrical malocclusion with the mandibular midline to the right of the maxillary midline (Fig. 6e). The incisal opening exceeded 40 mm and the patient has symmetrical and full lateral excursive movements and protrusive movement. It is hypothesized that the child fractured a condyle (left) very early in life.

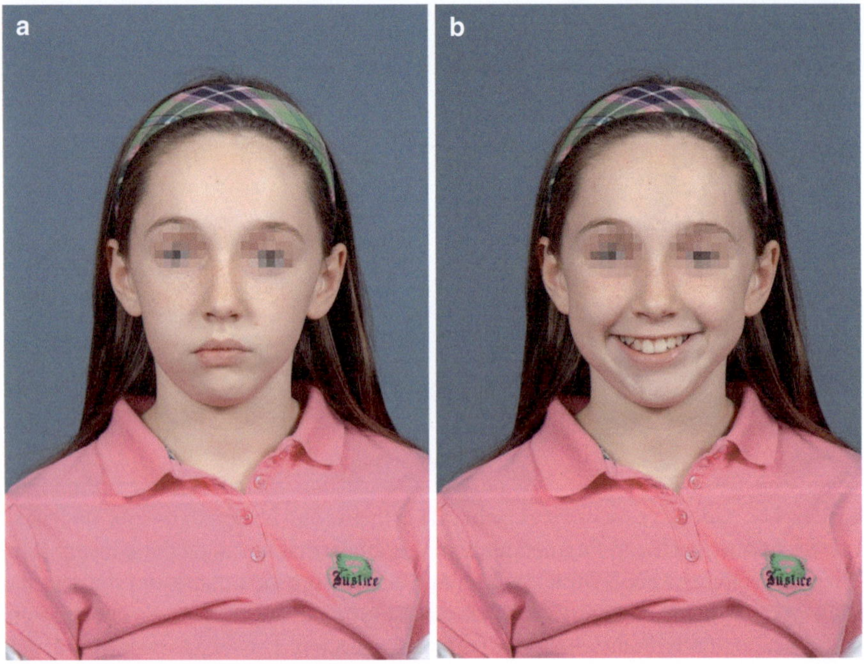

Fig. 6 (**a** and **b**) Full-face views at age 9 demonstrating lower facial asymmetry with the mandible deviated to the left, canted lip commissures, and a cant to the maxilla with the right side down. (**c** and **d**) Left and right profiles consistent with convexity secondary to mandibular deficiency and retrogenia. Notice the left posterior face is shorter. (**e**) Occlusion views demonstrating severe midline discrepancy with the mandibular incisor midline to the right. This is the opposite of the skeletal deviation. (**f**) Preoperative radiographs (age 12 years). Notice the abnormally shaped condyles. The right condyle is positioned in the fossa but is flattened. The left condyle is very short and is anterior to where the glenoid fossa should be. The ramus on the left is short and the glenoid fossa has flattened. The lateral cephalometric radiograph demonstrates the differences in mandibular inferior border heights. (**g**) Hybrid functional appliance designed to center the maxillary and mandibular midlines and to allow the left maxilla to level. (**h**) The postoperative radiographs following inverted L osteotomy on the left with split-thickness interpositional cranial bone grafts to support the advancement and elongation of the left mandible. This was conducted via a neck incision. The right mandible was advanced with a sagittal osteotomy. An advancement genioplasty was also performed. The surgery was completed at age 12. (**i** and **j**) Facial and profile views at age 13 after mandibular surgery. (**j**) Views of the occlusion 9 months following surgery demonstrating centered midlines and bilateral class I cuspids and molars. (**k**) Composite facial and occlusal photos at age 18 (6 years post-surgery). The improved facial symmetry with chin position coincident with the facial midline and the maxilla leveled. Improved chin projection has been maintained. The occlusion remains class I with coincident midlines. (**l**) Superimposition cephalometric tracing demonstrating postsurgical growth

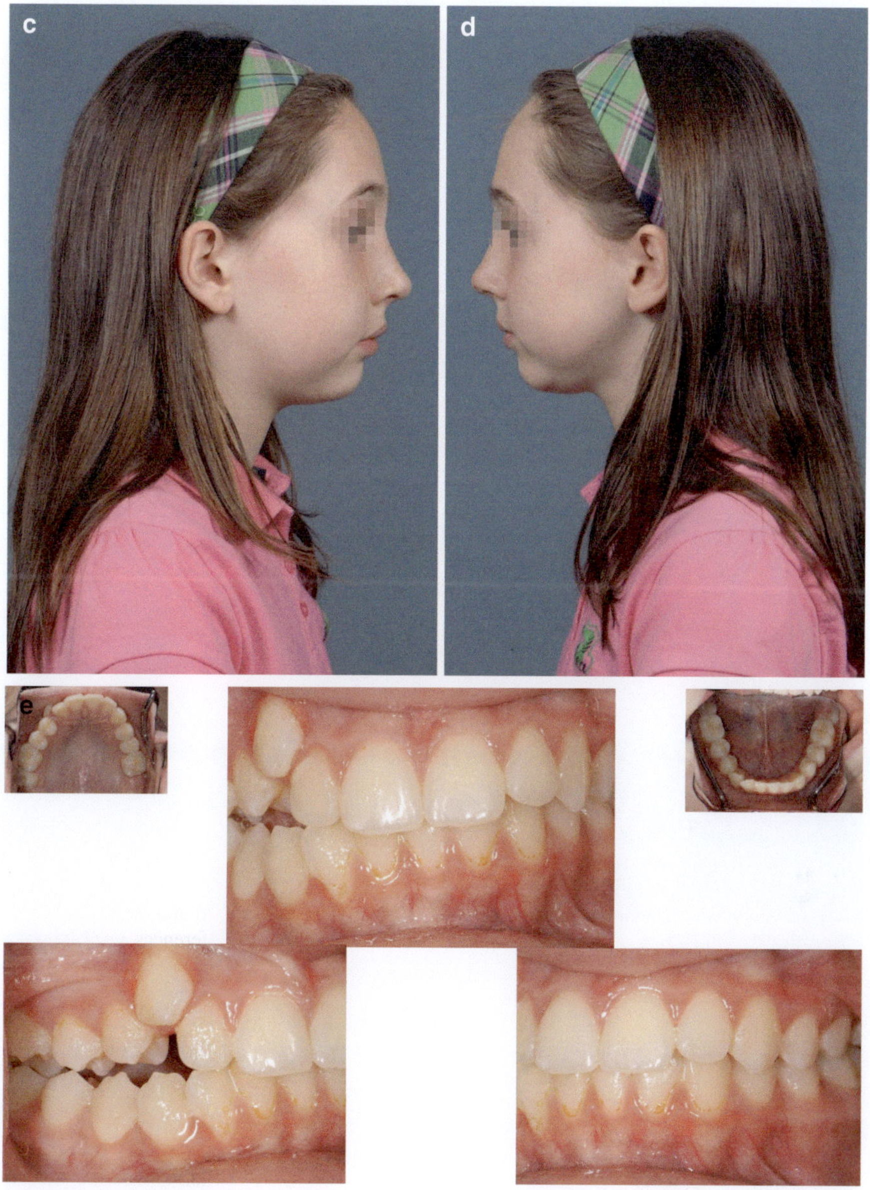

Fig. 6 (continued)

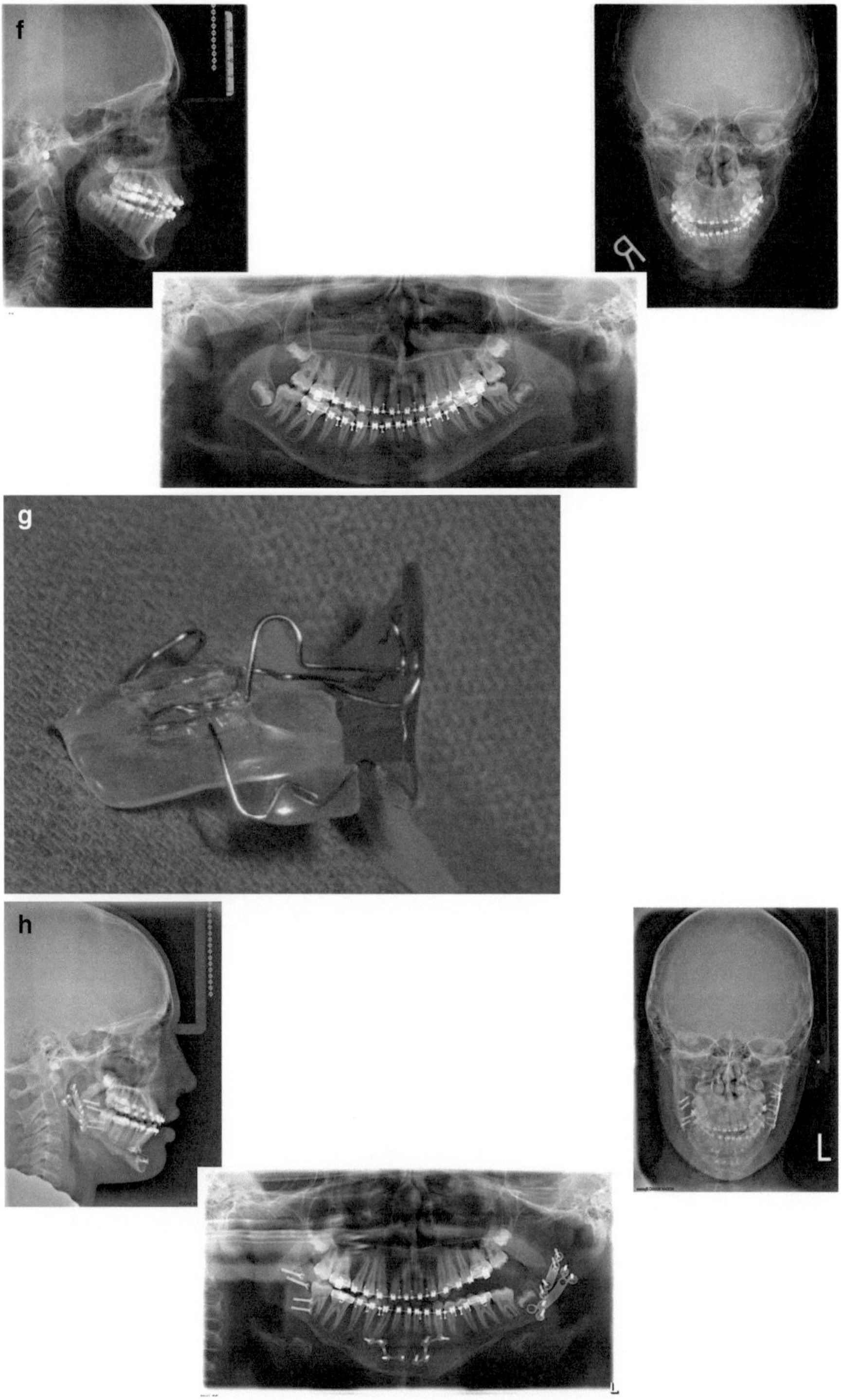

Fig. 6 (continued)

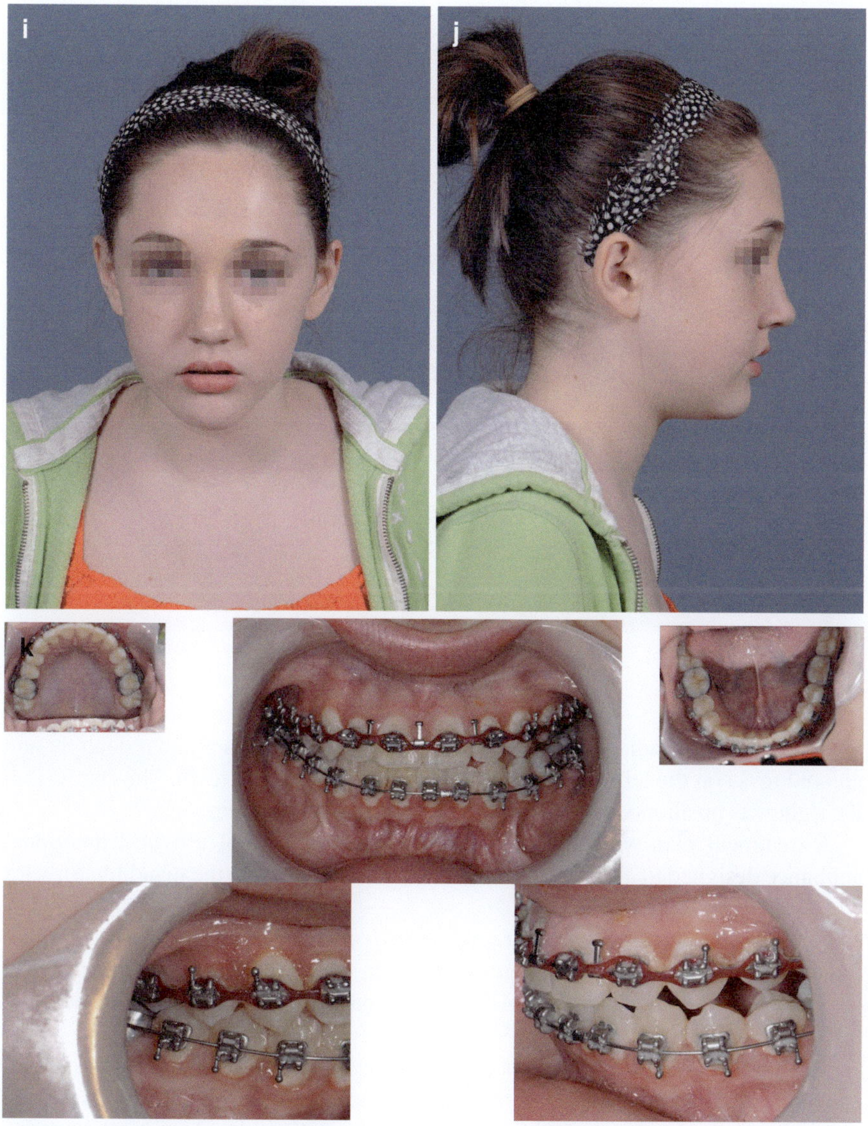

Fig. 6 (continued)

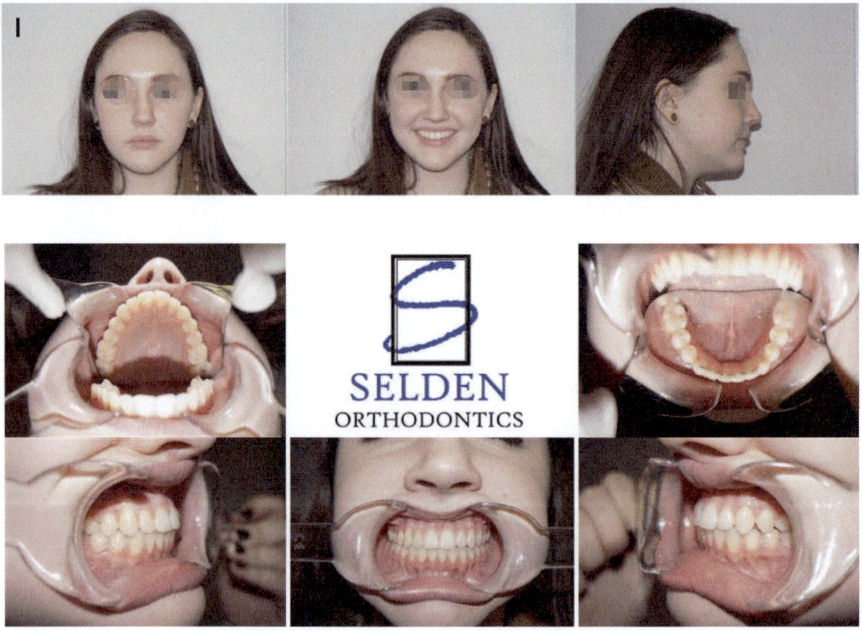

Fig. 6 (continued)

The panoramic radiograph demonstrated a dysmorphic mandibular condyle and glenoid fossa on the left and a full complement of permanent teeth. The condyle on the right was positioned well in the fossa but was flattened (Fig. 6f).

A treatment plan was developed that included the use of a hybrid functional appliance designed to allow the maxilla to level and to posture the mandible forward with centered midlines (Fig. 6g).

After 2 years of appliance therapy, the patient was reevaluated. The mandible remained asymmetrical and deficient; however, the maxillary occlusal plane had improved but not completely. At this point, the mandible was deviated to the left and very deficient in projection.

The family indicated that their impression was that at best, the asymmetrical appearances were unchanged in spite of significant growth. They also expressed concern over peer teasing which was having a toll on their daughter's self-esteem.

It was agreed that orthodontic appliances would be placed with the intention of preparing her for early mandibular advancement and elongation of the left mandibular ramus.

At age 12, the patient underwent surgery to improve the position of the mandible. A sagittal osteotomy was conducted on the right and an inverted L osteotomy on the left. The left coronoid process was removed and used as an interpositional bone graft. Bone screws were used to stabilize the right and bone plates and screws were used on the left. The impacted third molars were removed simultaneously. A genioplasty was also performed to advance and position the chin to the left. Bone screws stabilized the chin segment (Fig. 6h).

The surgical splint was designed to level the mandibular occlusal plane and advance the mandibular position with coincident midlines. This was left in place for 9 months and the patient functioned into it with guiding elastics. At 9 months post-operative, the maxillary arch wire was sectioned and the maxillary surface of the splint was reduced to allow the maxillary occlusal plane to level. By one year post-surgery, the occlusal splint was discontinued as the maxilla leveled. (Fig. 6i and j).

The patient's treatment was completed at age 13 and she has been followed since. Her remaining growth has been favorable and she has maintained improvable facial symmetry and projection. Her function remains excellent and occlusion remains class I. The occlusal splint was left in place for 9 months to assure complete bone healing before the posterior open bite was closed. Without a posterior occlusal to stop on the left, the muscle activity would place additional strain on the immature bone and a tendency to shorten the ramus (Fig. 6k and l).

References

1. Proffit WR, Turvey TA. Dentofacial asymmetry in profit. In: White RP, Savere DM, editors. Contemporary treatment of dentofacial deformity. St. Louis: Mosley; 2003.
2. Severt TR, Proffit WR. The prevalence of facial asymmetry in the dentofacial deformities population at the University of North Carolina. Int J Adult Orthodontics Orthodontic Surg. 1997;12:171–6.
3. Al Sharif AA, et al. Standardization of quantitative single photon emission, computed tomography in control individuals and in patients with condyle hyperplasia. Nu Med Commun. 2014;35(12):1268–76.
4. Obwegeser HC, Makek MS. Hemimandibular hyperplasia and hemimandibular elongation. J Maxillofac Surg. 1986;14:183.
5. Obwegeser HL. Mandibular growth anomalies. Berlin: Springer; 2001.
6. Gateno J, Xia JI, Techgraeber JF, et al. Clinical feasibility of computer aided surgical simulation (CASS) in the treatment of complex cranio-maxillofacial deformities. J Oral Maxillofac Surg. 2007;65:728–34.
7. Swennen GR, Malhaous W, Schutyser F. Three dimensional treatment planning of orthognathic surgery with area of virtual imaging. J Oral Maxillofac Surg. 2009;67:2080–92.
8. Sailer HF, et al. The value of stereolithographic models for preoperative diagnosis of craniofacial deformities and planning of surgical corrections. Int J Oral Maxillofacial Surg. 1998;27:327–33.
9. Ghawai S, Aagaard E, Thygesen TH. High condylectomy for the treatment of mandibular condylar hyperplasia: a systemic review of the literature. Int J Oral Maxillofac Surg. 2016;45:60–71.
10. Wolford LM, Mehra P. Efficacy of high condylectomy for management of condylar hyperplasia. Am J Orthod Dentofac Orthop. 2002;121:136–50, discussion 150–151.
11. Brusati R, Pedrazzole M, Colletti G. Functional results after condylectomy in active laterognathia. J Craniomaxillofac Surg. 2010;38:179–84.

MIX
Papier aus verantwortungsvollen Quellen
Paper from responsible sources
FSC® C105338

If you have any concerns about our products, you can contact us on
ProductSafety@springernature.com

In case Publisher is established outside the EU, the EU authorized representative is:
Springer Nature Customer Service Center GmbH
Europaplatz 3, 69115 Heidelberg, Germany

Printed by Libri Plureos GmbH
in Hamburg, Germany